A PRACTICAL MANUAL OF

Thyroid and Parathyroid Disease

A PRACTICAL MANUAL OF

Thyroid and Parathyroid Disease

Edited by

Asit Arora MRCS, DOHNS
ENT Research SpR
St Mary's Hospital, Imperial College Healthcare NHS Trust
London, UK

Neil S. Tolley MD, FRCS, DLO
Consultant ENT–Thyroid Surgeon
St Mary's Hospital, Imperial College Healthcare NHS Trust
London, UK

R. Michael Tuttle MD
Associate Professor of Medicine
Joan and Sanford I. Weill Medical College of Cornell University,
Memorial Sloan Kettering Cancer Center
New York, USA

WILEY-BLACKWELL
A John Wiley & Sons, Ltd., Publication

Blackwell Publishing was acquired by John Wiley & Sons in February 2007. Blackwell's publishing program has been merged with Wiley's global Scientific, Technical and Medical business to form Wiley-Blackwell.

Registered office: John Wiley & Sons Ltd, The Atrium, Southern Gate, Chichester, West Sussex PO19 8SQ, UK

Editorial offices: 9600 Garsington Road, Oxford OX4 2DQ, UK
The Atrium, Southern Gate, Chichester, West Sussex PO19 8SQ, UK
111 River Street, Hoboken, NJ 07030-5774, USA

For details of our global editorial offices, for customer services and for information about how to apply for permission to reuse the copyright material in this book please see our website at www.wiley.com/wiley-blackwell

Library of Congress Cataloging-in-Publication Data

A practical manual of thyroid and parathyroid disease / edited by Asit Arora, Neil Tolley, R. Michael Tuttle.
p. ; cm.
Includes bibliographical references and index.
ISBN 978-1-4051-7034-5
1. Thyroid gland–Diseases–Handbooks, manuals, etc. 2. Parathyroid glands–Diseases–Handbooks, manuals, etc. I. Arora, Asit. II. Tolley, Neil. III. Tuttle, R. Michael.
[DNLM: 1. Thyroid Diseases–therapy. 2. Parathyroid Diseases–diagnosis. 3. Parathyroid Diseases–therapy. 4. Thyroid Diseases–diagnosis. WK 200 P895 2010]
RC655.P84 2010
616.4′4--dc22

2009004443

ISBN: 978-14051-7034-5

A catalogue record for this book is available from the British Library.

Set in 9.25 on 11.5 pt Minion by Toppan Best-set Premedia Limited
Printed and bound in Singapore by Fabulous Printers Pte Ltd

1 2010

Contents

Cover images

Image 1 (left): Cytological appearance of low grade B Cell Non Hodgkin's lymphoma in the thyroid gland.

Image 2 (centre): Thyroid FNA shows intranuclear inclusions and longitudinal grooves consistent with papillary thyroid cancer.

Image 3 (right): Thyroid FNA demonstrates large follicular cells with a repetitive microfollicular pattern and scanty colloid (Thy 3 lesion). Following surgical excison, histopathological assessment revealed a mixed follicular thyroid cancer with capsular breach.

Contributors

Asit Arora MRCS DOHNS
ENT Research SpR
St Mary's Hospital, Imperial College Healthcare NHS Trust
London, UK

Piero Berti MD
Associate Professor
Department of Surgery
University of Pisa
Pisa, Italy

Jorge A. Carrasquillo MD
Director, Targeted Radionuclide Therapy
Attending Physician, Nuclear Medicine Service
Radiology Department
Memorial Sloan-Kettering Cancer Center
New York, New York, USA

Jeremy Cox MD FRCP
Consultant Endocrinologist
St Mary's
Hospital, Imperial College Healthcare NHS Trust
London, UK

Glen Dixon FRCPath
Consultant Cytopathologist
St Mary's Hospital, Imperial College Healthcare NHS Trust
London, UK

Christos Georgalas PhD, MRCS, DLO, FRCS (ORL-HNS)
Consultant Otolaryngologist-Head and Neck Surgeon,
Academic Medical Centre
Amsterdam, The Netherlands

Ravinder K. Grewal MD
Assistant Attending Physician
Nuclear Medicine Service
Department of Radiology
Memorial Sloan-Kettering Cancer Center;
Professor of Radiology
Weill Medical College of Cornell University
New York, New York, USA

Masud Haq BSc MRCP MD
Consultant Endocrinologist
Maidstone & Tunbridge Wells NHS Trust
Kent, UK

Clive Harmer FRCP, FRCR
Consultant Oncologist
Former Head of the Thyroid Unit
Royal Marsden Hospital
London, UK

Graham Hornett MA, MB, BChir (Cantab), MRCS, FRCGP
General Practitioner with Special Interest in ENT
Surrey PCT
Wonersh, Guildford
Surrey, UK

Steven M. Larson MD, FACNP, FACR
Donna and Benjamin M. Rosen Chair in Radiology
Chief of Nuclear Medicine Service
Department of Radiology
Memorial Sloan-Kettering Cancer Center;
Professor of Radiology
Weill Medical College of Cornell University
New York, New York, USA

David J. Lesnik MD
Otolaryngologist
Division of Thyroid and Parathyroid Surgery
Department of Laryngology and Otology
Harvard Medical School
Massachusetts Eye and Ear Infirmary
Boston, Massachusetts, USA

Paul Lewis MD, DSc, FRCP, FRCPath
Endocrine Pathologist
BUPA Cromwell Hospital
London, UK

John Lynn MS, FRCS
Endocrine Surgeon
BUPA Cromwell Hospital
London, UK

Gitta Madani FDSRCS MRCS FRCR
Consultant Radiologist
St Mary's Hospital, Imperial College Healthcare NHS Trust
London, UK

Vishy Mahadevan PhD, FRCS(Ed) FRCS
Professor of Surgical Anatomy and Barber's Company Reader in Anatomy
Raven Department of Education
The Royal College of Surgeons of England
London, UK

Gabriele Materazzi MD
Researcher
Department of Surgery
University of Pisa, Italy

Julie McCarthy PhD, FRCPath
Consultant Cytopathologist
St Mary's Hospital, Imperial College Healthcare NHS Trust
London, UK

Paolo Miccoli MD
Chief of the Department of Surgery
University of Pisa
Pisa, Italy

J. Pieter Noordzij MD
Otolaryngologist
Department of Otolaryngology
Boston Medical Center
Boston, Massachusetts, USA

Miriam A. O'Leary MD
Otolaryngologist
Department of Otolaryngology
Boston Medical Center
Boston, Massachusetts, USA

Nick Oliver BSc, MBBS, MRCP
Clinical Research Fellow
St Mary's Hospital, Imperial College Healthcare NHS Trust
London, UK

Kepal N. Patel MD
Assistant Professor of Surgery and Biochemistry
Division of Endocrine Surgery
New York University School of Medicine
New York, New York, USA

Gregory W. Randolph MD, FACS
Director General of Thyroid Surgical
Division, Massachusetts Eye and Ear Infirmary
Member Endocrine Surgical Service
Massachusetts General Hospital
Associate Professor
Department of Laryngology and Otology
Harvard Medical School
Boston, Massachusetts, USA

Stephen Robinson MD, FRCP
Consultant Physician
St Mary's Hospital, Imperial College Healthcare NHS Trust
London, UK

Bhuvanesh Singh MD, PhD
Director, Laboratory of Epithelial Cancer Biology
Associate Attending Surgeon, Head and Neck Service
Memorial Sloan-Kettering Cancer Center;
Associate Professor of Otolaryngology
Weill Medical College of Cornell University
New York, New York, USA

Brendan C. Stack MD, FACS, FACE
Professor and Vice Chairman
Department of Otolaryngology-HNS
University of Arkansas for Medical Sciences
Little Rock, Arkansas, USA

Mike Stearns MB, BS, BDS, FRCS
Consultant ENT-Thyroid Surgeon,
Royal Free Hospital,
London, UK

Tim Stephenson MA, MD, MBA, FRCPath
Consultant Histopathologist;
Clinical Director of Laboratory Medicine
Sheffield Teaching Hospitals NHS Foundation Trust;
Honorary Professor
Faculty of Health and Wellbeing
Sheffield Hallam University
Sheffield, UK

Neil S. Tolley MD, FRCS, DLO
Consultant ENT-Thyroid Surgeon
St Mary's Hospital
Imperial College Healthcare NHS Trust
London, UK

R. Michael Tuttle MD
Associate Professor of Medicine
Joan and Sanford I. Weill Medical College of Cornell University;
Memorial Sloan Kettering Cancer Center
New York, New York, USA

Malcolm H. Wheeler MD, FRCS
Formerly
Professor of Endocrine Surgery
University Hospital of Wales
Heath Park
Cardiff, Wales

Foreword

It is a special honour for us to endorse this text book edited by Neil Tolley, Asit Arora, and R. Michael Tuttle. The title *A Practical Manual Of Thyroid and Parathyroid Surgery* is apropos for this well-written and informative volume on thyroid and parathyroid disease. The authors have succinctly covered all the major aspects of clinical disease related to the thyroid and parathyroid glands.

There has been great interest in thyroid disease for the past two decades because it is common and unlike most other cancers, the incidence of thyroid cancer has been rising rapidly. This nearly 3-fold rise in the last 3 decades has been noted worldwide. The increase is primarily due to findings from routine thyroid evaluation by clinical examination and technologically advanced imaging studies. Most of these tumors are smaller than 2 cm and they generally have an excellent prognosis. Similarly, the rising incidence of parathyroid disease has principally been due to findings from routine serum calcium analysis and subsequent investigation by internists and endocrinologists. Non-neoplastic thyroid disorders such as hypothyroidism, hyperthyroidism, and Hashimoto's thyroiditis are also diagnosed more frequently and need to be treated efficiently. This book covers all aspects of thyroid and parathyroid disease with a special focus on the surgical and medical management of well differentiated thyroid cancer. The authors discuss recent advances and risk group stratification to individualize treatment. They also expand on the philosophy of the extent of thyroidectomy and use of radioactive iodine ablation.

The editors are well known specialists in the field of thyroid and parathyroid disease and have made a commendable effort to gather international experts for a broad view of the topic. Chapters are well planned and the information provided is important because it is clinically relevant and directly relates to the optimal standards of care for patients with thyroid and parathyroid disease. The structure of each chapter differs from most of the other textbooks on this subject. An evidence appraisal section is included at the end of most chapters. Key points and multiple choice questions are also included which reinforce important points and ensures the reader re-address their understanding of the disease. The book as a whole is easy to read, with highlighted case studies included where appropriate that are informative and educational. As there are no randomized controlled trials for this pathology, most conclusions are based on large non-randomized retrospective data analyses and the personal philosophy of the individual treating physician. Large databases, such as the SEER database and the National Cancer Database (NCDB), are quite helpful in correlating one's personal philosophy to the 'best practices' shown in the large data that is available.

Primary care physicians will find this an excellent resource for reference purposes, and it will update the endocrinologist, endocrine surgeon and specialist treating thyroid cancer. We wholeheartedly recommend this book as a practical manual and handy reference.

Barney Harrison MS, FRCS
Consultant Endocrine Surgeon
Sheffield Teaching Hospitals NHS Foundation Trust
Sheffield
UK

Ashok R. Shaha, MD, FACS
Professor of Surgery
Memorial Sloan-Kettering Cancer Center New York,
New York
USA

Preface: A Practical Manual of Thyroid and Parathyroid Disease

A rapid advance in the management of patients with thyroid and parathyroid disease has necessitated a multidisciplinary approach. This is crucial to deliver the highest standards of care for our patients and we hope this book adequately reflects the input provided by the various specialities involved. We are extremely grateful to the contributors who, as leaders in their individual areas of expertise, have provided authority, experience and invaluable insight.

Demands placed upon a clinician's time are both unrelenting and enormous. As busy specialists in this field, we believe that there was a genuine need for an up to date, evidence based overview which was both concise and practically orientated. The aim of the book is to serve as a succinct guide to the clinical management of common Thyroid and Parathyroid conditions. Indeed, because these disorders are so common and their pathological spectrum affects virtually every medical specialty, it was considered appropriate that the book begin in the context of the primary care setting. Specialists in General Practice will find this useful as a clinical guide, particularly as guidelines for referral to secondary care become more stringent and political directives emerge which increasingly place the onus of care in the community setting.

The book will also be relevant to the medical undergraduate, postgraduate and clinical nurse specialist. It is intended to serve as a primary source of knowledge, reference and self assessment. Multiple choice questions have been included at the end of each chapter for this purpose. Regarding our colleagues in secondary care, we hope that specialists in the fields of Pathology, Radiology, Oncology, Endocrinology and Surgery find the content both informative and pertinent to their daily clinical practice.

Finally, we would like to thank Wiley-Blackwell for having the trust, determination and encouragement to see this project to fruition.

Neil S. Tolley MD, FRCS, DLO
Asit Arora MRCS, DOHNS
R. Mike Tuttle MD
December 2009

Section 1 Thyroid disease

1 Symptoms, assessment and guidelines for primary care referral

Graham Hornett[1], Stephen Robinson[2] & Asit Arora[2]

[1]Wonersh, Guildford, Surrey, UK
[2]St Mary's Hospital, Imperial College Healthcare NHS Trust, London, UK

KEY POINTS

- Thyroid function disorders are common in the general population and can cause significant morbidity. Primary care physicians should therefore have a low threshold for checking thyroid-stimulating hormone (TSH) as a screening test for thyroid disease
- Hypothyroidism can be insidious and may be associated with other conditions. It should be screened for in this setting and in the whole population over the age of 65 years. Most patients with hypothyroidism can be diagnosed and managed within the primary care setting
- Hyperthyroidism is less common than hypothyroidism. It is associated with atrial fibrillation and osteoporosis, and should always be considered when these conditions are present. Patients should be referred to an endocrine specialist for diagnosis of the cause and continued management
- Thyroid goitre is common. Worldwide, it is often associated with insufficient iodine consumption
- Thyroid nodules are also common. Solitary or clinically obvious nodules should be investigated as they carry a small but significant malignant potential. Thyroid cancer is rare and, with appropriate early diagnosis and management, survival rates are generally very good.

INTRODUCTION

This chapter gives a brief overview of the salient features of hypothyroidism, hyperthyroidism and thyroid swellings, with particular emphasis on the primary care management of these conditions. Case studies have been used to highlight specific clinical scenarios which the primary healthcare physician may encounter when managing patients with thyroid disease. This introductory chapter serves to outline some of the pertinent features of thyroid disease which will be expanded in greater detail in subsequent chapters.

A Practical Manual of Thyroid and Parathyroid Disease, 1st Edition. Edited by Asit Arora, Neil Tolley & R. Michael Tuttle.

HYPOTHYROIDISM

Hypothyroidism is a condition in which the body lacks sufficient thyroid hormone. Lack of thyroid hormone affects many organs or systems and results in a slow body metabolism. It is common in western populations. In the UK, primary hypothyroidism is found in 3.5 per 1000 women and in 0.6 per 1000 men. A brief outline is given below, and further details of this condition are described in Chapters 2 and 6.

Clinical diagnosis

Hypothyroidism is notoriously difficult to diagnose in its early stages due to its variable and gradual presentation. The presence of other conditions may detract the primary care clinician from appreciating that hypothyroidism is associated with, or indeed is the primary cause of, these symptoms. Initially, the diagnosis may be easily overlooked (see Case study 1). In view of this, it is important for the clinician to be familiar with its incidence and aetiology, particularly in the primary care setting.

Aetiology (Table 1.1)

Primary hypothyroidism occurs due to intrinsic failure of the thyroid gland which is characterized by a rise in thyroid-stimulating hormone (TSH). The most common cause of chronic hypothyroidism in the UK is autoimmune thyroiditis (Hashimoto's thyroiditis). Worldwide, iodine deficiency is common and in older individuals thyroid atrophy is a well-recognized cause. In the long term, autoimmune thyrotoxicosis is often associated with hypothyroidism. The latter arises following treatment with radioactive iodine or thyroidectomy, or eventually results from the natural history of the condition itself. Iatrogenic hypothyroidism occurs due to inappropriately monitored thionamide therapy and is also precipitated by amiodarone, lithium and other immune-modulating medications.

Table 1.1 Aetiology of hypothyroidism

Cause of hypothyroidism	Comments
Autoimmune (Hashimoto's disease)	Most common cause: The patient may present with a goitre
Atrophic (idiopathic)	Common in the elderly
Congenital	One in 4000 births either absence of the thyroid or absence of enzyme in thyroid hormone synthesis
Iodine deficiency	Common on a worldwide basis
Iatrogenic	Following inappropriately monitored thionamides, radioactive iodine, amiodarone, lithium, interferon α
Previous thyroid surgery or neck irradiation	
Secondary	Following pituitary tumour

Temporary hypothyroidism (which sometimes progresses to permanent deficiency) occurs with thyroiditis. Post-viral, subacute or De Quervain thyroiditis are usually temporary. Lymphocytic and post-partum thyroiditis account for the vast majority of cases, and the associated hypothyroidism is usually permanent.

Congenital hypothyroidism occurs due to the anatomical absence of the thyroid gland or absence of one the enzymes required for thyroid hormone biosynthesis. Infants may also be born with the condition due to thyroid-suppressing drugs taken by the mother during pregnancy which cross the placenta. Hypothyroidism is screened for in all neonates in the UK by a heel-prick blood test which is usually performed 6 days after birth. By the age of 25, one-third of individuals with Down syndrome develop hypothyroidism[1]. Annual TSH screening is therefore recommended in this group.

Secondary hypothyroidism is caused by pituitary failure leading to an absence of TSH secretion and resulting atrophy of the thyroid gland. Pan-hypopituitarism was first described by Simmonds (Simmond's syndrome) in 1914. When it rises in the peri-partum period, it is referred to as Sheehan's syndrome. Secondary hypothyroidism following a pituitary tumour (or its treatment) is usually one of the later hormone deficiencies from the anterior pituitary gland.

Presenting symptoms

In infants it is important to recognize the condition as early as possible because, when left untreated, it causes growth and mental retardation. Signs of hypothyroidism in the newborn include prolonged periods of sleep, puffy myxoedematous facies, protruding tongue, hoarse cry, hypothermia, prolonged neonatal jaundice, constipation, feeding difficulties and abdominal distension (see Fig. 1.1). In adults, there may be no symptoms at all in the early stages of hypothyroidism. Speed of onset is variable and symptoms may take many months to develop. Classically these include fatigue, generalized aches and pains, weight gain, constipation, heat sensitivity, dry skin and hair, fluid retention, mental slowing and depression. Patients with sleep apnoea and persistent hoarseness should always have their thyroid function checked.

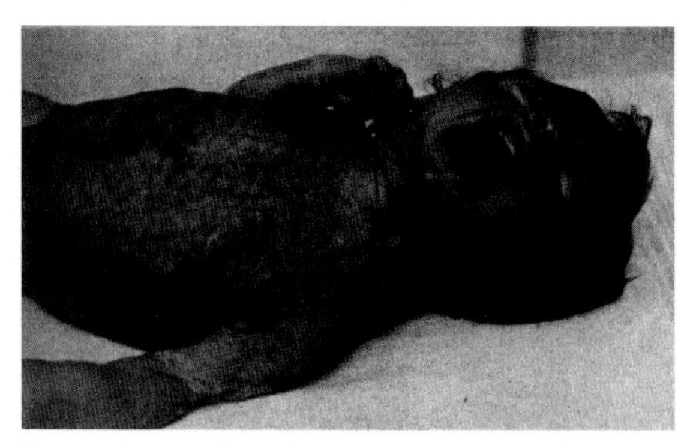

Fig. 1.1 Features of cretinism.

Clinical signs and conditions associated with hypothyroidism

Clinical findings associated with hypothyroidism are outlined in Table 1.2.

Examination may reveal a thyroid swelling, oedema of the eyes, hands or lower limbs, dry skin and hair, hair loss and sluggish reflexes, particularly the ankle jerk (see Fig 1.2). Cardiovascular manifestations include hypertension, sinus bradycardia and hyperlipidaemia. Neuropsychiatric sequelae also occur.

Case study 1

A 54-year-old female patient underwent routine cholesterol screening which was elevated (>8.5 mmol/l). Following commencement of a statin by the primary healthcare physician, the cholesterol level dropped to 6.0 mmol/l. The following year, she reported significant weight gain and became increasingly lethargic. Concentration and memory were noticeably impaired and her husband was unable to sleep in the same room due to her prolific snoring. She was subsequently referred to a respiratory specialist. A sleep study confirmed moderate sleep apnoea and, following commencement of continuous positive airways pressure (CPAP), symptoms improved. Twelve months later, she presented to her local A&E Department with chest pain. Blood pressure was persistently elevated and an abnormally raised cholesterol level was again noted. Six months later, she presented with a thyroid swelling to the primary care physician, who organized thyroid function tests, thyroid autoantibodies and a neck ultrasound scan. Serum TSH was greater than 100 μU/l (normal TSH 0.4–4.5 μU/ml), indicative of hypothyroidism. The patient was referred to an endocrine specialist.

Comment. This case illustrates how the presence of other pathology can significantly delay diagnosis of hypothyroidism, which in turn may have a profound effect on the patient's quality of life. Hypercholesterolaemia, weight gain, lethargy, sleep apnoea and hypertension may all, individually, be indicators of hypothyroidism. The primary care physician should have a low threshold for organizing thyroid function tests in a patient with these symptoms.

Clinical investigations in primary care

TSH measurement is the most universally accepted standard for assessing thyroid function. The normal TSH range is 0.4–4.5 μIU/ml. When the TSH is abnormal, the free hormones should be assessed. Usually free thyroxine (T4) is measured when the TSH is elevated to confirm hypothyroidism or investigate subclinical hypothyroidism. When the TSH is suppressed, the free tri-iodothyronine (T3) can be used to investigate thyrotoxicosis. Thyroid function tests should be requested to determine the thyroid status before further investigation to identify the cause of thyroid dysfunction[3] (Level IV) (Table 1.3).

TSH levels will often be raised when thyroxine levels are normal and the patient is clinically euthyroid. This biochemical finding, termed 'subclinical hypothyroidism', may herald the development of hypothyroidism. If the clinician suspects that thyroxine supplementation has been prescribed inappropriately, it should be reduced or discontinued and thyroid function re-evaluated after an interval of 4–6 weeks.

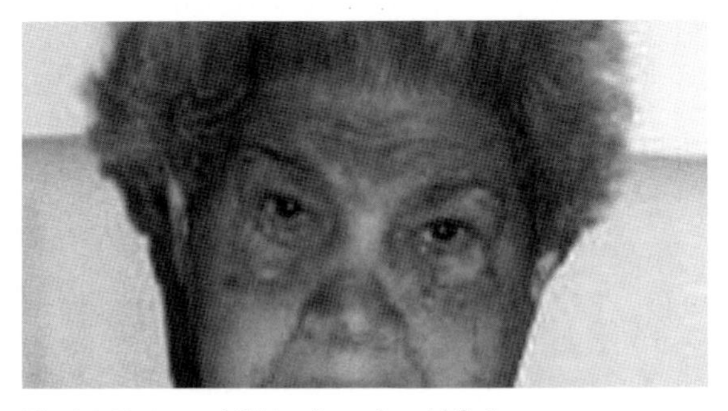

Fig. 1.2 Patient exhibiting hypothyroid facies.

Table 1.2 Symptoms and signs of hypothyroidism

General
Weight gain
Intolerance of cold weather
Goitre
Gastrointestinal
Constipation
Nervous system
Poor central nervous system development in children
Loss of intellectual function
Lethargy
Slow relaxing reflexes
Dermatology
Dry skin
Hair loss (in severe untreated hypothyroidism)
Myxoedema (rare)
Cardiovascular
Reduced cardiac output
Reduced exercise tolerance
Angina pectoris (uncommon but may appear during treatment)
Reproductive
Menorrhagia in women
Subfertility in men and women
Haematological
Macrocytosis and anaemia
Hypercholesterolaemia (common and improves following thyroxine replacement)

Hypothyroidism can affect any system within the body, and a range of common symptoms are listed above. Although most patients with hypothyroidism in the UK are diagnosed before overt symptomatic presentation occurs, the clinical diagnosis is sometimes easily overlooked (see Case study 1).

Table 1.3 Differential diagnosis of abnormal thyroid function tests

TSH	T4	T4	T4
	Normal	Decreased	Increased
Increased >4.5 μIU/ml	Subclinical hypothyroidism	Hypothyroidism	**Hyperthyroidism** (very rarely related either to TSH-producing adenoma or thyroid hormone resistance)
Decreased <0.4 μIU/ml	Subclinical hyperthyroidism	Hypothyroidism (pituitary failure)	**Hyperthyroidism**

When thyroid function is abnormal, thyroid antibodies can be measured to investigate the possibility of autoimmune thyroiditis (Hashimoto's). Thyroid antibodies should not be measured in patients with normal thyroid function. Hashimoto's thyroiditis occurs due to an autoimmune inflammatory reaction resulting in an underactive thyroid. The condition is outlined in greater detail in Chapters 2 and 6. It is important to exclude Hashimoto's in pregnant women with abnormal thyroid function because thyroid antibodies cross the placenta, leading to congenital hypothyroidism.

Abnormal findings in screening tests for certain conditions should prompt the primary care clinician to check for thyroid disease. These include hypercholesterolaemia (manifest by a raised low-density lipoprotein), macrocytosis and anaemia.

Management of hypothyroidism in primary care

Diagnosis of thyroid dysfunction must be confirmed biochemically. There is no evidence base for the use of thyroxine in tired patients with normal thyroid function. The aim of treatment is to suppress the TSH to normal levels and render the patient symptom free, which can take several months. Treatment in affected patients is life-long. The ideal treatment range of TSH is 0.4–4.5 μIU/ml. Thyroxine (in the form of levothyroxine) is prescribed, initially at a single dose of 50 μg. The dose is increased by increments of 50 μg every 4 weeks until the TSH level becomes normal and the T4 level is within or slightly above its reference range. In elderly patients or those with cardiac disease, the incremental dose increase should be halved to 25 μg. Following an alteration in thyroxine dose it takes at least 2 months for thyroid function to stabilize. Therefore, repeat thyroid function tests should only be performed after this timeframe.

It may be desirable to obtain lower levels if the patient has no symptoms of hyperthyroidism. Undetectable TSH levels may indicate overtreatment even if the serum thyroxine is normal. Even with appropriate thyroid hormone treatment, TSH suppression may be associated with osteoporosis, atrial fibrillation and possibly increased mortality.

Subclinical hypothyroidism

Subclinical hypothyroidism is not uncommon, affecting up to 10% of the adult population. The diagnosis is made in the asymptomatic patient who has a raised TSH level with normal free T4 and T3 levels. It is associated with potentially increased cardiovascular risk, hyperlipidaemia and neuropsychiatric effects. Up to 20% of patients progress to overt hypothyroidism. The management of subclinical hypothyroidism is somewhat controversial.[4,5] The British Thyroid Association (BTA) recommends that thyroxine supplementation should be commenced if the serum T4 is normal and the TSH level is greater than 10 μIU/ml.[3] (Level IV) When thyroxine is prescribed, subsequent management is the same as for hypothyroid patients.

When the TSH is slightly raised but is less than 10 μIU/ml, there is no evidence base for initiating thyroxine supplementation. A mild alteration in TSH levels is common in a wide range of acute and chronic illnesses, often referred to as 'sick euthyroid' syndrome (outlined in further detail in Chapter 6). As TSH suppression may be associated with atrial fibrillation and osteoporosis, repeating TSH measurement in 3–6 months, in addition to thyroid autoantibodies, is advocated in the first instance.

Screening for thyroid dysfunction

Screening for congenital hypothyroidism is appropriate, cost-effective and well established in the UK. However, evidence from community studies suggests that 'carte blanche' adult population screening only detects a few cases of overt thyroid disease and is therefore unjustified except in the elderly and in patients with Down syndrome. In addition, patients treated with thyroid surgery or radioiodine have an increased risk of developing hypothyroidism and should also undergo routine surveillance. There is no consensus for screening women for post-partum thyroiditis, although those with type 1 diabetes mellitus have a higher risk and should therefore be followed-up after pregnancy. Patients treated with lithium or amiodarone are also at higher risk of thyroid dysfunction. TSH levels must be routinely screened before and after treatment. An abnormal result should prompt specialist referral, particularly as difficulties may arise in the interpretation of biochemical abnormalities in this group.

Follow-up

In the UK, the recommendation is that patients commenced on thyroxine in primary care should have their TSH monitored annually to ensure optimal dosage. TSH levels should be maintained between 0.4 and 4.5 μIU/ml.

Specialist referral

Referral to an endocrinology specialist is not usually required unless there is an unusual presentation or associated feature. A patient presenting with hypothyroidism associated with a long-standing nodular goitre is unlikely to have thyroid cancer and can be referred routinely to an endocrinologist rather than the thyroid oncology multidisciplinary team (MDT). In contrast, a patient who presents with a thyroid lump which is new or enlarging should be referred to the thyroid MDT or to a clinician with a special interest in thyroid cancer[6] (Level IV).

HYPERTHYROIDISM

Hyperthyroidism is a condition characterized by excess thyroid hormone which results in an overactive body metabolism. This is described in greater detail in subsequent chapters (Chapter 2 and 6), and a brief overview follows below.

Clinical diagnosis

In many cases the diagnosis is clear-cut, but sometimes the condition is difficult to recognize due to the insidious onset of symptoms. The primary care clinician should always be alert to the possibility of hyperthyroidism in patients with certain symptoms which do not appear overtly endocrine, e.g. atrial fibrillation, dyslipidaemia, osteoporosis and subfertility.[3] (Level IV).

Aetiology

Hyperthyroidism has an annual incidence of 0.5 cases per 1000 people and, as with hypothyroidism, there is a significant female preponderance (the female:male ratio is roughly 5:1). There may be a family history of thyroid disease, particularly Graves' disease, which is associated with a diffuse thyroid swelling and exophthalmos. Hyperthyroidism can be classified in terms of adenosine uptake (usually technetium is used). 'High uptake' thyrotoxicosis, in which the thyroid traps too much iodine and produces excessive thyroid hormone, accounts for 85% of thyrotoxic patients. This group includes autoimmune thyroid disease with thyrotoxicosis (known as Graves' disease in the UK or Jod Basedow in Europe), multinodular goitre with thyrotoxicosis, an autonomously functioning thyroid nodule or single toxic adenoma.

'Low uptake' thyrotoxicosis, in which the thyroid gland prematurely releases thyroid hormone following an insult, accounts for the minority. This group includes post-viral, post-partum and lymphocytic thyroiditis. In each of these conditions there is a thyrotoxic phase which typically lasts a few weeks, followed by a hypothyroid phase.

Fewer drugs cause hyperthyroidism compared with the hypothyroid patient. As with hypothyroidism, amiodarone causes thyroid dysfunction in 18–20% of patients. Therefore, TSH should be assessed before it is commenced and at a minimum of 6-monthly intervals. Excessive consumption of iodine preparations or thyroxine may also precipitate the condition. Other causes arise from excess TSH secretion either directly by the pituitary or from rare tumours which contain thyroid tissue, such as hydatidiform mole.

Presenting symptoms

As with hypothyroidism, hyperthyroidism may develop insidiously. Patients present with wide-ranging symptoms relevant to different specialties including cardiology, gastroenterology, gynaecology, ophthalmology and dermatology.

It is unusual for hyperthyroidism to occur before puberty. A thyroid disorder should be suspected in children with an enlarged thyroid, weight loss, behavioural disorders (including attention deficit disorder) and premature growth or development. It is equally unusual for cardiac symptoms to occur at an early age so the presence of palpitations should alert the clinician to the possibility of hyperthyroidism.

In adults, symptoms include heat sensitivity, increased appetite and weight loss, mood change, palpitations and neck swelling. Eye symptoms include protrusion, pain, excessive lacrimation and blurred vision.

Clinical signs and clinical conditions associated with hyperthyroidism

Typical findings on clinical examination are outlined in Table 1.4. The clinician should check for a thyroid swelling, hand tremor, anorexia, tachycardia and hypertension. There may be excessive sweating, brisk reflexes and eye signs. The latter includes lid retraction, proptosis, peri-orbital or conjunctival oedema, papilloedema and reduced visual acuity (although these may all be absent in children and the elderly). Atrial fibrillation, infertility and osteoporosis can all arise secondary to thyrotoxicosis (Fig. 1.3).

Table 1.4 Symptoms and signs of hyperthyroidism

General
Heat intolerance/sweating
Weight loss (despite increased appetite)
Cardiac
Palpitations with resting tachycardia
Respiratory
Shortness of breath
Central nervous system
Agitation and low temper threshold
Reflexes. (fatigue and muscle weakness)
Gastrointestinal
Increased bowel frequency
Features of autoimmune thyroid disease
Diffuse goitre
Exophthalmos
Ophthalmoplegia (lid lag and retraction occur with thyrotoxicosis of any aetiology)
Pre-tibial myxoedema
Vitiligo

Thyrotoxic patients may have one or more of the symptoms and/or signs listed. Even in the absence of symptoms, it is important to treat patients with hyperthyroidism to reduce their risk of atrial fibrillation and osteoporosis.

Case study 2

A 55-year-old woman was found to be tachycardic during investigations for osteoporosis. Her thyroid function was subsequently requested. This revealed an undetectable TSH and an elevated free T3 at 9.4. Thyroid autoantibodies revealed mildly positive thyroid peroxidase antibodies. In view of this, she was referred to an endocrinology specialist who requested a technetium scan. This demonstrated an autonomously functioning thyroid nodule (AFTN or 'single hot nodule'). She was treated with carbimazole until she became euthyroid and was then given radioactive iodine treatment. Following this, she remained euthyroid and did not require thyroxine therapy.

Comment. This case illustrates the importance of assessing thyroid function in patients with osteopenia osteoporosis. The rationale for treatment is to improve her thyrotoxic symptoms and reduce the future risk of osteoporosis, atrial fibrillation and stroke. Thyroid peroxidase and TSH receptor antibodies have a relatively poor sensitivity. A technetium scan is indicated (rather than an ultrasound scan) as this will detect even a small nodule and successfully illustrate the abnormal toxic adenoma. This guides further management as radioactive iodine is the ideal treatment in

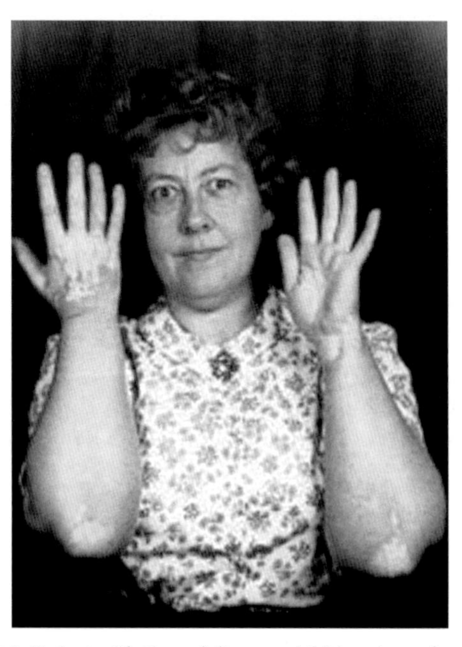

Fig. 1.3 Patient with Graves' disease exhibiting signs of exophthalmos and vitiligo.

this scenario. Once the patient has been protected from thyrotoxicosis with thionamide, she can receive radioactive iodine, which only affects the functioning nodule. The rest of the thyroid gland returns to normal and the patient becomes euthyroid with no need for subsequent thyroxine therapy.

Clinical investigations in primary care

Hyperthyroidism is diagnosed by a suppressed TSH concentration and an elevated serum free T4 and/or free T3 level which may be due to exogenous or endogenous causes. The former is prevented by optimizing levothyroxine dosage. The treatment of endogenous subclinical thyrotoxicosis depends on the clinical situation and existing co-morbidity (see 'Subclinical hyperthyroidism' below).

An ultrasound scan is not indicated in most hyperthyroid patients. However, euthyroid patients with a thyroid swelling require referral to the thyroid MDT. The primary care physician should not organize imaging in these cases due to the delay that may arise[6] (Level IV).

Management of hyperthyroidism in primary care

There are three treatments for hyperthyroidism: antithyroid drugs, radioiodine (^{131}I) and surgery. All patients, particularly the young and old, should be considered for treatment with β-blockers (in the absence of asthma) to protect against the risk of atrial fibrillation. The Royal College of Physicians and other guidelines recommend that patients are referred to an endocrinologist for further management.[7]

Subclinical hyperthyroidism

This is uncommon, affecting less than 2% in the adult population. Patients are usually asymptomatic and diagnosed biochemically; the TSH level is less than 0.4 μIU/ml, with normal T4 and T3 levels. It is of clinical significance because of the associated risks of atrial fibrillation and osteoporosis.[8] Furthermore, it may progress to overt hyperthyroidism.

Treatment is decided on an individual basis and it is advisable to monitor thyroid function every 3–6 months.[2,4,5] (Level IV). Patients with a persistently low TSH and normal T4 levels should be referred for specialist endocrinology opinion.

Specialist referral

In view of the uncertain clinical course and variety of treatment options (see Chapters 6 and 8), patients should be referred to an endocrinologist rather than managed in the primary care setting. Other indications for specialist endocrinology input include patients with persistent subclinical hyperthyroidism and thyrotoxic patients with single or multiple thyroid nodules[6] (Level IV).

THYROID TUMOURS

Clinical diagnosis

The term goitre means swelling in the neck and, although this is common, non-thyroid causes should always be entertained. A thyroid goitre may be diffuse, nodular or mulitnodular (Fig. 1.4) Once the clinical diagnosis has been made, further investigation is necessary to determine the nature of the lesion (see Chapters 2–5).

Aetiology

The most common causes are benign hypertrophy or degeneration. The thyroid can be diffusely enlarged in both hyperthyroid conditions (Graves' disease) and hypothyroid states (Hashimoto's disease). There may be a family history of thyroid goitre or it can arise during puberty and pregnancy. It can also arise in later years and is possibly associated with the ageing process. Deficient dietary iodine intake causes goitre formation, which may have a geographical association. This is particularly evident in hilly regions where the drinking water contains

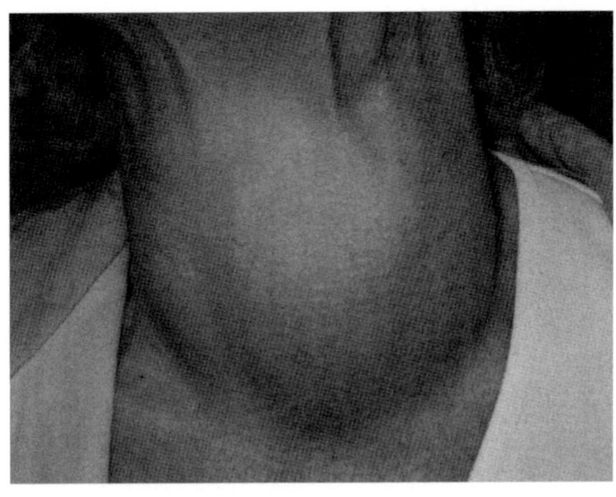

Fig. 1.4 Patient with a multinodular goitre.

low levels of iodine (endemic goitre). Conversely, too much iodine can also produce a goitre in susceptible individuals. Iodine occurs in a variety of foods and medications, e.g. iodine-containing cough remedies and artificial colouring such as E127.

Solitary nodules are prevalent in 5% of the population, and this figure increases with age. Autopsy studies have detected nodules in up to 50% of the population. Benign nodules are four times more common in females compared with males. A toxic or 'hot' nodule is an uncommon cause of hyperthyroidism.

Malignant nodules are rare, with a prevalence of 25 per million, a male:female ratio of 3:1 and an incidence of 1–2 per 100 000 per annum. Thyroid cancer usually presents as a solitary nodule and is more prevalent in children and those over 50 years of age. The patient is usually clinically and biochemically euthyroid.

Thyroid nodules may be multiple, and it is unusual for these to be malignant. The incidence of thyroid cancer is higher in patients with a long-standing thyroid goitre or thyroiditis. Solitary thyroid nodules have a 10–30% risk of malignancy (this increases to 50% in children). Radiation is a well recognized risk factor, such as radiation exposure from atomic fallout and radiotherapy to the neck. There is a genetic predisposition to thyroid cancer in families with the *RET* gene. The presence of this gene may result in families suffering multiple endocrine neoplasia (MEN) syndrome (see Chapters 9, 12, 13 and 15).

Presenting symptoms

Features that raise suspicion of malignancy are listed in Table 1.5.

Table 1.5 Clinical features which suggest thyroid malignancy

- Sudden or rapid growth of a nodule over a period of weeks, particularly in a pre-existing goitre or in a patient on long-term thyroid suppression
- Hard, fixed or irregular thyroid swelling
- Pain
- Hoarseness, or voice change
- Haemoptysis
- Dysphagia/globus
- Stridor
- Cervical lymphadenopathy
- Thyroid nodule or a goitre in a child
- Cervical lymphadenopathy associated with a thyroid lump
- Horner's syndrome (see Fig. 1.5)

Clinical signs

There is usually no evidence of thyroid dysfunction, but pulse and blood pressure should be recorded. Neck examination may reveal a firm thyroid lump. Not all cases of thyroid malignancy fit the classical description of a hard fixed swelling; over-reliance on the consistency of a thyroid lesion can be misleading. The primary care clinician should also palpate the cervical lymph node chain for associated enlargement.

Clinical investigations in primary care

Thyroid function and thyroid autoantibodies (thyroid peroxidase antibodies) must be assessed, as the management of a hypo- or hyperthyroid goitre is entirely different to that of a euthyroid goitre. An abnormal result warrants an endocrinology referral. If the results are normal and the patient has a palpable firm thyroid nodule, consideration should be given to referring the patient to a thyroid lump clinic.

Management of thyroid cancer in primary care

Recognition and referral (see below) is the role of the primary care physician. Specialist endocrinology input following treatment is important to monitor subsequent thyroxine replacement. The aim in these cases is to maintain TSH suppression to a level less than 0.1 μIU/ml[6] (Level IV) (see Chapters 5, 11 and 12 for further details).

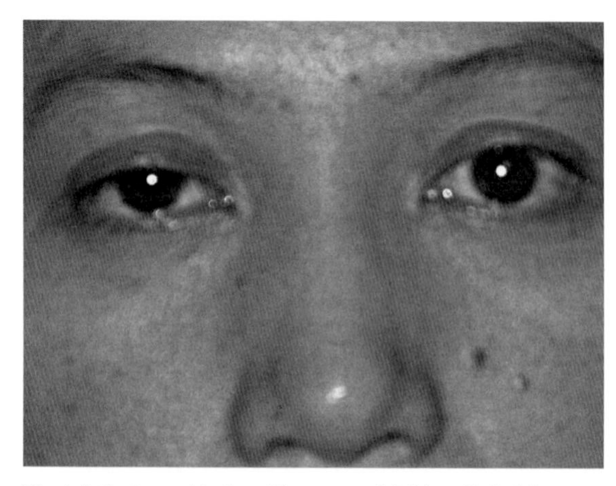

Fig. 1.5 Patient with thyroid cancer exhibiting clinical features of a right Horner's syndrome.

The overall 10-year survival for middle-aged adults is between 80 and 90%. Up to 20% of patients will develop locoregional recurrence, and 10–15% distant metastasis. Important poor prognostic factors include:

1. Age: <10 years or >40 years.
2. Male gender.
3. Grade: poorly differentiated tumours.
4. Histology: poorer prognosis is associated with particular papillary subtypes such as tall cell and columnar variants. Follicular variants associated with poorer prognosis include an insular pattern and Hurthle cell carcinoma.
5. Tumour extent: size of the primary tumour, extracapsular invasion, cervical lymph node metastases and distant metastases.
6. Completeness of resection.

Specialist referral

The updated BTA guidelines 2007 suggest that an urgent 'same day' referral to secondary care (A&E Department, Head and Neck or General Surgical emergency services) is warranted for any patient with stridor associated with a thyroid swelling.[6] Urgent referral to a specialist in thyroid cancer or to a member of the thyroid MDT is indicated in the following circumstances.

- Unexplained hoarseness or voice change
- Thyroid nodule/goitre in a child
- Cervical lymphadenopathy associated with a thyroid lump (usually deep cervical or supraclavicular region)
- A rapidly enlarging painless thyroid mass over a period of weeks (a rare presentation of thyroid cancer and usually associated with anaplastic thyroid cancer or thyroid lymphoma).

Non-urgent referrals include patients who have abnormal thyroid function as cancer is very rare in these cases. Ideally, patients should be referred to an endocrinologist. Other indications include sudden onset of pain in a thyroid lump as this is likely to represent haemorrhage within a benign thyroid cyst. Non-urgent referral is also warranted when the thyroid lump has been increasing in size slowly over many months or years.

Case study 3

A 63-year-old male smoker with a previous history of neck irradiation presented to his primary care physician with non-productive cough, noisy breathing and hoarseness. He had run out of salbutomol and becotide inhalers several months earlier. On examination, the patient was found to have biphasic transmitted breath sounds and an incidental firm thyroid swelling. Thyroid function was requested and the patient commenced on a course of oral antibiotics, steroid and salbutomol inhalers. The patient was reviewed 2 weeks later. His hoarseness persisted and it was now apparent that there was biphasic stridor at rest. The thyroid function test was normal. Immediate referral to the local Head and Neck Department was organized and the patient was admitted into hospital the same day. The patient was commenced on intravenous steroids and regular adrenaline nebulizers, and the stridor resolved over the next 24 h. Flexible nasoendoscopy revealed a unilateral vocal cord palsy. Subsequent investigation was organized including cytology, ultrasound and non-contrast computed tomography (CT) scan head and neck.

Comment. This case illustrates that it is important for the primary care physician to be alert to the risk factors of thyroid cancer, i.e. previous history of irradiation. The 'patient factors' also suggest an increased likelihood of thyroid cancer. The presence of the chest infection may account for hoarseness but, in view of the other clinical information, thyroid malignancy should be suspected immediately. Stridor suggests advanced thyroid malignancy with recurrent laryngeal involvement. Same day referral, as previously outlined, is imperative.

Screening for thyroid cancer[9] (Level IV)

Risk-directed screening, usually by a specialist secondary team, should be considered in patients with:

- Familial thyroid cancer, including medullary thyroid cancer (MTC)
- History of neck irradiation in childhood
- Family history of multiple endocrine neoplasia type 2 (MEN2).

The following carry a statistically increased risk of thyroid malignancy but screening is not recommended in the UK:

- Endemic goitre
- Hashimoto's thyroiditis (risk of lymphoma)
- Family or previous history of thyroid adenoma
- Cowden's syndrome (macrocephaly, mild learning difficulties, carpet-pile tongue, with benign or malignant breast disease)
- Familial adenomatous polyposis.

EVIDENCE APPRAISAL

Much of the evidence of this chapter has been taken from the most recent national guidelines. Where appropriate within the text, references have been classified into the definition of types of evidence based on Agency for Health Care Policy and Research (1992).

Level	Type of evidence
Ia	Evidence obtained from meta-analysis of randomized controlled trials
Ib	Evidence obtained from at least one randomized controlled trial
IIa	Evidence obtained from at least one well-designed controlled study without randomization
IIb	Evidence obtained from at least on other type of well-designed quasi-experimental study
III	Evidence obtained from well designed non-experimental descriptive studies
IV	Evidence obtained from expert committee reports or opinions and/or clinical experience of respected authorities

REFERENCES

1. Karlson B, Gustafsson J, Hedov G, *et al.* Thyroid dysfunction in Down's syndrome. Arch Dis Childhood 1998;79:242–6.
2. American Association of Clinical Endocrinologists. Medical guidelines for the evaluation and treatment of hyperthyroidism and hypothyroidism. Endocr Pract 2002;8:457–69.
3. British Thyroid Association. UK guidelines for the use of thyroid function tests. London: British Thyroid Association, 2006.
4. Chu JN, Crapo LM. The treatment of subclinical hypothyroidism is seldom necessary. J Clin Endocrinol Metab 2001; 86:4591–5.
5. McDermott MT, Ridgway EC. Subclinical hypothyroidism is mild thyroid failure and should be treated. J Clin Endocrinol Metab 2001;86:4585–90.
6. British Thyroid Association and Royal College of Physicians. Guidelines for the management of thyroid cancer in adults. London: British Thyroid Association and Royal College of Physicians, 2007.
7. Vanderpump MPJ, Ahlquist JAO, Franklyn JA, *et al.* Consensus statement of good practice and audit measures in the management of hypothyroidism and hyperthyroidism. BMJ 1996;313:539–44.
8. Sawin CT, Geller A, Wolf PA, *et al.* Low serum thyrotrophin concentration as a risk factor for atrial fibrillation in older patients. N Engl J Med 1994;81:4224–8.
9. Wilson GR, Curry RW Jr. Subclinical thyroid disease. Am Fam Physician 2005;72:1517–24.

MULTIPLE CHOICE QUESTIONS

Select the single most appropriate option.

1. Thyroid hormone levels
A. Free T4 is the ideal screening test for thyroid function
B. TSH should be used to screen for thyroid disease and T3 or T4 used if the TSH is abnormal
C. In subclinical hypothyroidism TSH levels are within the normal range
D. A mild alteration in TSH levels is uncommon in acute and chronic illnesses
E. A TSH level greater than 4.5 μU/l confirms clinical hypothyroidism

2. Thyroid disease
A. Lethargy is a feature of both hyper- and hypothyroidism
B. Hyperthyroidism is obvious to diagnose clinically
C. Subclinical hyperthyroidism requires no treatment
D. Hypothyroidism is screened for in all neonates in the UK by a heel-prick blood test which is usually performed 6 weeks after birth
E. 'High uptake' thyrotoxicosis accounts for a minority of thyrotoxic patients.

3. Thyroid swellings
A. The thyroid can be diffusely enlarged in both hyperthyroid conditions and hypothyroid states
B. Autopsy studies have detected nodules in up to 20% of the population
C. A toxic or 'hot' nodule is a common cause of hyperthyroidism.
D. Solitary thyroid nodules have a 5% risk of malignancy
E. The management of a hypo- or hyperthyroid goitre is the same to that of a euthyroid goitre

4. Thyroid cancer
A. Patients with thyroid cancer usually show clinical signs of thyrotoxicosis
B. The overall 10-year survival for differentiated thyroid cancer is 80–90%
C. Multiple thyroid nodules have no significant malignant risk
D. Important poor prognostic factors include female gender and age >40 years

E. The incidence of thyroid cancer is not significantly raised in patients with a long-standing thyroid goitre

5. In the UK, risk-directed screening:
A. Is recommended in patients with Hashimoto's thyroiditis
B. Is recommended in patients with familial adenomatous polyposis
C. Is usually performed by the primary care physician
D. Recommendations are based on high level evidence
E. Should be considered in patients with a history of neck irradiation in childhood

Answers

1. B
2. A
3. A
4. B
5. E

2 Pathological spectrum of thyroid disease

Tim Stephenson
Department of Pathology, Royal Hallamshire Hospital, Sheffield, UK

KEY POINTS

- The thyroid is subject to two organ-specific autoimmune diseases. The presence of either increases the likelihood of developing other organ-specific autoimmune disease
- Benign thyroid masses are far more common than malignant tumours
- The thyroid develops several distinct malignant tumour types which must be correctly distinguished to enable accurate prognosis and treatment planning
- Accurate staging of thyroid cancer is essential to treatment planning
- A number of benign and physiological conditions simulate malignancy including post-fine needle aspiration cytology. Interpretation by experienced pathologists is therefore essential

The thyroid gland normally weighs 20–30 g and is composed of follicles (Fig. 2.1) containing colloid which is a proteinaceous stored secretion.[1] The follicles are lined by cuboidal epithelial cells which synthesize iodinated amino acids, thyroxine (T4) and tri-iodothyronine (T3). The secretion of T3 and T4 is under negative feedback control by thyroid-stimulating hormone (TSH) from the anterior pituitary. A fall in the plasma level of these thyroid hormones causes increased TSH secretion by their effects on the adenohypophysis and hypothalamus.[2]

The thyroid also contains a population of cells known as C cells. These are sparsely scattered throughout the gland and secrete calcitonin, a peptide hormone involved in calcium metabolism. Medullary carcinoma[3] can arise from these cells and is discussed later in this chapter.

There are three main types of clinical thyroid disease:

1. Secretory malfunction: hyper-/hypothyroidism
2. Swelling of the entire gland: goitre
3. Solitary masses: a dominant nodule within a multinodular goitre, adenoma or carcinoma.

A Practical Manual of Thyroid and Parathyroid Disease, 1st Edition. Edited by Asit Arora, Neil Tolley & R. Michael Tuttle.

SECRETORY MALFUNCTION

Hyperthyroidism

- Syndrome due to excess T3 and T4
- Most common cause is Graves' disease in which there is a long-acting thyroid-stimulating immunoglobulin (LATS)
- May be due to functioning adenoma
- Very rarely due to excess TSH.

Thyrotoxicosis is the clinical syndrome resulting from the effect of excess circulating T3 and T4 which ultimately causes an increased metabolic rate.[1] The source of circulating T3 and T4 is usually the thyroid gland affected by hyperthyroidism which arises due to a variety of pathological processes. The most common of these are:

1. Graves' thyroiditis
2. Functioning adenoma
3. Toxic nodular goitre (Plummer's disease).

Hyperthyroidism can also develop in a previously non-toxic multinodular goitre if the patient has taken unusually large amounts of iodine.[2] This probably arises due to autonomous foci within the goitre previously restricted in their capacity to synthesize thyroxine due to a lack of iodine. The increased iodine supply triggers the cuboidal epithelial cells abruptly to achieve their thyroxine-producing potential.

Thyrotoxicosis also occurs when excess exogenous thyroid supplementation is taken by the patient. More rarely, it arises from ectopic TSH secretion by certain tumours or is due to excess thyroxine secretion by struma ovarii, a monophyletic teratoma of the ovary comprising thyroid tissue.

Graves' thyroiditis

The most common cause of thyrotoxicosis is Graves thyroiditis[1] which is often associated with a diffuse goitre. The thyroid is moderately enlarged, firm and has a 'beefy-red' appearance reflecting increased gland vascularity. Histologically, there is hyperplasia of the

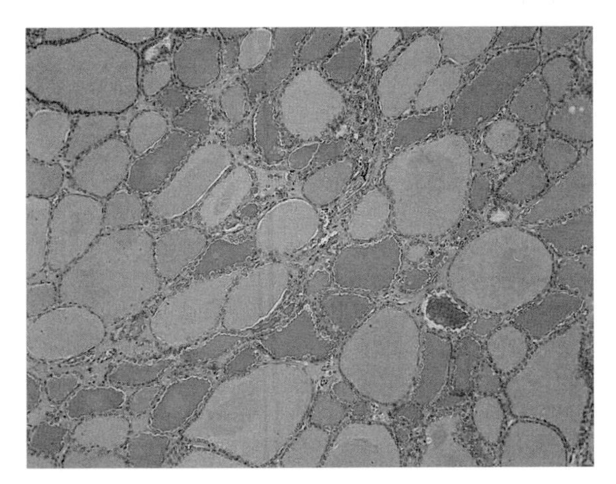

Fig. 2.1 Normal thyroid showing follicular epithelial cells and colloid.

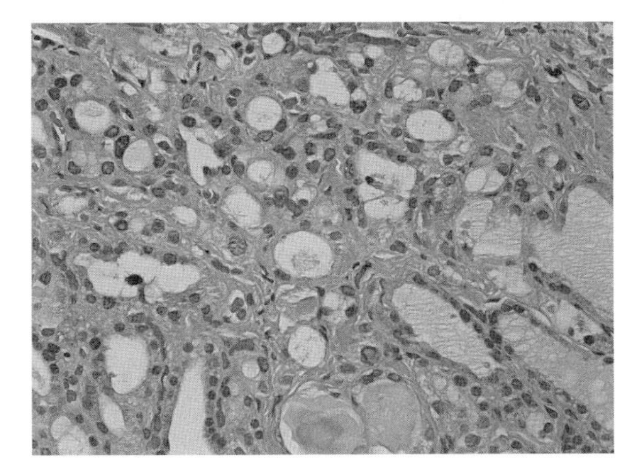

Fig. 2.2 Nuclear atypia in carbimazole-treated Graves' thyroiditis.

acinar epithelium, reduction of stored colloid and a local accumulation of lymphocytes with lymphoid follicle formation. The complete spectrum of classical features is rarely seen now due to the effect of anti-thyroid drugs given to the patient before surgery. Reaching the correct histological diagnosis can sometimes be hindered by the effects of medical therapy. For instance, the effects of carbimazole can mask important diagnostic clues such as lymphocytic infiltration. Carbimazole induces nuclear pleomorphism (Fig. 2.2) in the follicular epithelium which may be mistaken for follicular carcinoma. ^{131}Iodine therapy also induces long-lasting severe nuclear pleomorphism which mimics several tumour types, is associated with mild fibrosis and can be confused with invasive growth. Marked fibrosis is more typically a feature of external beam radiotherapy.

Graves' thyroiditis is an organ-specific autoimmune disease. The underlying pathogenesis involves immunoglobulin G (IgG) autoantibody which binds to thyroid epithelial cells and mimics the stimulatory action of TSH. Its effect on the thyroid is considered a 'stimulatory' hypersensitivity reaction because it stimulates the function and growth of thyroid follicular epithelium. In addition to the usual features of thyrotoxicosis, Graves' disease is associated with exophthalmos, pre-tibial myxoedema (due to accumulation of mucopolysaccharides in the deep dermis of the skin) and finger-clubbing. The latter two signs are rare effects compared with exophthalmos, which occurs due to fat infiltration of the orbital tissues (interestingly, adipocytes possess cell surface TSH receptors). Mucopolysaccharide and lymphocyte infiltration also occur, which may be due to an additional autoantibody reaction in the orbital tissue.

Functioning adenoma

Functioning adenomas[3] of the thyroid may cause thyrotoxicosis, although less than 1% possess sufficient secretory activity to do so. Histologically, the tumour is composed of thyroid follicles and is sometimes so small that it can only be visualized with an ^{131}I radioisotope scan. Occasionally the lesion presents as a solitary thyroid mass.

Toxic nodular goitre

Rarely one or two nodules in a nodular goitre develop hypersecretory activity.[2] This condition is called 'toxic' nodular goitre (Plummer's disease) and an ^{131}I radioisotope scan is usually required to demonstrate which nodule(s) demonstrate hypersecretory activity.

It is difficult or impossible to determine the relative functional state of the nodules based on histological analysis of the excised gland.

Hypothyroidism

- Syndrome due to insufficient circulating T3 and T4
- Most common cause is Hashimoto's thyroiditis which is an autoimmune disorder
- Other causes are: iatrogenic (thyroid excision, thyroid suppression by drugs), thyroid atrophy (can be due to anterior pituitary destruction with failure of TSH secretion) and peripheral T3/T4 resistance
- Congenital hypothyroidism causes cretinism.

The clinical syndrome resulting from inadequate levels of circulating T3 and T4 is called hypothyroidism. The metabolic rate is lowered and mucopolysaccharides accumulate in the dermal connective tissues, producing the typical myxoedematous facies. The most common cause of acquired hypothyroidism in adults is Hashimoto's thyroiditis. Iatrogenic causes are less common, e.g. following thyroidectomy or due to drugs such as sulphonylureas, resorcinol, lithium and amiodarone.

When hypothyroidism is present in the newborn, physical growth and mental development are impaired, sometimes irreversibly. The condition is known as cretinism and may be endemic in geographical areas where there is dietary iodine insufficiency. Sporadic cases are usually due to congenital absence of thyroid tissue or enzyme defects which block hormone synthesis.

Hashimoto's thyroiditis

In the early stages of Hashimoto's thyroiditis the gland is enlarged and appears firm, fleshy and pale. Damage to the thyroid follicles may cause thyroglobulin release into the circulation, resulting in a transient phase of thyrotoxicosis. Gland atrophy and fibrosis develop over time. Histologically, the gland is densely infiltrated by lymphocytes and plasma cells, with lymphoid follicle formation (Fig. 2.3). Colloid content is reduced and the thyroid epithelial cells typically enlarge, developing eosinophilic granular cytoplasm due to mitochondrial proliferation. These cells are variously termed Askanazy cells, Hurthle cells or oncocytes.[2]

Hashimoto's thyroiditis is another example of an organ-specific autoimmune disease. Two serum autoantibodies are detected in most patients. One reacts with thyroid peroxidase, the other with thyroglobulin. These autoantibodies are probably formed locally by plasma cells which infiltrate the thyroid gland and may be the result of a loss of specific suppressor T lymphocytes. As with other organ-specific autoimmune diseases there is a female preponderance, and certain human leucocyte antigens (HLAs) are commonly found in affected individuals, e.g. HLA-B8 and HLA-DR5.

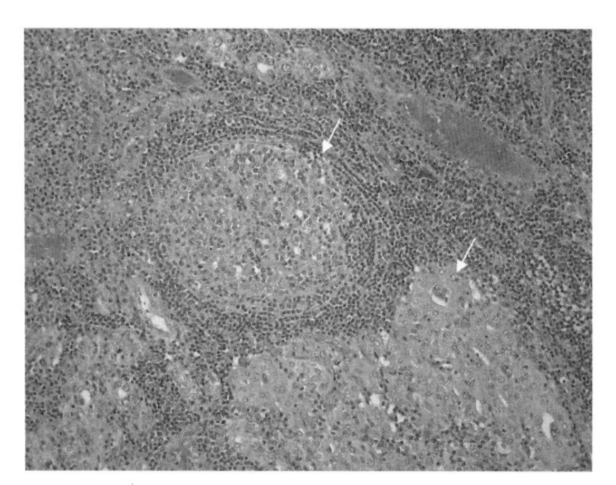

Fig. 2.3 Hashimoto's thyroiditis showing lymphoid follicles and enlarged thyroid epithelial cells due to Hurthle cell metaplasia.

GOITRE (ENLARGEMENT OF THE WHOLE GLAND)

The term goitre denotes an enlargement of the thyroid without hyper-/hypothyroidism.

Simple goitre

A spectrum of pathological changes occurs, ranging from parenchymatous to colloid goitre.

The former is characterized by hyperplasia of the thyroid epithelium with loss of stored colloid. Eventually less active areas appear and become compressed by the hyperplastic foci.

Tracts of fibrosis separate these areas, resulting in a multinodular goitre. The multiple nodules in this type of goitre are often clinically palpable. Occasionally one large nodule becomes 'dominant', giving rise to suspicion of neoplasia.

In colloid goitre the follicles accumulate large volumes of colloid and coalesce to form colloid-filled cysts (Fig. 2.4). There may be areas of haemorrhage, fibrosis and dystrophic calcification, but epithelial hyperplasia does not occur, unlike the parenchymatous type. The thyroid may be diffusely enlarged or multinodular. A complication of this condition is haemorrhage into a cyst, which causes rapid enlargement, potential tracheal compression and stridor.

Aetiology

It is thought to involve a phase of relative lack of T3 and T4 which causes a rise in TSH with subsequent hyperplasia of the thyroid epithelium. Lack of T3 and T4 is usually the result of three mechanisms:

1. Iodine deficiency due to endemic goitre or food faddism
2. Rare inherited enzyme defects in T3 and T4 synthesis
3. Drugs which induce hypothyroidism.

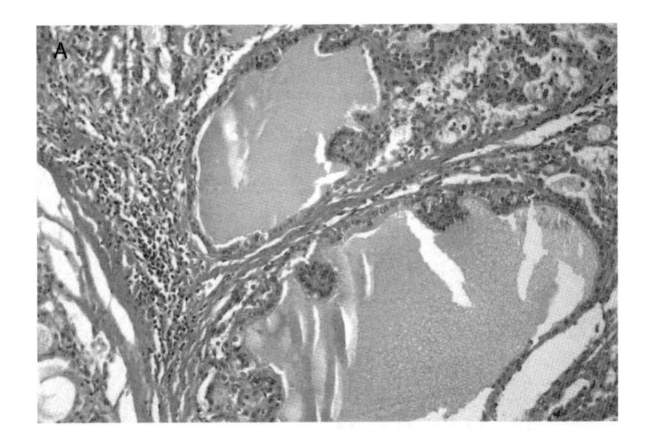

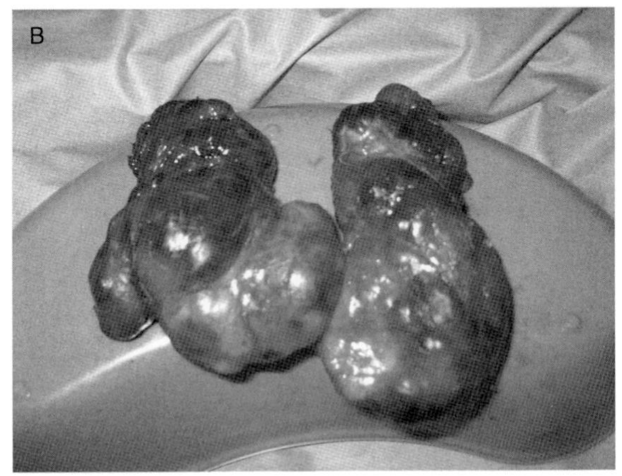

Fig. 2.4 **A** Variation in follicular size and colloid accumulation in dilated follicles in colloid goitre. **B** Excised multinodular goitre specimen.

Endemic goitre was formerly common in areas remote from the sea where the soil contains little iodine, e.g. the Derbyshire hills in the UK, parts of Switzerland and mountainous regions. The addition of iodine to the diet by iodination of table salt has reduced its incidence in some areas.

Rare causes of thyroiditis

Giant cell thyroiditis

Subacute/giant cell thyroiditis[1] (de Quervain's thyroiditis) is a distinctive form characterized by slight thyroid swelling with tenderness on palpation and abrupt onset of fever. Histologically, the gland is infiltrated by a mixture of neutrophil polymorphs and lymphocytes. There is a focal giant cell reaction which is probably due to epithelial cell fusion or histiocytic giant cells. It is thought to be induced by viral infections such as mumps, although the reason why only a few individuals develop this rare disease remains unclear.

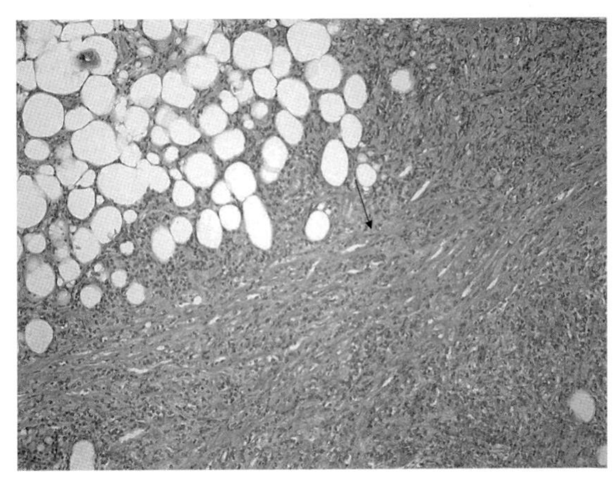

Fig. 2.5 Diffuse destructive fibrosis extending from the thyroid gland into surrounding connective tissue in Riedel's thyroiditis.

De Quervain's thyroiditis presenting as a spontaneous and diffuse condition should be distinguished from so-called 'palpation thyroiditis' in which there is focal lymphocytic infiltration and occasional giant cells. This latter condition is thought to be iatrogenic arising due to recent palpation of the thyroid gland.

Riedel's thyroiditis

Riedel's thyroiditis is an exceptionally rare cause of thyroid enlargement[1] characterized by dense fibrosis which may involve adjacent muscles. This renders the thyroid firm and immobile on palpation, thus mimicking carcinoma. Histologically, there is dense and somewhat diffuse fibrous replacement of the gland which causes characteristic occlusion of thyroid veins (Fig. 2.5) The aetiology is unknown but the condition is associated with retroperitoneal fibrosis. Hashimoto's thyroiditis has a fibrous variant in which there is early coarse fibrosis, although this condition lacks the obliterative vascular change seen in Riedel's thyroiditis. Fibrous variant Hashimoto's thyroiditis is considered distinct from Riedel's thyroiditis as the latter lacks the association with fibromatoses and occurs in individuals with a different HLA type. In fibrous variant Hashimoto's thyroiditis, destructive thyroid autoantibodies are particularly elevated.

Post-partum thyroiditis

A period of thyrotoxicosis may develop 3–12 months post-partum. Sometimes this is followed by a period of hypothyroidism which can last several months before the patient eventually becomes euthyroid.[1] It occurs in up to 10% of the population and is more common in women with the thyroid peroxidase autoantibody. The true histological picture is not known (due to a lack of biopsy data) although autoimmune thyroiditis with overlapping or sequential features of Graves'/Hashimoto's is postulated.

SOLITARY MASSES

Cytology, often targeted by ultrasound, has revolutionized the management of thyroid nodules (see Chapters 3 and 4). It allows the clinician to make a pre-operative diagnosis of thyroid neoplasia. Many of the clinically diagnosed solitary nodules are actually a dominant nodule within a multinodular goitre.

Tumours

- Usually benign (follicular adenoma)
- Malignant forms include carcinomas and lymphoma:
  - papillary adenocarcinoma (often multifocal, lymphatic spread)
  - follicular adenocarcinoma (usually solitary, haematogenous spread)
  - anaplastic carcinoma (aggressive local spread)
  - medullary carcinoma (derived from calcitonin-producing C cells, sometimes associated with multiple endocrine neoplasia syndromes)
  - lymphoma (usually non-Hodgkin's lymphoma of B cell type)
  - metastatic tumours.

Thyroid tumours are mostly benign. Carcinomas are rare and lymphomas even less common. Malignant thyroid tumours have a variable behaviour which dictates their clinical management.[4] Histological classification is therefore of vital importance.[5]

Benign tumours

Follicular adenoma[3] is a common cause of a solitary thyroid nodule. It usually consists of a solid mass within a fibrous capsule which compresses the adjacent gland. The centre of the lesion may contain areas of haemorrhage and cystic change. Microscopically, a range of appearances is seen. The most common architecture consists of compact follicles containing little colloid lined by epithelial cells with slight nuclear hyperchromatism. The surrounding fibrous capsule is not breached by the tumour. Rarely, a follicular adenoma may synthesize excess T3 and T4 and appear 'hot' on a radioisotope scan.

Malignant tumours

Thyroid cancer comprises only 1.3% of all malignancies and accounts for 0.4% of cancer deaths.[6] Because of the relatively low case-load, acquiring sufficient familiarity with the necessary criteria to establish thyroid malignancy is a challenge.[2] Accurate pathological diagnosis, including subclassification, is important because the clinical behaviour of thyroid cancer spans a broad spectrum. The indolent papillary microcarcinoma is virtually never associated with mortality,[2,7] in contrast to anaplastic carcinoma which is almost invariably fatal within 1 year of diagnosis.[8] Accurate staging is particularly important, and for certain histological subtypes it is the most important prognostic feature. The UK Endocrine Pathology Society recommends the 5th edition UICC TNM staging system[9] (rather than the latest 6th edition) because the earlier edition applies a pT1 cut-off of 10 mm which allows separation of papillary microcarcinomas into a distinct group with different treatment.[4] The 6th edition groups all tumours under 20 mm together as pT1.

Papillary adenocarcinoma

Classical type.

Classical papillary thyroid carcinoma is a well-differentiated form of adenocarcinoma most commonly found in younger (<45 years old) patients.[3] It presents as a non-encapsulated infiltrative mass which may be firm and white due to fibrosis. Histologically, it consists of epithelial papillary projections between which calcified spherules (psammoma bodies) may be present. The epithelial cell nuclei are characteristically large with central clear areas (Plate 2.1). It is for this reason that they are sometimes termed 'orphan Annie' nuclei. Optically clear nuclei, instrumental for establishing the diagnosis of papillary carcinoma, are also a consistent artefact of formalin fixation and paraffin processing. Frozen sections need to be used with caution in thyroid pathology because they usually fail to show the nuclear clearing typical of papillary carcinoma. Nuclear clearing occurs because papillary carcinoma cell nuclei have a cytoplasmic invagination and are often markedly hypodiploid, explaining their lack of chromatin. Air-dried Giemsa cytology preparations also fail to demonstrate nuclear clearing reliably although there may be partial grooving. The latter is better demonstrated in alcohol-fixed Papanicolaou-stained cytospin preparations.

Papillary adenocarcinoma metastasizes via the lymphatics within the thyroid gland (which may result in multifocal disease) and to the cervical lymph nodes.

Well-differentiated classical papillary carcinoma generally runs an indolent course with reported 5-year survival rates of 90% in males and 94% in females. Papillary microcarcinoma, by definition less than 10 mm diameter,[10] has an outstanding prognosis.[2] This is confirmed by post-mortem studies which detect papillary microcarcinoma in up to 35% of post-mortems.[11] Even the subset of microcarcinomas (11% of cases) which exhibits lymph node metastases or local recurrence[12] generally conform to an indolent long-term course.[13] Papillary microcarcinoma is usually diagnosed in the context of an incidental histological finding in a thyroidectomy specimen when surgery has been performed for benign disease.[14] In this clinical setting, the finding is of no prognostic significance[15]. Surgical treatment does not extend beyond thyroid lobectomy and isthmusectomy unless the microcarcinoma is multifocal. In this case total thyroidectomy is advocated due to the greater incidence of lymph node metastases and local recurrence associated with multifocal disease.[12] The surgical management of thyroid cancer is outlined in further detail in Chapter 10.

Benign conditions which mimic papillary cancer and its variants.

Classical papillary cancer shows true papillae with fibrovascular cores[13] rather than the epithelial multilayering typical of hyperplasia.[11] Follicular variant papillary carcinoma (FVPC) is diagnosed on nuclear appearances supplemented by scalloping of the colloid[16] and the finding of cells with dark nuclei. Grading of papillary carcinoma is not currently recommended by the UK Endocrine Pathology Society because most papillary carcinomas are well differentiated, and their classification based on histological variant probably contributes more prognostic information.

Follicular variant papillary carcinoma.

FVCP has three recognized variants. The encapsulated variant is surrounded by a capsule and the nuclear clearing is typically clonal and subcapsular.[17] Problems in diagnosis occur because benign follicular neoplasms may also exhibit focal nuclear clearing.[18] The nuclei are round, small and often centrally located in benign follicular neoplasms, which allows the two conditions to be differentiated.[19,20] Although encapsulated FVPC has a very good prognosis, its malignant potential should not be underestimated as bone metastasis has been reported in the occasional FVCP misdiagnosed as follicular adenomas.[3] The macrofollicular variant of FVPC exhibits focal distribution of diagnostic nuclear features and has large distorted follicles which can be easily mistaken for macrofollicular adenoma or adenomatous goitre. Correct differentiation is important as some studies suggest that the macrofollicular variant of FVPC is associated with an adverse prognosis.

Variants of papillary carcinoma associated with adverse prognosis.

The tall cell variant, the very rare columnar cell variant, the solid variant and the diffuse sclerosing variant are all considered to have an adverse prognosis. The demographic and clinical–pathological features of these relatively rare variants differ from those of papillary carcinoma, although there is some controversy concerning their true prognostic significance.[20] Hurthle cell variants of papillary carcinoma[21] are discussed later in this chapter.

Follicular adenocarcinoma

Follicular adenocarcinoma (Plate 2.2) presents in a similar fashion to follicular adenoma, often appearing as a round encapsulated nodule on 'naked-eye' inspection. Diagnosis of carcinoma is made by the demonstration of full-thickness capsular transgression by the tumour or genuine (extracapsular) vascular invasion. If either feature exists, the tumour is, by definition, a follicular carcinoma.[2] Previous fine needle aspiration cytology can create a range of artefactual appearances which mimic genuine capsular invasion.[22,23] The diagnosis is therefore not always straightforward and this is reflected in the widely disparate incidence of follicular carcinoma reported in the literature. Indeed, when thyroid pathologists co-review cases, follicular carcinoma is invariably the most poorly concordant diagnosis.[24]

Assigning prognosis.

Prognostic evidence suggests that it is important to differentiate between follicular carcinomas which are encapsulated and minimally invasive (associated with good outcome) and widely invasive tumours where it can be difficult to find the original capsule. The importance of this distinction is underlined by the observation that most of the latter group are poorly differentiated tumours.

Powerful prognostic information emerges from the finding of genuine vascular invasion and therefore this should always be categorized in encapsulated minimally invasive carcinoma. When there is capsular invasion without vascular invasion, an indolent course is probable similar to benign disease.[25] The number of instances of vascular invasion is also prognostic. Minimally invasive carcinoma with four or more instances of vascular invasion has a significantly worse prognosis than those with fewer.[26]

Capsular invasion can sometimes be incomplete. This occurs when there is inner 'partial thickness' capsular invasion or if tumour islands lie within the capsule but do not traverse it. The Chernobyl Pathologists Group suggested that a lesion with these findings can be classified using the term 'follicular tumour of uncertain malignant potential' (FT-UMP). However, several studies (subsequently formalized into new classifications[3]) suggest that full-thickness capsular invasion is a prerequisite for malignant behaviour. Even when this feature exists, adverse prognosis is highly dependent upon the occurrence and incidence of vascular invasion. It is our opinion that terminology such as FT-UMP is confusing and should be abandoned. The prognostic classification of follicular carcinoma compliant with existing best evidence is as follows:

- Encapsulated
  - with capsular invasion only
  - with infrequent (<4 instances) vascular invasion
  - with extensive (≥4 instances) vascular invasion
- Widely invasive.

Sampling for follicular tumours.
As previously outlined, the frequency of focal histological features such as vascular invasion has important prognostic use and therefore tumour sampling must be thorough. Usually this involves blocking out the entire capsule to ensure vascular invasion is not missed. The minimum sampling required for encapsulated follicular lesions is to process small lesions (up to 30 mm) in total and to take 10 blocks from larger lesions.[27] Some authorities suggest that all follicular lesions should have their entire capsule processed into blocks.

When the previously outlined diagnostic criteria are fulfilled, follicular carcinoma accounts for 5–15% of thyroid cancer. Patients with minimally invasive encapsulated tumours have 10-year survival rates ranging from 100% (cases without vascular invasion) to 70% (extensive vascular invasion present). The 10-year survival drops to 25–45% for widely invasive follicular thyroid carcinoma.[28]

Metastasis characteristically occurs via the bloodstream to the bones and lungs which represent the most common sites of secondary spread. Many follicular metastases retain their ability to take up ^{131}I. This iodine avidity can be exploited to deliver a highly effective targeted form of radiotherapy. The prognosis is therefore generally good.

Hurthle cell tumours

Hurthle cells tumours are considered to be variants of other tumour types rather than a truly distinct entity. They have voluminous eosinophilic cytoplasm rich in mitochondria which is readily demonstrated with special stains and by electron microscopy.[21] The term Hurthle cell tumour is applicable when it comprises more than 75% oncocytic cells.[3]

Diagnosing malignancy.
The defining criteria for malignancy is the same as for differentiated thyroid neoplasms.[29] The process involves correct recognition of the basic type of thyroid tumour (e.g. papillary, follicular) of which the Hurthle cell tumour is a variant before deploying the relevant diagnostic and prognostic rules according to appropriate tumour categorization.[21] There are a few cautionary points as Hurthle cell tumours are more likely than ordinary follicular neoplasms to demonstrate invasion and tumour necrosis.[30] Thorough sampling of Hurthle cell neoplasms is therefore important and any cystic, necrotic thyroid tumour should be carefully assessed for Hurthle cell elements. The Hurthle cell has an innate degree of nuclear atypia which does not predict malignancy. The same is true for the mitotic count and presence of multinucleation.[21] A proportion of Hurthle cell tumours are variants of papillary carcinoma, including its follicular variant. It is probably the Hurthle cell variant FVPC which accounts for the notoriety of encapsulated Hürthle cell tumours in relation to its propensity for lymph nodes metastasis.

Diagnosing Hurthle cell variant of papillary carcinoma.
Special care is required when diagnosing Hurthle cell variants of papillary carcinoma.

- Hurthle cell change is seen in thyroid hyperplasia and degeneration which also produces benign pseudopapillary appearances in the thyroid.[21]
- Hurthle cell papillary carcinomas sometimes have solid, pleomorphic nuclei rather than the characteristic optically clear nuclei.[10]
- Immunohistochemistry of Hurthle cells is hindered by their non-specific imbibition, irrelevant antibodies and abundant endogenous peroxidase which is difficult to block.

- Some of the most reliable markers of papillary carcinoma, e.g. cytokeratin 19 and HBME-1, do not routinely stain the Hurthle cell variant well.[31]

Prognosis of Hurthle cell tumours.
The prognosis of patients with Hurthle cell papillary carcinoma and follicular carcinoma is probably worse than those with standard tumours. Hurthle cell variants of follicular carcinomas are generally more resistant to radioiodine therapy due to their poor uptake of this.[3] In Hurthle cell papillary carcinoma, the worse prognosis may be explained by the presence of tall cell variants which are mixed in with this group.

Poorly differentiated, insular and anaplastic carcinoma

A useful approach in tumours which appear poorly differentiated is to assess multiple blocks for areas of better differentiation which may betray their origin. Careful observation and special techniques are required to re-classify them into the existing categories of thyroid carcinoma, invariably at the less differentiated end of the spectrum.

Insular carcinoma is a well-defined entity[32] with a distinct histological appearance characterized by well-formed nests and islands. It is positive for thyroglobulin on immunohistochemistry,[2] indicating follicular cell origin. These tumours occur in a slightly younger age group than anaplastic carcinoma and behave in an aggressive fashion due to early metastatic spread.[2]

Anaplastic carcinoma (Fig. 2.6) is thought to arise by de-differentiation of well-differentiated neoplasms.[33]

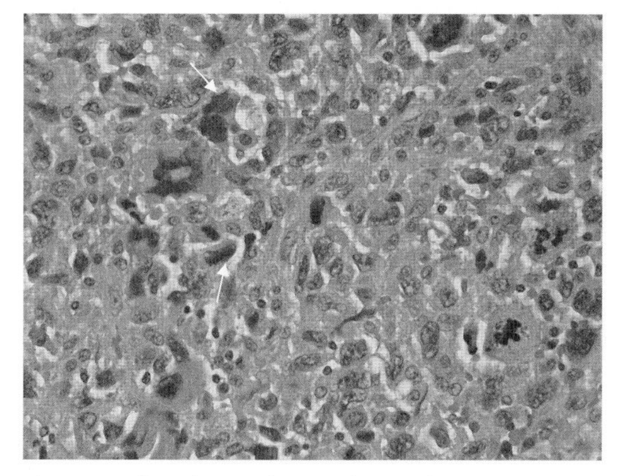

Fig. 2.6 Nuclear pleomorphism and atypical mitoses in anaplastic carcinoma.

Areas of poorly differentiated follicular or papillary carcinoma can sometimes be found within these tumours. Adverse prognostic histological variants may also be demonstrated by sampling a large number of blocks.

Prognosis.
Anaplastic carcinoma accounts for 5–10% of thyroid cancers, is seen principally in the elderly and has a notoriously appalling prognosis due to aggressive local spread to adjacent structures. The finding of anaplastic carcinoma within a differentiated tumour automatically upgrades the tumour stage to a T4 cancer.[9]

Medullary carcinoma

Several different growth patterns are possible in medullary carcinoma (Plate 2.3), and when it is suspected special techniques should be employed to investigate this tumour.[34] Usually this involves immunohistochemical confirmation rather than using argyrophil stains. Immunohistochemistry for calcitonin is the appropriate initial technique as only a small proportion of medullary carcinomas do not stain for it. Alternative markers include calcitonin gene-related product (CGRP) which is positive in most medullary carcinomas,[34] and neuroendocrine markers, e.g. chromogranin A, synaptophysin and carcinoembryonic antigen (CEA). The latter is almost always strongly present. Amyloid is evident in up to 80% of cases, and its presence may be associated with an indolent clinical course.[35]

C-cell hyperplasia.
To determine whether a patient with medullary cancer has familial disease, non-tumoural thyroid tissue may be scrutinized for C-cell hyperplasia.[36] Calcitonin immunohistochemistry assists the process but demonstration of C-cell hyperplasia is tricky and knowledge of the specific location of background thyroid blocks is helpful (C cells are most frequent in the lateral regions of the upper poles of the thyroid). Fortunately genetic testing for *RET* mutations to detect MEN type 2 syndromes is now possible.[37] This technique is recommended in preference to the less reliable process of demonstrating C-cell hyperplasia.

Prognosis.
Prognosis depends largely on tumour stage, age and sex. The best prognosis is seen in women younger than 40 years who present with early stage disease.[38] Familial cases generally have a poorer prognosis. This includes cases arising within the context of MEN type 2B which is associated with C-cell hyperplasia, phaeochromocytoma,

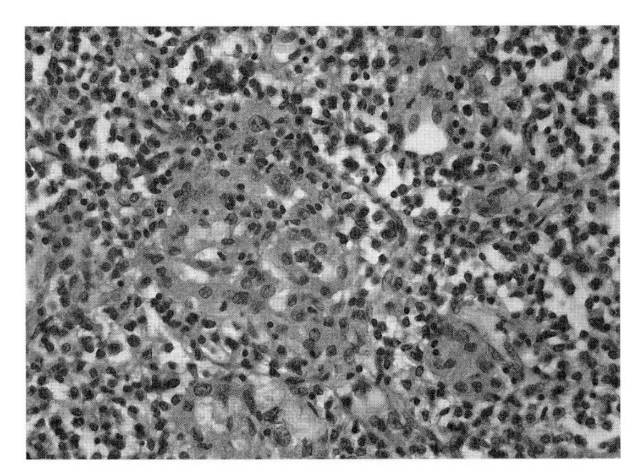

Fig. 2.7 Over-running of thyroid follicules by destructive lymphocytic infiltrate in thyroid lymphoma.

adrenal medullary hyperplasia, mucosal neuromas, gastrointestinal ganglioneuromas and musculoskeletal abnormalities. It may be that the percentage of cells staining for calcitonin acts as a marker of tumour differentiation. Less than 25% of cells staining positive for calcitonin and concurrent CEA-positive staining is associated with an adverse clinical outcome.[38]

Lymphoma

Thyroid tumours which were classified as anaplastic carcinoma in previous years are now recognized, on the basis of electron microscopy and immunohistochemistry, mostly to comprise non-Hodgkin's lymphoma. There is an increased incidence of this lymphoma type originating in the thyroid in Hashimoto's thyroiditis.[39] Most thyroid lymphomas are neoplasms of mucosa-associated lymphoid tissue and termed marginal zone lymphoma (Fig. 2.7).

Correct differentiation between Hashimoto's thyroiditis (a common antecedent of lymphoma) and lymphoma can be difficult, particularly on frozen section. Features suggestive of marginal zone lymphoma rather than Hashimoto's thyroiditis include penetration of the lymphocytic infiltrate through venous walls, lack of Hurthle cell metaplasia, extensive follicular destruction with formation of lymphoepithelial lesions and diffuse distribution of the lymphocytic infiltrate.[39] Immunohistochemistry is required to assist the differential diagnosis from other types of thyroid lymphoma, including mantle cell lymphoma and diffuse large B-cell lymphoma. The latter conditions have a worse prognosis and require a treatment different from that of the common marginal zone lymphoma. Clonality studies[40] such as molecular biological techniques for IgH gene rearrangement assist the differentiation of early lymphoma from Hashimoto's thyroiditis.

Metastatic tumours

The thyroid is a surprisingly frequent recipient of metastatic deposits beyond what might be expected in view of its small size. Autopsy studies in patients with disseminated malignancy demonstrate metastatic thyroid tumour in up to 20% of cases.[3] Certain tumours are more likely to metastasize to the thyroid gland, such as renal cell carcinoma. Metastatic colorectal carcinoma involving the thyroid mimics the tall cell and columnar cell variants of papillary cancer.

REFERENCES

1. Lloyd RV, Douglas BR, Young WF. Endocrine diseases. Fascicle 1 in atlas of nontumor pathology. Washington: American Registry of Pathology and Armed Forces Institute of Pathology, 2002.
2. LiVolsi VA, Asa SL. Endocrine Pathology. Edinburgh: Churchill Livingstone, 2002.
3. Rosai J, Carcangiu ML, DeLellis RA. Tumors of the thyroid gland. Atlas of tumor pathology, Third series fascicle 5. Washington: Armed Forces Institute of Pathology, 1992.
4. British Thyroid Association and Royal College of Physicians. Guidelines for the management of thyroid cancer in adults. London, 2002.
5. Royal College of Pathologists. Dataset for thyroid cancer histopathology reports. London, 2006,
6. Chu KC, Kramer BS. Cancer patterns in the United States. In: Greenwald P, Kramer BS, Weed DL, eds. Cancer prevention and control. New York: Marcel Dekker, 1995:37.
7. Sipponen P, Louhimo J, Nordling S, *et al.* Prognostic factors in papillary thyroid cancer: an evaluation of 601 consecutive patients. Tumor Biol 2005;26:57–61.
8. Hadar T, Mor C, Shvero J, *et al.* Anaplastic carcinoma of the thyroid. Eur J Surg Oncol 1993;19:511–6.
9. International Union Against Cancer. TNM classification of malignant tumours, 5th edn. New York: Springer-Verlag, 1997:47–50.
10. Hedinger C, Williams ED, Sobin LH. Histological typing of thyroid tumours: WHO international histological classification of tumours, 4th edn. Berlin: Springer-Verlag, 1988.
11. Hubert JP, Kiernan PD, Beahrs OH, *et al.* Occult papillary carcinoma of the thyroid. Arch Surg 1980;115:394–8.
12. Strate SM, Lee EL, Childers JH. Occult papillary carcinoma of the thyroid with distant metastases. Cancer 1984;54: 1093–1100.

13. Stephenson TJ. Commentary: papillary carcinoma of the thyroid—difficult yet fascinating model of oncogenesis and tumour progression. Histopathology 2004;44:498–500.
14. Baudin E, Travagli JP, Ropers J, *et al.* Microcarcinoma of the thyroid gland: the Gustave-Roussy Institute experience. Cancer 1998;83:553–9.
15. Anderson CE, McLaren KM. Best practice in thyroid pathology. J Clin Pathol 2003;56:401–5.
16. Rosai J, Kuhn E, Carcangiu ML. Pitfalls in thyroid tumour pathology. Histopathology 2006;49:107–20.
17. Stephenson TJ. Benign lesions and mimics of malignancy in the thyroid gland. CPD Bull-Cell Pathol 2003;4:139–44.
18. Stephenson TJ. Endocrine. In: Al-Sam S, Lakhani SR, Davies JD, eds. A practical atlas of pseudomalignancy. London: Edward Arnold, 1998:1–19.
19. Stephenson TJ. Prognostic and predictive factors in endocrine neoplasia. Histopathology 2006;48:629–43.
20. Stephenson TJ. Criteria for malignancy in endocrine tumours. In: Anthony PP, MacSween RNM, Lowe D, eds. Recent advances in histopathology 17. Edinburgh: Churchill Livingstone, 1997:93–111.
21. Asa SL. My approach to oncocytic tumours of the thyroid. J Clin Pathol 2004;57:225–32.
22. LiVolsi VA, Merino MJ. Worrisome histologic alterations following fine-needle aspiration of the thyroid (WHAFFT). In: Sommers SC, Rosen PP, eds. Pathology annual. Connecticut: Appleton-Century-Crofts, 1994;29:99–120.
23. Baloch ZW, LiVolsi VA. Post fine-needle aspiration histologic alterations of thyroid revisited. Am J Clin Pathol 1999;112:311–6.
24. Khan NF, Perzin KH. Follicular carcinoma of the thyroid: an evaluation of the histologic criteria used for diagnosis. In: Sommers SC, Rosen PP, eds. Pathology annual. Connecticut: Appleton-Century-Crofts, 1983;18:221–53.
25. Baloch ZW, LiVolsi VA. Our approach to follicular-patterned lesions of the thyroid. J Clin Pathol 2007;60: 244–50.
26. Lang W, Choritz H, Hundeshagen H. Risk factors in follicular thyroid carcinomas. A retrospective follow-up study covering a 14-year period with emphasis on morphological findings. Am J Surg Pathol 1986;10:246–55.
27. Franssila KO, Ackerman LV, Brown CL, Hendinger CE. Follicular carcinoma. Semin Diagn Pathol 1985;2:101–22.
28. Brennan MD, Bergstrahl EJ, van Heerden JA, *et al.* Follicular thyroid cancer treated at the Mayo Clinic, 1946 through 1970: initial manifestations, pathologic findings, therapy and outcome. Mayo Clin Proc 1991;66:105–11.
29. Carcangiu ML, Bianchiu S, Savino D, *et al.* Follicular Hürthle cell tumors of the thyroid gland. Cancer 1991;68: 1944–53.
30. Bronner MP, LiVolsi VA. Oxyphilic (Askenazy/Hürthle cell tumors of the thyroid. Microscopic features predict malignant behaviour. Surg Pathol 1988;1:137–50.
31. Mai KT, Bokkary R, Yazdi HM, *et al.* Reduced HBME-1 immunoreactivity of papillary thyroid carcinoma and papillary thyroid carcinoma-related neoplastic lesions with Hürthle cell and/or apocrine like changes. Histopathology 2002;40:133–42.
32. Carcangiu ML, Zampi G, Rosai J. Poorly differentiated (insular) thyroid carcinoma: a reinterpretation of Langhan's 'wuchernde Struma'. Am J Surg Pathol 1984;8:655–68.
33. Kapp DS, LiVolsi VA, Sanders MM. Anaplastic carcinoma following well-differentiated thyroid cancer: etiologic considerations. Yale J Biol Med 1982;55:521–8.
34. Sikri KL, Varndell IM, Hamid QA, *et al.* Medullary carcinoma of the thyroid gland: an immunocytochemical and histochemical study of 25 cases using eight separate markers. Cancer 1985;56:2481–91.
35. Scopsi L, Sampietro G, Boracchi P, *et al.* Multivariate analysis of prognostic factors in sporadic medullary carcinoma of the thyroid. A retrospective study of 109 consecutive patients. Cancer 1996;78:2173–83.
36. Perry A, Molberg K, Albores-Saavedra J. Physiologic versus neoplastic c-cell hyperplasia of the thyroid. Cancer 1996;77:750–6.
37. Bugalho MJ, Domingues R, Sobrinho L. Molecular diagnosis of multiple endocrine neoplasia Type 2. Expert Rev Mol Diagn 2003;3:769–79.
38. Shroder S, Bocker W, Baisch H, *et al.* Prognostic factors in medullary thyroid carcinoma: survival in relation to age, sex, stage, histology, immunohistochemistry and DNA content. Cancer 1988;61:806–16.
39. Thompson LDR. Primary thyroid lymphoma. In: Thompson LDR, ed. Endocrine pathology. Philadelphia: Elsevier, 2006:123–31.
40. Widder S, Pasieka JL. Primary thyroid lymphomas. Curr Treat Options Oncol 2004;5:307–13.

MULTIPLE CHOICE QUESTIONS

Select the single most appropriate option.

1. Which of the following thyroid tumours has the best prognosis?
A. Anaplastic carcinoma
B. Follicular variant papillary carcinoma
C. Follicular carcinoma
D. Insular carcinoma
E. Medullary carcinoma

2. Why does frozen section lead to non-recognition of papillary carcinoma and its variants?
A. Papillae disappear on freezing
B. Frozen sections are impossible to cut from thyroid tissue
C. Cancer can never be diagnosed reliably on any frozen section

D. Optically clear nuclei feature only in paraffin sections
E. Frozen sections make cells look smaller than in paraffin sections

3. Which pair of conditions are both candidates for considering ^{131}I therapy?
A. Hashimoto's thyroiditis and follicular carcinoma
B. Riedel's thyroiditis and Hashimoto's thyroiditis
C. Graves thyroiditis and follicular carcinoma
D. Thyroid lymphoma and Graves thyroiditis
E. Granulomatous thyroiditis and post-partum thyroiditis

4. Which of the following types of thyroiditis is usually associated with thyrotoxicosis?
A. Hashimoto's thyroiditis
B. Granulomatous thyroiditis
C. Graves thyroiditis
D. Palpation thyroiditis
E. Riedel's thyroiditis

5. Which of the following is true of Hurthle cell tumours?
A. Hurthle cell follicular tumours are less likely to show invasion than ordinary follicular tumours
B. They are exclusively derived from follicular tumors
C. They take up radioiodine better than non-Hurthle cell tumours
D. Their chance of malignant behaviour is impossible to predict
E. By definition, at least 75% of the cells within this tumour demonstrate oncocytic change

Answers

1. B
2. D
3. C
4. C
5. E

3 Thyroid cytopathology

Glen Dixon & Julie McCarthy
St Mary's Hospital, Imperial College Healthcare NHS Trust, London, UK

KEY POINTS

- Fine needle aspiration (FNA) of the thyroid is best performed free-hand by an experienced cytopathologist with immediate staining for assessment of adequacy and interpretation
- The use of thyroid FNA reduces the use of surgery by approximately one-third (70–40%)
- An adequate thyroid FNA is one which is truly representative of the lesion
- One repeat FNA 6–12 months after an initial benign aspiration reduces the false-negative rate
- There is currently no magic marker which preoperatively differentiates benign follicular neoplasia from follicular carcinoma.

The modern use of fine needle aspiration (FNA) cytology of the thyroid gland was developed in Europe during the 1950s and 1960s, with the major developments occurring in Scandinavia.[1,2] In the latter part of the 20th century, FNA secured its rightful position as an essential first step in the assessment of a thyroid nodule. Thyroid FNA is now well established as a first-line diagnostic test in the evaluation of all thyroid swellings and is the single most effective test for pre-operative assessment and diagnosis of solitary thyroid nodules.

Thyroid nodules are common. Within the general population, palpable thyroid nodules are present in 4–7% of adults and non-palpable nodules in up to 70% of individuals. At least 90% of thyroid nodules are benign and often do not require treatment. The incidence of thyroid malignancy in the UK is 1.2 per 100 000 of the population in men and 3.0 per 100 000 in women. There are 900 new thyroid cancer cases and 250 disease-specific deaths every year.[3] FNA acts as an effective screening test by identifying nodules likely to be malignant and require surgery from the larger group of individuals with benign nodules which can be managed conservatively.

WHO SHOULD PERFORM THYROID FNA?

There is good evidence to suggest that cytopathologists are best placed to aspirate palpable lesions.[4–7] In some centres, radiologists perform a significant proportion of thyroid FNA under ultrasound guidance. While they may perform sufficient numbers to gain experience and expertise, there is no doubt that palpable nodules should be aspirated by a cytopathologist performing the technique free-hand. This is the most cost-effective way of obtaining a fast and accurate pre-operative diagnosis. In our practice, once FNA has been performed by the cytopathologist, thyroid ultrasound is carried out on the vast majority of thyroid nodules. This provides invaluable information about cystic areas, calcification and lesion size, and is useful for monitoring the growth of a nodule (see Chapter 4). For smaller nodules which are difficult to palpate, ultrasound-guided FNA with cytopathologist support is recommended. This has the advantage of confirming that the sample is from the nodule in question and allows targeted sampling of solid areas within cystic nodules. Impalpable lymph nodes are also best sampled by ultrasound-guided FNA. The cytology report assists with staging thyroid malignancy and subsequent surgical management.

In the absence of a dedicated cytopathologist, a radiologist or surgeon who performs aspirations routinely can achieve high levels of adequacy.[5,8] Sample preparation should be performed according to guidelines outlined by the cytopathology laboratory to maximize the diagnostic potential of every aspiration. This ideally involves a member of the laboratory staff to assist in sample spreading and preparation.

HOW IS THYROID FNA PERFORMED AND PROCESSED?

The technique can be performed on ambulatory patients in an outpatient setting or at the bedside with inpatients. A chaperone is usually required during the procedure. This can be a nurse, clinic assistant or trained member of the cytopathology laboratory staff.

Following a brief clinical history that should include the patient's sex, age, family history of thyroid disease and history of previous radiotherapy to the neck, a full examination of the neck and thyroid is performed. This allows identification of additional nodules and palpable lymph nodes.

The patient is consented (either verbal or written) for the procedure and asked to lie supine with a pillow

A Practical Manual of Thyroid and Parathyroid Disease, 1st Edition. Edited by Asit Arora, Neil Tolley & R. Michael Tuttle.

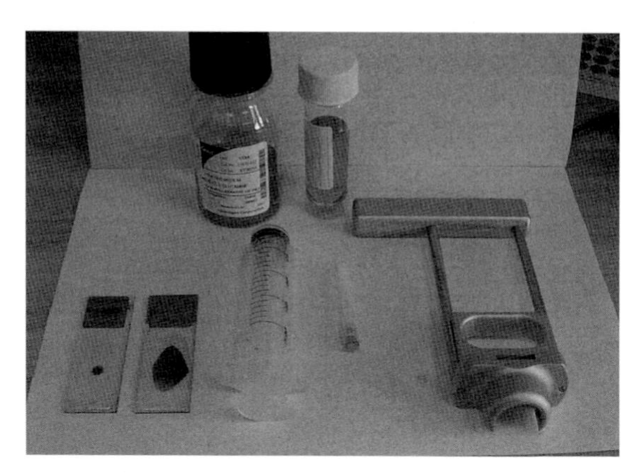

Fig. 3.1 The equipment required to perform thyroid FNA is inexpensive and readily available. The pistol shown is the Cameco syringe pistol (Cameco AB, Taby, Sweden). The fluid used may be culture medium (shown here) or commercially available cell fixative solution such as Cytolyt.

supporting the shoulders to extend the neck such that the sternocleidomastoid muscles are splayed laterally. The patient is requested not to swallow or speak during the aspiration procedure. The skin is cleaned with an alcohol swab, the nodule is 'fixed' with one hand while the overlying skin is stretched between finger and thumb. Local anaesthesia is not necessary.

A 22 or 23 gauge needle attached to a 10 or 20 ml syringe within a syringe holder (Cameco syringe pistol; Fig. 3.1) is passed into the nodule. Once the needle tip is within the nodule, suction is applied and the needle is advanced through the nodule in different directions for approximately 10–20 s. The needle is withdrawn after suction is released and a sterile gauze or cotton wool ball used to apply pressure to the puncture site. Some guidelines advocate the use of capillary aspiration to prevent excessive blood contamination.[9] In our experience, this technique is not superior to using a syringe and pistol particularly as many thyroid lesions have a cystic component. The degree of blood contamination can be minimized by rapid spreading and the use of a fluid-based collection system that lyses red blood cells. Loss of vacuum in the syringe during aspiration is usually due to puncture of the trachea with the needle which causes the patient to cough. The presence of ciliated respiratory epithelial cells and mucus in the cytological preparations confirms this.

Pressure must be applied to the puncture site following withdrawal of the needle to prevent a haematoma forming. The patient or clinic assistant can perform this task using a sterile gauze or cotton wool for a few minutes. This allows the aspirator to prepare the sample rapidly. It is at this point that the game is won or lost. Obtaining material from thyroid nodules is relatively easy. Submitting well-spread, good quality slides that facilitate diagnosis is the tricky part. Speed is of the essence as even a short delay results in sample clotting with diagnostic material trapped in and obscured by fibrin strands. The needle and syringe are disengaged from the holder. There is usually sufficient air in the syringe to expel a small amount of material onto the upper one-third of two glass slides which are labelled with three patient identifiers. If material is not expelled and the syringe is empty of air, the needle should be detached and air sucked into the barrel prior to re-attaching the needle and repeating the process.

The sample is spread evenly along the length of two slides using a third slide which is then discarded. Material remaining in the needle hub or syringe (whether visible or not) is flushed into fluid to provide a liquid-based sample. Appropriate fluid medium includes a preservative solution such as Cytolyt which is methanol based, haemolytic cell culture fluid such as RPMI 1640 or sterile saline. The cytology laboratory determines the specific fluid medium. There are several benefits to providing two air-dried slides and a fluid sample. First, the time taken to screen two slides and a fluid sample is far shorter than screening the large number of slides often submitted by less experienced clinicians. It is not the case that more is better in this situation; quality supersedes quantity. Providing a fluid sample allows further laboratory processing to be undertaken as this sample is ideal for multiple slides for immunocytochemistry and other special stains.

Immediate assessment of direct smears in the outpatient setting is advisable to ensure adequate sampling. It also provides an initial impression of the likely cytological diagnosis so that further investigations such as immunocytochemistry and microbiology can be initiated. More than one pass is sometimes necessary, particularly for larger thyroid nodules, to increase the likelihood of obtaining a representative sample. The importance of the macroscopic description of aspirated material is often forgotten in pathology reports. The macroscopic appearance of the aspiration is extremely useful to record. For instance, water clear fluid is only ever aspirated from parathyroid cysts.

The patient may use a mild non-aspirin analgesic following the procedure, although in our experience this is not usually required. It is important to inform the patient how and when the FNA results will become available.

HOW IS THYROID FNA INTERPRETED?

Cytopathology plays a central role within the thyroid multidisciplinary team (MDT) framework. A structured, regular multidisciplinary meeting is the best way to arrange thyroid cancer care.[10] Given that FNA cytology of thyroid nodules is the mainstay of pre-operative assessment, accurate cytological interpretation and thorough case review is paramount to maintain high sensitivity and specificity and prevent unnecessary surgery.

> It is estimated that the use of FNA with interpretation by specialist cytopathologists has reduced the number of patients requiring thyroid surgery from approximately 70% to 40%.[11]

FNA results are reported according to the 'Thy 1–5' classification system in the UK (see Table 3.1).[3] This allows the MDT to plan the patient's management. The classification includes: inadequate, benign, indeterminate, suspicious and malignant categories.

There is good evidence validating the need for a five-tier system, and published data suggest that the positive predictive value (PPV) of an indeterminate (Thy 3), suspicious (Thy 4) and malignant (Thy 5) cytological diagnosis is 50, 71 and 100% respectively.[12] Other centres use a four-tier classification system.[13]

Thyroid FNA remains the most sensitive and specific non-surgical investigation available for thyroid cancer.[14–17] Accuracy has been reported as greater than 95% in adequate samples. Sensitivity ranges from 43 to 98%, specificity is between 72 and 100%, PPV between 89 and 98% and negative predictive value (NPV) between 94 and 99%.[11] False-negative rates of 1–11% and false-positive rates of 0–7% have been reported. High test accuracy can be consistently achieved by an experienced aspirator and specialist cytopathologist interpreting the specimen. The broad range of sensitivities and specificities reported in the literature reflects the variability of these factors.

False-negative cytological diagnoses usually reflect inadequate sampling, poor technique or errors of diagnostic interpretation. The principal cause of false positives reflects the cytological diagnosis of follicular neoplasms in colloid nodules with follicular hyperplasia and neoplasms in thyroiditis.[18]

Thy 1: inadequate

Samples may be considered inadequate due to poor cellularity, cystic aspirates, aspirates obscured by blood, extensive air-drying artefact and poor technique when spreading material on slides. Thyroid FNA is inadequate in approximately 10–20% of cases.[19,20] Limiting thyroid sampling to experienced aspirators improves this figure. In our experience, Thy 1 samples can be reduced to less

Table 3.1 Thy 1–5 classification

Thy 1: non-diagnostic (inadequate or when technical artefact precludes interpretation). Smears must contain six or more groups of at least 10 thyroid follicular cells to be considered adequate.
Action: FNA should be repeated. Ultrasound guidance may permit more targeted sampling.
Thy 2: non-neoplastic (features consistent with a nodular goitre or thyroiditis)
Action: two diagnostic benign results 3–6 months apart are required to exclude neoplasia. In patients in a high clinical risk group (e.g. male gender, extremes of age, other features suggestive of tumour, family history or history of irradiation) the decision to proceed to lobectomy is justified even with a benign FNA diagnosis. Surgery is also indicated if there are pressure symptoms or when there is rapid growth in a thyroid lesion. In addition, patient choice regarding management is important.
Thy 3
(i) All follicular lesions (indeterminate).
Action: lobectomy. Completion thyroidectomy will be necessary if the histology proves malignant.
(ii) There may be a very small number of cases where the cytological findings warrant inclusion in this category rather than in Thy 2 or Thy 4. The text of the report will indicate the suspicious findings.
Action: these cases should be discussed at MDT meetings to decide on the appropriate course of action.
Thy 4: abnormal, suspicious of malignancy (suspicious, but not diagnostic of papillary, medullary, anaplastic carcinoma or lymphoma).
Action: surgical intervention is indicated for differentiated tumour. Further treatment will depend on the pathology report. Further investigation indicated for anaplastic thyroid carcinoma, lymphoma or metastatic tumour.
Thy 5: diagnostic of malignancy (unequivocal features of: papillary, medullary, anaplastic carcinoma, lymphoma or metastatic tumour).
Action: surgical intervention indicated for differentiated thyroid cancer, depending on tumour size, clinical stage and other risk factors such as gender and extremes of age. Indication for appropriate further investigation, radiotherapy or chemotherapy for anaplastic thyroid carcinoma, lymphoma or metastatic tumour.

than 5% by performing immediate microscopic assessment of cytopathologist-obtained FNA samples in the outpatient setting.

When assessing whether a thyroid FNA is adequate, the degree of cellularity is an important factor. Adequacy is traditionally defined as a minimum of six groups of well-preserved follicular epithelial cells with each group containing at least 10 cells. However, we believe that this is somewhat arbitrary and prefer the notion that an adequate sample should be representative of the lesion. Samples containing scanty atypical cells are not necessarily considered inadequate. Benign thyroid cysts include macrophages and thin colloid with scanty or no epithelial cells. These may be classified as benign (Thy 2) provided that follow-up and repeat aspiration of the remaining lesion is performed within 6 months. Cystic lesions contribute to a significant false-negative rate so the possibility of missing a papillary or follicular carcinoma with cystic change should always be considered. The sensitivity of FNA diagnosis in cystic neoplasms may be as low as 40%.[21,22] In this setting, ultrasound evaluation is particularly helpful to target re-aspiration of the solid component within a cystic lesion.

Thy 2: benign

The most common entity within this diagnostic category is the colloid nodule or nodular colloid goitre. Aspiration of a colloid nodule results in abundant colloid, usually in association with flat sheets of benign follicular epithelial cells, foamy macrophages and occasional Hurthle cells. The cytoplasm of follicular cells in nodular colloid goitre frequently shows involutional changes such as small paravacuolar granules which represent lysosomal debris or lipofuscin. Colloid nodules may undergo cystic or haemorrhagic degeneration. Generally, the ratio of colloid to the degree of cellularity is high in these lesions. Abundant colloid is a reassuring cytological feature.

While the degree of cellularity is usually low in benign conditions, hyperplastic nodules may be highly cellular. A macrofollicular architecture is suggestive of a benign lesion. The presence of large flat sheets of uniformly spaced thyroid follicular cells indicates the presence of macrofollicles.

Highly cellular samples may be seen in other benign conditions, including Graves' disease and Hashimoto's thyroiditis. In both conditions, colloid may be scanty and the degree of cellularity worrying. Treated Graves' disease is associated with marked nuclear pleomorphism, and adequate, accurate clinical information is essential to avoid misinterpretation. Hashimoto's thyroiditis (defined by the presence of anti-microsomal anti-thyroid antibodies) is associated with florid lymphocytic infiltration and Hurthle cell metaplasia with multinucleate histiocytic giant cells and lymphoid follicle fragments in the background. A florid lymphocytic thyroiditis may mimic reactive lymphadenopathy or low-grade lymphoma within the thyroid gland. Immunocytochemistry may be required to reach the correct diagnosis.

> One repeat FNA 6–12 months after an initial benign aspiration increases the sensitivity for malignancy and decreases the false-negative rate.

Guidelines recommend that a minimum of two aspirates showing benign features be performed 6–12 months apart before opting for conservative management.[23] Surgery may be warranted for other reasons regardless of the FNA result, e.g. clinical suspicion, local pressure effects or cosmetic reasons.

Thy 3: all follicular lesions (indeterminate)

The most problematic area in thyroid aspiration interpretation is that of follicular lesions. These include benign hyperplastic (adenomatous) nodules, follicular adenomas, follicular carcinomas and the follicular variant of papillary thyroid carcinoma. Cytologically, there can be a significant overlap in these conditions, and other parameters and ancillary tests help to define these lesions further pre-operatively.

> **Case study 1**
> A 63-year-old female presented with symptoms of tracheal obstruction and superior vena caval (SVC) compression. An ultrasound scan revealed a large mass arising from the inferior pole of the left thyroid lobe extending into the mediastinum. CT scan confirmed a large retrosternal thyroid mass with SVC, oesophageal and tracheal compression.
> FNA was performed.
> Diagnosis: Thy 3 follicular neoplasm (Fig 3.2).
> Action: surgical excision of the thyroid revealed a haemorrhagic, necrotic tumour measuring 90 × 60 × 50 mm arising from the left lower pole of the thyroid. Microscopically, the tumour was follicular carcinoma with evidence of capsular breach.

A follicular pattern is characterized by the formation of rosettes of follicular epithelial cells around a central space. The space may be filled with colloid or appear empty. Normofollicular and macrofollicular lesions are usually

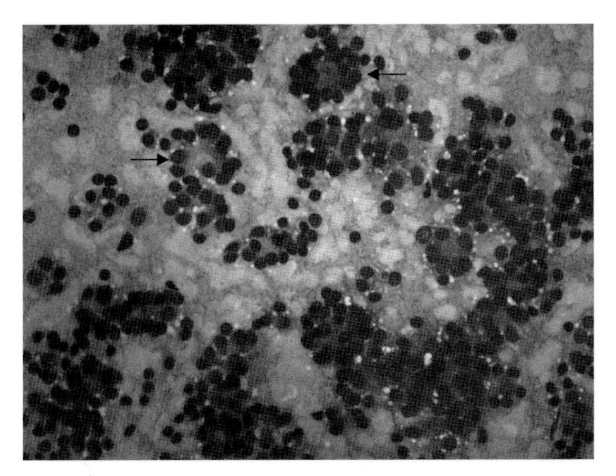

Fig. 3.2 Follicular lesion, Thy 3. A repetitive pattern of empty microfollicles characterizes a follicular lesion.

part of the same benign hyperplastic spectrum. Hyperplastic nodules within an otherwise unremarkable multinodular goitre may yield intact small follicular structures reminiscent of a follicular neoplasm. The presence of large flat sheets and an abundance of colloid make the diagnosis relatively straightforward. However, the appearance of repetitive microfollicles, which may contain inspissated colloid, is associated with follicular adenomas and carcinomas. Such aspirates are usually reported as 'follicular lesion, neoplasm cannot be excluded' and designated Thy 3. In carcinoma, nuclei tend to be larger with coarser chromatin and more prominent nucleoli than in adenomas.[24–26] In the majority of cases, cytology alone cannot reliably discriminate between follicular adenomas and carcinomas. This distinction requires histological examination of the capsule of the excised nodule and evidence of vascular invasion (see Chapter 2).

Lobectomy is the management of choice for Thy 3 lesions, with completion thyroidectomy performed depending on the histological outcome.

Thy 4: suspicious

A relatively low proportion of thyroid FNA is reported as 'suspicious of malignancy'. The PPV of Thy 4 classification is at least 70%.[12] This category is used when the aspirate is clearly abnormal but lacks features diagnostic of malignancy. Usually the aspirate is poorly cellular or does not include well-preserved cells showing typical features of malignancy. A confident diagnosis of papillary carcinoma can only be made when several criteria have been fulfilled. The most important of these are the presence of papillary structures with or without adherent blood vessels, intranuclear pseudoinclusions and dense 'metaplastic' cytoplasm. A combination of two of these features yields 100% PPV.[27] Cases which do not display these features but contain other atypical features should be classified as suspicious. The presence of papillary structures alone is insufficient for a diagnosis of papillary carcinoma.

Primary low-grade lymphoma within the thyroid can be difficult to diagnose. Lymphocytic infiltration within the thyroid is abnormal and may be associated with autoimmune thyroiditis (Hashimoto's thyroiditis) or de Quervain's thyroiditis. In autoimmune thyroiditis, a florid lymphocytic infiltrate may be present with few residual epithelial cells. This makes it difficult to distinguish from a lymphomatous process particularly in the elderly. Lymphoma of the thyroid arises on a background of autoimmune disease in approximately 75% of cases, which compounds the problem.

Case study 2

A 67-year-old man presented with a 6-month history of a left thyroid swelling. Previous FNA was reported as benign (Thy 2). His free thyroxine (T4) and triiodothyronine (T3) were within the normal range but throid-stimulating hormone (TSH) was reduced at 0.18 mU/l (range 0.35–4.00 mU/l).

FNA was performed (see Plate 3.1).

Diagnosis: low-grade B-cell non-Hodgkin's lymphoma.

Action: a surgical biopsy was performed to confirm the diagnosis. This was reported as low-grade non-Hodgkin's lymphoma, extranodal marginal zone MALT (mucosa-associated lymphoid tissue) type. A staging CT scan confirmed thyroid enlargement with prominence of the left lobe and several small lymph nodes (<9 mm short axis) in the left carotid sheath. There was no evidence of systemic disease.

High-grade lymphoma is easier to recognize as it usually presents with a short clinical history and a rapidly enlarging gland. High-grade lymphomas are mainly diffuse high-grade B-cell non-Hodgkin's lymphoma. This is easier to recognize cytologically due to diffuse sheets of large atypical lymphoid cells. Immunocytochemistry and flow cytometric immunophenotyping are useful to confirm the diagnosis. Hodgkin's lymphoma is extremely rare in the thyroid gland.

In the relatively small number of cases when FNA is reported as suspicious of malignancy, frozen section combined with intraoperative cytology has been shown to be of value in preventing two-step surgical excision (lobectomy followed by total thyroidectomy).[28] Frozen section is of no value in the diagnosis of follicular carcinoma.

Thy 5: malignant

This category includes aspirates with unequivocal features of malignancy. The main features of papillary carcinoma have already been outlined. Additional findings include longitudinal nuclear grooves, multinucleate giant cells, 'chewing gum' colloid, psammomatous calcifications and lymphocytic infiltration. Nuclear pseudoinclusions are also found in medullary carcinoma, anaplastic carcinoma, hyalinizing trabecular adenoma, metastatic malignant melanoma and in some follicular neoplasms.[29–31] Nuclear grooves are less specific as this finding may be encountered in many non-neoplastic thyroid lesions.[32]

The degree of accuracy for diagnosis of papillary carcinoma is reported to range between 60 and over 90% in several large series.[27,33,34]

Case study 3

A 34-year-old female presented with a lateral neck swelling. She was 18 weeks pregnant and ultrasound scan revealed an 18 × 14 × 12 mm solitary left thyroid nodule.
FNA was performed under ultrasound guidance.
Diagnosis: papillary carcinoma (Thy 5).
Action: surgical excision deferred until the post-partum period.

Medullary carcinoma usually yields very cellular aspirates. Cells are arranged in loose clusters, sheets or syncytial aggregates and sometimes the pattern is reminiscent of follicular or papillary tumours (Plates 3.2 and 3.3).

Cell morphology is variable and often includes plasmacytoid cells together with spindle cells. Other common features include hyperchromasia, binucleation and multinucleation. Neurosecretory granules may be seen within the cytoplasm of malignant cells and intranuclear inclusions are also frequently observed. Amyloid may be demonstrated using Congo red staining. Immunocytochemistry is very helpful to confirm the diagnosis. Tumour cells are positive for calcitonin, CEA (carcinoembryonic antigen) and chromogranin, but do not contain thyroglobulin.

Case study 4

An 88-year-old female presented with a solitary thyroid nodule. Thyroid function tests revealed a normal free T4 of 15.2 pmol/l (range 10.3–24.5) and an elevated TSH of 8.7 mU/l (range 0.35–4.00). Ultrasound revealed a well-defined solitary nodule measuring 22 × 13 mm with peripheral and central vascularity.
FNA was performed (see Fig. 3.3 and Plate 3.4).
Diagnosis: medullary carcinoma (Thy 5).
Action: total thyroidectomy and right neck dissection. Histopathology confirmed a 20 mm medullary carcinoma with no evidence of lymph node metastases.

Anaplastic carcinoma may be difficult to diagnose due to fibrosis and inflammation. Malignant cells are typically large and bizarre. They may also appear spindled or rounded. A small cell variant exists but this is rare. Anaplastic cells show high mitotic activity and tumour necrosis in keeping with rapid growth and a short clinical history. Many cells contain intranuclear inclusions which can sometimes create diagnostic confusion with papillary carcinoma. Areas of residual papillary, medullary or follicular carcinoma have all been sampled from anaplastic tumours which may pre-exist in these neoplasms. The presence of necrosis and loss of thyroglobulin immune reactivity usually prevent an erroneous diagnosis.

The thyroid is not an uncommon site for metastases in patients with disseminated malignancy. The most frequent primary sites metastasizing to the thyroid include lung, gastrointestinal tract, breast, kidney, melanoma and lymphoma. Cytological features suggestive of metastatic disease include an admixture of benign macrofollicles and colloid with the malignant cells and a background tumour diathesis. Immunocytochemistry can be very helpful in confirming the diagnosis. With the exception of anaplastic carcinoma, primary thyroid tumours are thyroglobulin positive. Tumours from other sites display a variety of immunoprofiles. Tumours arising from adjacent structures, such as laryngeal or tracheal squamous cell carcinoma, can directly invade the thyroid gland.

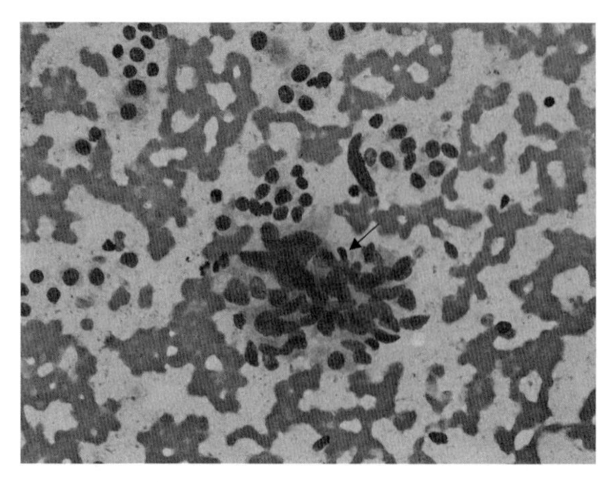

Fig. 3.3 Medullary carcinoma of thyroid. Cohesive clusters of atypical, hyperchromatic spindle and plasmacytoid cells.

ANCILLARY INVESTIGATIONS

> There is currently no 'magic marker' which pre-operatively differentiates malignant follicular thyroid tumours from adenomas.

Immunocytochemistry is useful to characterize known or suspected malignancy and is particularly useful in the diagnosis of medullary carcinoma, lymphoma and metastasis.

Recent advances in molecular diagnostics raise the possibility of being able to differentiate cytologically between benign and malignant thyroid lesions. At the present time, however, no sensitive and specific molecular or imunocytochemical test exists which reliably distinguishes follicular adenoma from carcinoma (Table 3.2). Markers that have shown promise include galectin-3, CK19 and HBME-1.

Galectin-3 is a carbohydrate-binding polypeptide involved in regulating cell–cell and cell–matrix interactions. In addition, galectins appear to play an important role in the initiation and regulation of cell growth and malignant transformation. A number of studies have assessed the diagnostic value of galectin-3 overexpression in determining the benign or malignant nature of thyroid tumours, particularly of follicular origin.[35–42] The results are somewhat conflicting and there are concerns regarding the specificity of galectin-3 due to the false-positive staining of galectin-3 in normal thyroid tissue, Hashimoto's thyroiditis and adenomas.

CK19 is a low molecular weight cytokeratin present in simple epithelia and basal cell layers of stratified epithelium. Analysis of cytological and surgical samples has shown that CK19 is strongly and diffusely expressed in papillary carcinoma, heterogeneously expressed in follicular carcinoma and absent or focally expressed in follicular adenomas.[43]

Table 3.2 Sensitivity and specificity of cytological molecular markers for thyroid cancer

Marker	Patients/controls	Sensitivity/specificity (%)	Study
Galectin-3	35/29	100/89	Orlandi *et al.* (1998)[54]
Galectin-3	83/86	100/100	Inohara *et al.* (1999)[42]
Galectin-3	226	100/98*	Bartolazzi *et al.* (2001)[55]
Galectin-3	17/52	100/92	Saggiorato *et al.* (2001)[41]
Galectin-3	45/20	98 (93)/45 (90)†	Giannini *et al.* (2003)[56]
CD44v6	16/14	88/93	Chieng *et al.* (1997)[57]
CD44v6	7/29	100/82	Takano *et al.* (1997b)[58]
CD44v6	12/17	75–91/41–72‡	Aogi *et al.* (1999)[46]
CD44v6/Gal-3§	53/104	85/98	Gasbarri *et al.* (1999)[59]
Oncofetal fibronectin	37/109	95/96	Takano *et al.* (1998b)[60]
Oncofetal fibronectin	45/20	98/60	Giannini *et al.* (2003)[56]
hTERT	12/17	67/71	Aogi *et al.* (1999)[46]
hTERT	19/18	79/72	Saji *et al.* (1999)[47]
hTERT	14/10	93/90	Zeiger *et al.* (1999)[61]
hTERT	14/13	93/39	Liou *et al.* (2003)[62]
hTERT	5/14	60/36	Sebesta *et al.* (2001)[63]
HMG1	126/232	96/81	Chiappetta *et al.* (1998)[64]
RET/PTC	33/40	52/100	Cheung *et al.* (2001)[65]
RET/PTC	39/4	54/100	Chiappetta *et al.* (2002)[66]
CT/CEA¶	11/24	100/100	Takano *et al.* (1999a)[67]
CT¶	6/5	100/100	Bugalho *et al.* (2000)[68]

Studies indicating sensitivity and specificity, respectively, are included. Control groups include patients without thyroid disease and patients with non-malignant thyroid disease. Some data are derived from subgroups of the studies.
* Data from the prospective analysis of the study.
† Data for RT-PCR-detected mRNA (for immunohistology).
‡ Range for different CD44 isoforms.
§ Data for combined parameters.
¶ Sensitivity and specificity for detecting medullary thyroid carcinoma.
CEA, carcinoembryonic antigen; CT, calcitonin; HMG1, high mobility group I proteins. hTERT, human telomerase reverse transcriptase.
Reproduced from Bojunga J and Zeuzem S,[51] with permission from Blackwell Publishing.

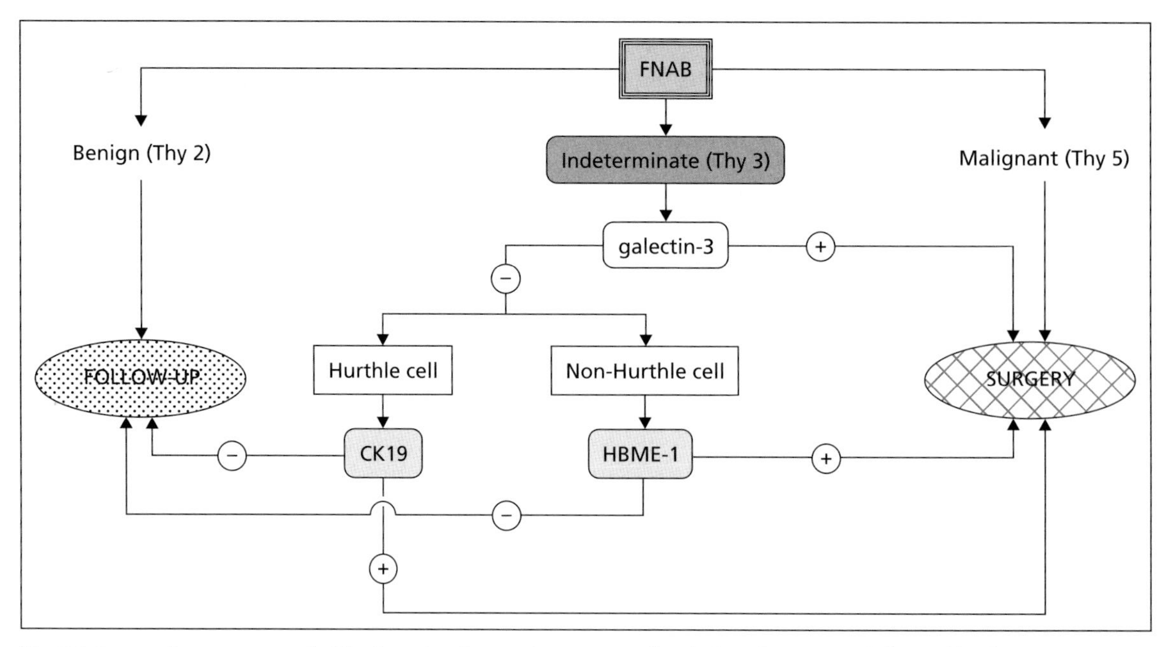

Fig. 3.4 Proposed management of a Thy 3 result using two immunocytochemical markers sequentially combined (galectin-3 + CK19 or galectin-3 + HMBE-1). From Saggiorato E *et al.*[43] © Society for Endocrinology (2005). Reproduced by permission.

HBME-1 is a monoclonal antibody directed against a membrane antigen of the microvillar surface of mesothelioma cells. This is positive in neoplastic cells, particularly papillary carcinoma, and negative in benign lesions.[43]

It is possible that combination assays utilizing two or more immunocytochemical markers can be developed to create an effective ancillary test. One suggested clinicopathological algorithm for the management of patients with an indeterminate FNA ('follicular neoplasm'—Thy 3) is outlined in Fig. 3.4. This uses a combination of galectin-3 and HBME-1 for conventional follicular lesions and galectin-3 with CK19 for Hurthle cell lesions.[43] Thyroid nodules with an indeterminate FNA and a positive galectin-3 test are directly referred for surgery without additional ancillary testing, regardless of clinical and ultrasound features. Galectin-3-negative cases require a second marker which is HBME-1 for the non-Hurthle cell neoplasms and CK19 for the Hurthle cell tumours. A negative test result with the second marker enables the clinician to recommend a conservative management policy with follow-up surveillance and repeat FNA in 6–12 months.

Other markers which have shown some promise as ancillary tests include human telomerase reverse transcriptase (hTERT) and 3p25 rearrangements of the *PPARG* gene. The catalytic component of telomerase, hTERT, is re-activated in immortalized cell lines. Several studies have demonstrated an intimate correlation between hTERT mRNA expression and telomerase activity in a number of human carcinomas including breast, testis, colon, ovary, pancreas, prostate and liver. The detection of the hTERT catalytic subunit of telomerase may be helpful in differentiating benign thyroid lesions from carcinoma.[44–50] Detection of the hTERT gene in thyroid carcinoma is also associated with poor prognosis.[52] However, it has been suggested that telomerase assays do not add any additional information to FNA alone and the presence of lymphocytes can give false-positive results.[47,51]

Among the numerous chromosomal changes described in follicular adenoma and carcinoma, chromosomal loss at 3p25 is most commonly found in both tumours. It was initially reported that 3p25 rearrangement of the *PPARG* gene may be specific for follicular carcinoma. Later studies showed that this rearrangement is also seen in follicular adenoma.[53] The use of panels of genetic markers or gene expression profiling may hold the key to the adenoma versus carcinoma conundrum in the future.

Papillary thyroid carcinomas may contain distinctive genetic features including chromosomal translocations involving the *RET* proto-oncogene on chromosome 10 (*RET/PTC*) and point mutations in the *BRAF* gene. *RET/*

PTC rearrangements have also been found in benign nodules and, to date, these potential markers have shown significant limitations in their predictive values. They are not routinely used in clinical practice.[51]

At the time of writing, routine FNA cytomorphology remains the gold standard in the pre-operative assessment of thyroid nodules. This should be performed in conjunction with radiology in selected cases.

EVIDENCE APPRAISAL

Research evidence referred to in this chapter is Level III, IV and V.

The Thy 1–5 classification forms part of the British Thyroid Association and Royal College of Physician guidelines for the management of thyroid cancer in adults which have been reviewed by leading international experts in thyroid cancer.

REFERENCES

1. Einhorn J, Franzen S. Thin-needle biopsy in the diagnosis of thyroid disease. Acta Radiol 1962;58:321–36.
2. Soderstrom N. Puncture of goitres for aspiration biopsy. A preliminary report. Acta Med Scand 1952;144:235–44.
3. British Thyroid Association. Guidelines for the management of thyroid cancer in adults. London: British Thyroid Association, Royal College of Physicians, 2002.
4. Hegedus L. Clinical practice: the thyroid nodule. N Engl J Med. 2004;351:1764–71.
5. Singh N, Ryan D, Berney D, *et al.* Inadequate rates are lower when FNA samples are taken by cytopathologists. Cytopathology 2003;14:327–32.
6. Hoda RS. Why pathologists should take needle aspiration specimens. Cytopathology 1995;6:419–20.
7. Padel AF, Coghill SB, Powis SJ. Evidence that the sensitivity is increased and the inadequacy rate decreased when pathologists take aspirates for cytodiagnosis. Cytopathology 1993; 4:161–5.
8. Kocjan G. Fine needle aspiration cytology: inadequate rates compromise success. Cytopathology 2003;14:307–8.
9. Bakshi NA, Mansoor I, Jones BA. Analysis of inconclusive fine-needle aspiration of thyroid follicular lesions. Endocr Pathol 2003;14:167–75.
10. Nix P, Nicolaides A, Coatesworth AP. Thyroid cancer review 1: presentation and investigation of thyroid cancer. Int J Clin Pract 2005;59:1340–4.
11. Gharib H, Goellner JR. Fine-needle aspiration biopsy of the thyroid: an appraisal. Ann Intern Med 1993;118:282–9.
12. Yoder BJ, Redman R, Massoll NA. Validation of a five-tier cytodiagnostic system for thyroid fine needle aspiration biopsies using cytohistologic correlation. Thyroid 2006;16: 781–6.
13. Gharib H, Papini E, Valcavi R, *et al.* American Association of Clinical Endocrinologists and Associazione Medici Endocrinoligi medical guidelines for clinical practice for the diagnosis and management of thyroid nodules. AACE/AME Task Force on Thyroid Nodules. Endocr Pract 2006;12:63–101.
14. Sangalli G, Serio G, Zampatti C, *et al.* Fine needle aspiration cytology of the thyroid: a comparison of 5469 cytological and final histological diagnoses. Cytopathology 2006;17: 245–50.
15. Schmitt FC. Thyroid cytology: FNA is still the best diagnostic approach. Cytopathology 2006;17:210–6.
16. Landsford CD. Evaluation of the thyroid nodule. Cancer Control 2006;13:89–98.
17. Nguyen G, Lee MW, Ginsburg J, *et al.* Fine-needle aspiration of the thyroid: an overview. Cytojournal 2005;2:12–25.
18. Gerhard R, da Cunha Santos G. Inter- and intraobserver reproducibility of thyroid fine needle aspiration cytology: an analysis of discrepant cases. Cytopathology 2007;18: 105–11.
19. Castro MR, Gharib H. Thyroid fine needle aspiration biopsy; progress, practice and pitfalls. Endoc Pract 2003;9:128–36.
20. Chow LS, Gharib H, Goellner JR, *et al.* Non-diagnostic thyroid fine needle aspiration cytology; management dilemmas. Thyroid 2001;11:1147–51.
21. Rosen IB, Provias JP, Walfish PG. Pathologic nature of cystic thyroid nodules selected for surgery by needle aspiration biopsy. Surgery 1986;100:606–16.
22. Sarda AK, Bal S, Dutta Gupta S, Kapur MM. Diagnosis and treatment of cystic disease of the thyroid by aspiration. Surgery 1988;103:593–6.
23. Flanagan MB, Ohori NP, Carty SE, *et al.* Repeat thyroid nodule fine-needle aspiration in patients with initial benign cytological results. Am J Clin Pathol 2006;125:698–702.
24. Kini SR. Thyroid. In: Kline TS, ed, Guides to clinical aspiration biopsy, 2nd edn. New York: Igaku-Shion, 1996:66–93.
25. Nunez C, Mendelsohn G. Fine needle aspiration and needle biopsy of the thyroid gland. Pathol Annu 1989;24:161–98.
26. Suen KC. How does one separate cellular follicular lesions of the thyroid by fine needle aspiration biopsy? Diagn Cytopathol 1988;4:78–81.
27. Miller TR, Bottles K, Holly EA, *et al.* A step-wise logistic regression analysis of papillary carcinoma of the thyroid. Acta Cytol 1986;30:285–93.
28. Deveci MS, Deveci G, LiVolsi VA, *et al.* Fine-needle aspiration of follicular lesions of the thyroid. Diagnosis and follow-up. Cytojournal 2006;3:9–14.
29. Glant MD, Berger EK, Davey DD. Intranuclear cytoplasmic inclusions in aspirates of follicular neoplasms of the thyroid. Acta Cytol 1989;28:576–9.
30. Goellner JR, Carnay JA. Cytological features of fine needle aspirates of hyalinizing trabecular adenoma of the thyroid. Am J Clin Pathol 1989;91:115–9.
31. Lew W, Orell SR, Henderson DW. Intranuclear vacuoles in non-papillary carcinoma of thyroid: a report of 3 cases. Acta Cytol 1984;28:581–6.

32. Gould E, Watzak L, Chamizo W, *et al.* Nuclear grooves in cytologic preparations. A study of the utility of this feature in the diagnosis of papillary carcinoma. Acta Cytol 1989;33: 16–20.
33. Hsu C, Boey J. Diagnostic pitfalls in the fine needle aspiration of thyroid nodules. A study of 555 cases in Chinese patients. Acta Cytol 1987;31:699–704.
34. Kini SR, Miller JM, Hamburger JI, *et al.* Cytopathology of papillary carcinoma of the thyroid by fine needle aspiration. Acta Cytol 1980;24:511–21.
35. Kovács RB, Földes J, Winkler G, *et al.* The investigation of galection-3 in disease of the thyroid gland. Eur J Endocrinol 2003;149:449–53.
36. Rossi ED, Raffaelli M, Minimo C, *et al.* Immunocytochemical evaluation of thyroid neoplasms on thin-layer smears from fine-needle aspiration biopsies. Cancer Cytopathol 2005;105:87–95.
37. Prasad MJ, Pellegata NS, Huang Y, *et al.* Galectin-3, fibronectin-1, CITED-1, HBME1 and cytokeratin-19 immunohistochemistry is useful for the differential diagnosis of thyroid tumors. Mod Pathol 2005;18: 48–57.
38. Jakubiak-Wielganowicz M, Kubiak R, *et al.* Usefulness of galectin-3 immunohistochemistry in differential diagnosis between thyroid follicular carcinoma and follicular adenoma. Pol J Pathol 2003;54:111–5.
39. Feilchenfeldt J, Tötsch M, Sheu SY, *et al.* Expression of galectin-3 in normal and malignant thyroid tissue by quantitative PCR and immunohistochemistry. Mod Pathol 2003;16:1117–23.
40. Papotti M, Volante M, Saggiorato E, *et al.* Role of galectin-3 immunodetection in the cytological diagnosis of thyroid cystic papillary carcinoma. Eur J Endocrinol 2002;147: 515–21.
41. Saggiorato E, Cappia S, De Giuli P, *et al.* Galectin-3 as a presurgical immunocytodiagnostic marker of minimally invasive follicular thyroid carcinoma. J Clin Endocrinol Metab 2001;86:5152–8.
42. Inohara H, Honjo Y, Yoshii T, *et al.* Expression of galectin-3 in fine-needle aspirates as a diagnostic marker differentiating benign from malignant thyroid neoplasms. Cancer 1999;85:2475–84.
43. Saggiorato E, De Pompa R, Volante M, *et al.* Characterisation of thyroid 'follicular neoplasms' in fine-needle aspiration cytological specimens using a panel of immunohistochemical markers: a proposal for clinical application. Endocr Relat Cancer 2005;12:305–17.
44. Siddiqui MT, Greene KL, Clark DP, *et al.* Human telomerase reverse transcriptase expression in Diff-Quik-stained FNA samples from thyroid nodules. Diagn Mol Pathol 2001;10:123–9.
45. Brousset P, Chaouche N, Leprat F, *et al.* Telomerase activity in human thyroid carcinomas originating from the follicular cells. J Clin Endocrinol Metab 1997;82: 4214–6.
46. Aogi K, Kitahara K, Buley I, *et al.* Telomerase activity in lesions of the thyroid: application to diagnosis of clinical samples including fine-needle aspirates. Clin Cancer Res 1998;4:1965–70.
47. Saji M, Xydas S, Westra WH, *et al.* Human telomerase reverse transcriptase (hTERT) gene expression in thyroid neoplasms. Clin Cancer Res 1999;5:1483–9.
48. Aogi K, Kitahara K, Urquidi V, *et al.* Comparison of telomerase and CD44 expression as diagnostic tumour markers in lesions of the thyroid. Clin Cancer Res 1999;5: 2790–7.
49. Lerma E, Mora J. Telomerase activity in 'suspicious' thyroid cytology. Cancer Cytopathol 2005;105:492–7.
50. Umbricht CB, Conrad GT, Clark DP, *et al.* Human telomerase reverse transcriptase gene expression and the surgical management of suspicious thyroid tumours. Clin Cancer Res 2004;10:5762–8.
51. Bojunga J, Zeuzem S. Molecular detection of thyroid cancer: an update. Clin Endocrinol 2004;61:523–30.
52. Asaad NY, abd El-Wahed MM, Mohammed AG. Human telomerase reverse transcriptase (hTERT) gene expression in thyroid carcinoma: diagnostic and prognostic role. J Egypt Natl Cancer Inst 2006;18(1):8–16.
53. Baloch ZW, LiVolsi VA. Our approach to follicular-patterned lesions of the thyroid. J Clin Pathol 2007;60: 244–50.
54. Orlandi F, Saggiorato E, Pivano G, *et al.* Galectin-3 is a presurgical marker of human thyroid carcinoma. Cancer Research 1998;58:3015–3020.
55. Bartolazzi A, Gasbarri A, Papotti M, *et al.* Application of an immunodiagnostic method for improving preoperative diagnosis of nodular thyroid lesions. Lancet 2001;357: 1644–1650.
56. Giannini R, Faviana P, Cavinato T, *et al.* Galectin-3 and oncofetalfibronectin expression in thyroid neoplasia as assessed by reverse transcriptionpolymerase chain reaction and immunochemistry in cytologic and pathologic specimens. Thyroid 2003;13:765–770.
57. Chieng DC, Ross JS & McKenna BJ. CD44 immunostaining of thyroid fine-needle aspirates differentiates thyroid papillary carcinoma from other lesions with nuclear grooves and inclusions. Cancer 1997;81:157–162.
58. Takano T, Sumizaki H & Amino N. (1997b) Detection of CD44 variants in fine-needle aspiration biopsies of thyroid tumor by RT-PCR. Journal of Experimental Clinical Cancer Research, 16, 267–271.
59. Gasbarri A, Martegani MP, Del Prete F, *et al.* Galectin-3 and CD44v6 isoforms in the preoperative evaluation of thyroid nodules. Journal of Clinical Oncology 1999;17: 3494–3502.
60. Takano T, Miyauchi A, Yokozawa T, *et al.* (1998b) Accurate and objective preoperative diagnosis of thyroid papillary carcinomas by reverse transcription-PCR detection of oncofetal fibronectin messenger RNA in fine-needle aspiration biopsies. Cancer Research, 58, 4913–4917.

61. Zeiger MA, Smallridge RC, Clark DP, *et al.* Human telomerase reverse transcriptase (hTERT) gene expression in FNA samples from thyroid neoplasms. Surgery 1999;126:1195–1198; discussion 1198–1199.
62. Liou MJ, Chan EC, Lin JD, *et al.* Human telomerase reverse transcriptase (hTERT) gene expression in FNA samples from thyroid neoplasms. Cancer Letters 2003;191: 223–227.
63. Sebesta J, Brown T, Williard W, *et al.* Does telomerase activity add to the value of fine-needle aspirations in evaluating thyroid nodules? American Journal of Surgery 2001;181:420–422.
64. Chiappetta GG, Tallini MC, De Biasio G, *et al.* Detection of high mobility Group I HMGI (Y) protein in the diagnosis of thyroid tumors: HMGI (Y) expression represents a potential diagnostic indicator of carcinoma. Cancer Research 1998;58:4193–4198.
65. Cheung CC, Carydis B, Ezzat S, Bedard YC & Asa SL. Analysis of ret/PTC gene rearrangements refines the fine-needle aspiration diagnosis of thyroid cancer. Journal of Clinical Endocrinology and Metabolism 2001;86:2187–2190.
66. Chiappetta G, Toti P, Cetta F, *et al.* The RET/PTC oncogene is frequently activated in oncocytic thyroid tumors (Hurthle cell adenomas and carcinomas), but not in oncocytic hyperplastic lesions. Journal of Clinical Endocrinology and Metabolism 2002;87:364–369.
67. Takano T, Miyauchi A, Matsuzuka F, *et al.* (1999a) Preoperative diagnosis of medullary thyroid carcinoma by RT-PCR using RNA extracted from leftover cells within a needle used for fine-needle aspiration biopsy. Journal of Clinical Endocrinology and Metabolism, 84, 951–955.
68. Bugalho MJ, Mendonca E & Sobrinho LG. Medullary thyroid carcinoma an accurate pre-operative diagnosis by reverse transcription–PCR. European Journal of Endocrinology 2000;143:335–338.

MULTIPLE CHOICE QUESTIONS

Select more than one option where appropriate.

1. A 35-year-old male presented with a solitary thyroid nodule. FNA cytology was cellular and intranuclear pseudoinclusions were a prominent feature. Which of the following lesions might be included in the differential diagnosis:
A. Hyalinizing trabecular adenoma
B. Adenomatous colloid nodule
C. Papillary thyroid carcinoma
D. Medullary thyroid carcinoma
E. Metastatic malignant melanoma.

2. The following statements are true regarding FNA thyroid procedure:
A. A local anaesthetic is often administered
B. Loss of vacuum in the syringe is usually due to tracheal puncture
C. Aspiration is usually performed with the patient lying in a semi-prone position
D. The patient is asked not to swallow or speak during the procedure
E. Aspiration should not be performed if the patient is anticoagulated

3. A 19-year-old female recently diagnosed with a phaeochromocytoma presented with a solitary thyroid nodule and a raised serum calcitonin. FNA of the thyroid nodule was undertaken. Which of the following cytological features might be seen in the aspirate:
A. Intranuclear pseudoinclusions
B. Plasmacytoid and spindled cells
C. Psammoma bodies
D. 'Salt and pepper' chromatin
E. Binucleation and multinucleation

4. With respect to thyroid FNA cytology, the following statements are true:
A. Cystic lesions cause false-negative results
B. Follicular carcinoma can be diagnosed as it is pleomorphic
C. A minimum of two Thy 2 diagnoses are required before malignancy can be confidently excluded
D. Core biopsy should be performed if an FNA is inadequate (Thy 1)
E. Palpable thyroid nodules require ultrasound-guided FNA for improved accuracy of diagnosis

5. The f]alse-negative rate of thyroid aspirates can be reduced by:
A. Repeating the FNA with ultrasound guidance
B. Using a larger needle to aspirate the thyroid
C. Discharging patients with a single benign FNA (Thy 2) from clinical follow-up
D. Having the slides reviewed by an experienced cytologist with an interest in thyroid cytology
E. Submitting at least six slides from any one aspiration for review

Answers

1. A, C, D, E
2. B, D
3. A, B, D, E
4. A, C
5. A, D

4 Thyroid imaging

Gitta Madani

St Mary's Hospital, Imperial College Healthcare NHS Trust, London, UK

KEY POINTS

- There is no single specific and sensitive radiological sign of malignancy
- The overall accuracy of ultrasound for the detection of papillary thyroid carcinoma is around 90%. Microcalcification is probably the most specific ultrasound sign, although this lacks sensitivity
- Fine needle aspiration of hypoechoic nodules with at least one suspicious ultrasound feature detects around 90% of thyroid malignancy
- Microinvasive follicular carcinoma may appear hyperechoic and exhibit relatively benign ultrasound features
- Cross-sectional imaging is superior to ultrasound in the assessment of extracapsular spread and involvement of adjacent structures. The main application of positron emission tomography is in previously treated differentiated thyroid cancer, when the serum thyroglobulin is persistently elevated despite negative ^{131}I scan and neck ultrasound.

INTRODUCTION

Although imaging is widely used in the management of thyroid nodules, its optimal role remains a matter of some controversy. Thyroid nodules are common and their incidence increases with age. Post-mortem studies have shown that as much as 50% of the population are affected.[1] The prevalence of malignancy in radiologically detected thyroid nodules is more difficult to quantify. The rate of malignancy in sonographically detected nodules is reported to range between 4 and 15%. There does not appear to be any difference between a multinodular goitre and a solitary nodule regarding the prevalence of malignancy.[2–5] Recent retrospective studies of incidental thyroid nodules detected on ultrasound have demonstrated a rate of malignancy approaching 30%.[6,7] Although these latter studies were performed in tertiary referral centres and are therefore prone to selection bias, it appears that incidental nodules detected on [^{18}F]fluorodeoxyglucose positron emission tomography (FDG-PET) have an even higher rate of malignancy, exceeding 40%.[8]

Papillary thyroid carcinoma (PTC) is the most common thyroid malignancy. It accounts for around 80% of cases and is associated with a good overall prognosis. Historically, patients with papillary microcarcinoma have an excellent prognosis.[9] This is largely because the vast majority are incidental tumours found within a thyroid gland which has been excised due to associated pressure symptoms. In view of the excellent prognosis of microcarcinoma, guidelines for the radiological management of thyroid nodules have been based on nodule size.[1] However, recent studies have shown that a significant number of papillary microcarcinomas are associated with extrathyroid extension and that microcarcinomas may have an increased long-term rate of nodal metastasis compared with larger tumours.[10] Nam-Goong *et al.* showed that a significant proportion of patients with incidental (small and impalpable) thyroid nodules actually fall within the high risk category. This was due to a high rate of extrathyroid tumour, regional lymph node involvement (69%) and multifocal disease (39%).[3] In addition, Berker *et al.* showed that the incidence of malignancy in subcentimetre nodules is not reduced compared with larger nodules.[11]

As all thyroid nodules initially arise from small lesions, the increased use of thyroid imaging is more likely to detect 'subclinical' nodules. The radiological management of thyroid nodules based on size alone therefore appears less logical than assumed earlier. The increased use of imaging is probably leading to the earlier detection of an entire spectrum of papillary cancers and incidentalomas which vary in histology and aggressiveness. Although their size is not a completely reliable indicator of biological behaviour, nodules measuring 5 mm or less do exhibit higher rates of false-positive ultrasound (US) findings coupled with lower rates of adequate fine needle aspiration (FNA) results.[12,13] Thus, imaging and fine needle aspiration cytology (FNAC) can sometimes confound the appropriate management of a thyroid nodule.

A Practical Manual of Thyroid and Parathyroid Disease, 1st Edition. Edited by Asit Arora, Neil Tolley & R. Michael Tuttle.

The increased incidence of PTC is not associated with a rise in disease-specific mortality which may, in part, reflect our increased use of thyroid imaging in recent times.[14] In the absence of randomized controlled trials, it is difficult to reconcile the relatively low mortality rates from PTC with the apparently high risk features of incidentalomas shown in recent studies. FNA of all thyroid nodules certainly has enormous resource implications. The diagnostic accuracy of FNAC for thyroid malignancy is around 95% with an inadequacy rate of 10%, so if all cytologically suspicious or inadequate nodules were excised, a substantial number of patients would undergo unnecessary thyroid surgery.[15]

US is the best primary imaging modality for the assessment of thyroid nodules. Although there is no single ultrasonographic feature with a high positive predictive value for malignancy, using a combination of suspicious features, US achieves an overall accuracy of around 90%.[6] Nevertheless, there is an overlap between the sonographic features of benign and malignant nodules. Thyroid US should be combined with the assessment of cervical lymph nodes and US-guided FNAC of sonographically or clinically suspicious nodules. The main role of cross-sectional imaging is in the assessment of the extent of locoregional spread and distant metastases. Cross-sectional imaging is probably superior to US in the assessment of extrathyroid disease. The main role of computed tomography (CT) and positron emission tomography (PET) co-registered imaging (PET-CT) is in the follow-up of dedifferentiated thyroid cancer.

ULTRASOUND FEATURES OF THYROID NODULES

Calcification

There are three types of pathological thyroid calcification on US; coarse calcification, microcalcification and peripheral calcification.

Coarse calcification manifests as echogenic foci with posterior acoustic shadowing and is most commonly seen in multinodular goitres where it is of no diagnostic significance. Conversely, coarse calcification in a solitary nodule is associated with a high rate of malignancy, as much as 75% in one study.[16] Up to 80% of cases of medullary carcinoma exhibit small foci of coarse calcification.[17] In PTC, coarse calcification may occur with co-existent microcalcification and exhibits a characteristically punctuate configuration which sometimes forms clusters (Fig. 4.1). Even a calcified spot, in the absence of a perceptible soft tissue component, is associated with malignancy and may warrant FNA.[18]

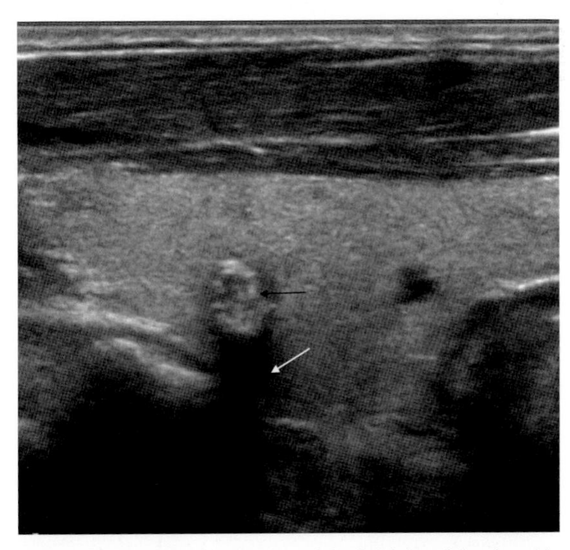

Fig. 4.1 Longitudinal sonogram of the left lobe of the thyroid demonstrating a papillary carcinoma. This exhibits clustered coarse calcification (black arrow). Note the posterior acoustic shadowing (white arrow) which masks the presence of extracapsular spread proven on histology.

Microcalcification is the presence of multiple tiny echogenic foci which do not cast acoustic shadows and is due to the presence of psammomma bodies (see Fig. 4.2A). Microcalcification is the most specific US sign of malignancy, with a specificity of 85–95% and positive predictive value of 42–94%. It is only present in 30–60% of malignant nodules and is therefore not a sensitive sign.[1] Microcalcification is most frequently observed in PTC but is also seen in follicular and anaplastic carcinomas and occasionally in follicular adenomas, multinodular goitres and Hashimoto's thyroiditis[19] (Fig. 4.2B).

Peripheral calcification is most commonly associated with chronic benign thyroid cysts. Its presence may result in acoustic shadowing, which prevents assessment of the internal architecture[18] (see Fig. 4.3). It does not exclude malignancy, and further assessment with FNAC may be warranted. In nodules which exhibit peripheral but no other calcification, a breach in the peripheral calcification may be the best indicator of malignancy.[20]

Echotexture

The majority of malignant nodules are predominantly solid. As an isolated finding this is of limited use because

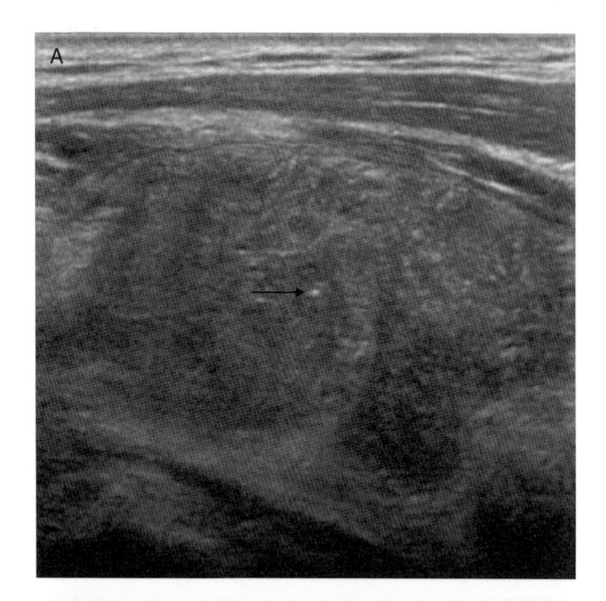

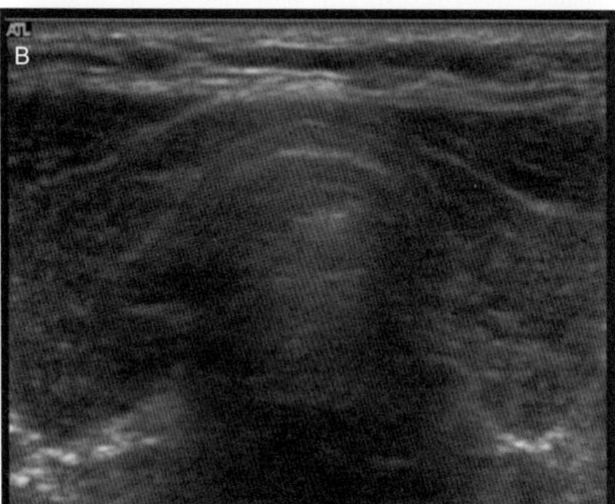

Fig. 4.2 A Longitudinal sonogram of the right lobe of the thyroid in a patient with diffuse PTC. It demonstrates a diffusely hypoechoic gland which contains small echogenic foci (arrow) consistent with microcalcification. **B** Transverse sonogram demonstrating a hypoechoic gland in a patient with thyroiditis.

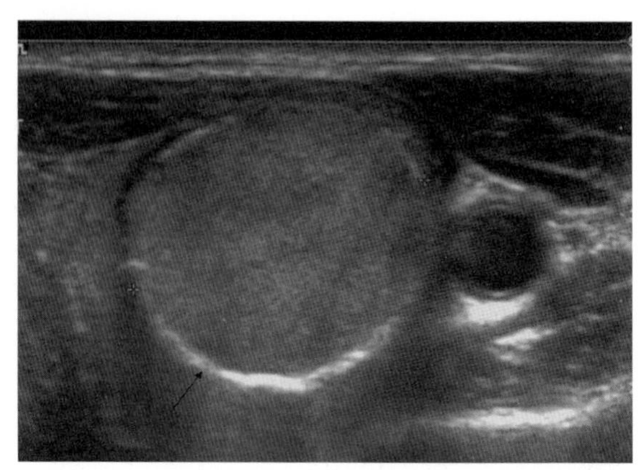

Fig. 4.3 Transverse sonogram demonstrating a benign nodule with discontinuous peripheral calcification (arrow).

at least 50% of benign nodules are also solid and malignancy occurs in cystic nodules too.[21,22] Cystic variants of PTC are well recognized, although a predominantly cystic appearance is uncommon. Even predominantly cystic papillary tumours are likely to possess other suspicious US features such as a solid component which exhibits vascularity or microcalcification.[22]

Hypoechogenicity is a characteristic feature of most malignant pathologies (papillary, medullary, anaplastic and some variants of follicular carcinomas, metastases to the thyroid and lymphoma) but is not a very sensitive sign. A large proportion of benign nodules are also hypoechoic.[21] Thyroiditis results in a hypoechoic gland which may be focal (similar to a malignant nodule) or diffuse and potentially indistinguishable from other diffuse infiltrative processes such as lymphoma or diffuse PTC (see Fig. 4.2A and B).

A prospective study of impalpable nodules by Papini *et al.* showed that FNA of hypoechoic nodules which exhibit an additional suspicious US feature detects around 87% of malignant nodules[23] (see Fig. 4.4A and B, and Plate 4.1).

Follicular tumours are typically hyperechoic and predominantly solid. From 60 to 70% of follicular carcinomas are associated with hyperplastic or adenomatous nodules. Malignant foci may be difficult to detect particularly when they exist within the background of a multinodular goitre. A microinvasive follicular carcinoma is sonographically indistinguishable from a follicular adenoma but frankly invasive follicular carcinoma tends to be hypoechoic.[24]

A spongiform or striated echotexture is a highly specific sign (99.7%) for a benign lesion but lacks sensitivity[12] (Fig. 4.5).

Margin and shape

An irregular, ill-defined nodule margin has a high specificity, approaching 92%. Unfortunately, it is not a very sensitive sign because many malignant tumours have well-defined margins.[12,22,25] A taller than wide dimension

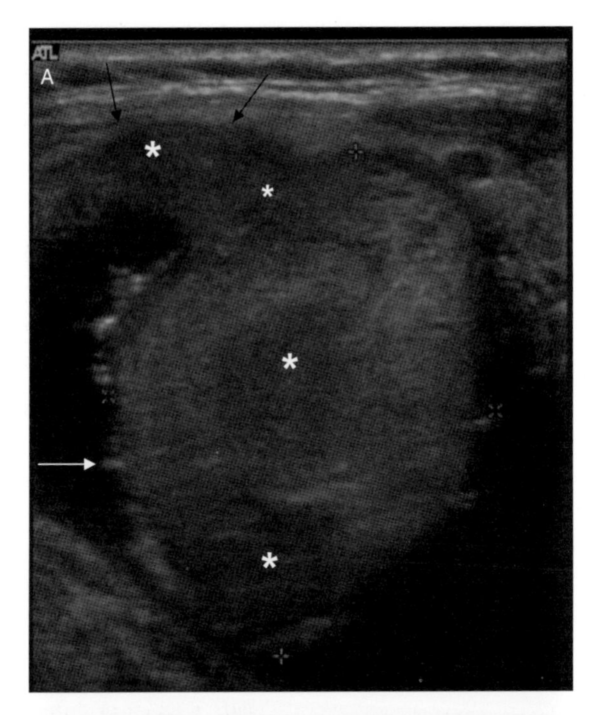

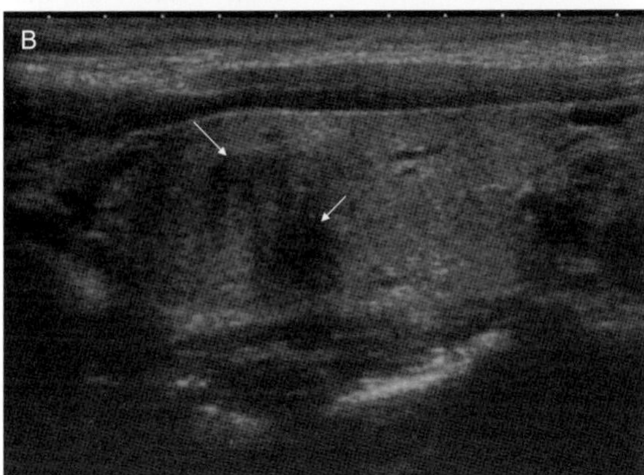

Fig. 4.4 **A** Transverse sonogram showing hypoechoic foci of PTC (asterisks) within a nodule, on a background of a multinodular goitre. Note the broad plane of contact of hypoechoic tumour with the capsule, suggestive of extracapsular spread (black arrows). The surrounding haemorrhagic cyst appears black and exhibits comet tail artefact (white arrow). **B** Longitudinal sonogram of the right lobe demonstrating an ill-defined hypoechoic nodule which was histologically proven to be medullary carcinoma.

is also a specific (92%) but poorly sensitive indicator of malignancy[12,25] (see Fig. 4B).

A completely hypoechoic or anechoic halo is an uncommon observation and is generally considered to be an unreliable sign of benign disease.[26] An incomplete halo is a common observation which has no diagnostic value.[22,25]

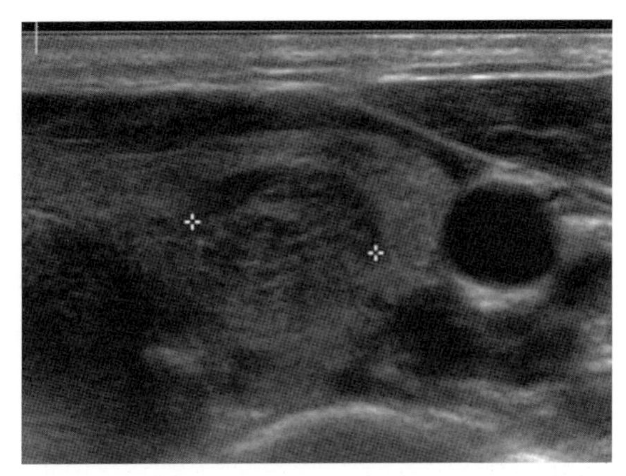

Fig. 4.5 Transverse sonogram of a nodule in the left lobe of the thyroid in a patient with a multinodular goitre. The spongiform appearance of the nodule is highly predictive of a benign lesion.

Vascularity

Most studies divide nodules into three patterns of Doppler flow: type I (avascular), type II (peripheral or peri-nodular vascularity) and type III (intranodular vascularity). In one study, intranodular vascularity had a specificity of 80% and sensitivity of 74% for malignancy[23] (Plate 4.1). Conversely, a complete lack of vascularity is highly predictive of benign disease. Frates *et al.*[27] showed that the prevalence of malignancy in solid hypervascular nodules was nearly 42% although 14% of malignant nodules were not hypervascular. Eighty percent of follicular lesions have a peri-nodular pattern of vascularity and 90% of follicular carcinomas exhibit intranodular flow.[24]

Size and number of nodules

Nodule size is not a predictor of malignancy.[11] Although the prevalence of malignancy per nodule is lower in a multinodular goitre, the overall risk of cancer is similar.[4] One study suggests that in patients with a follicular tumour, the presence of additional nodules is associated with a low risk of malignancy. However, this contrasts with reports that the majority of follicular tumours arise within a background of multinodular goitre.[24,28]

Lymph node metastases

The sensitivity of US in the detection of nodal metastases is very high (up to 96%) and its positive predictive value in the diagnosis of PTC nodal metastasis is around 89%.[29,30] The cervical lymph nodes should be assessed during US examination of the thyroid gland. Nodal involvement may be observed in papillary, anaplastic and medullary carcinomas, Hurthle cell tumours and lymphoma. The incidence of nodal metastases in PTC and anaplastic carcinoma is around 50%.[31] Lymphatic spread is uncommon in follicular carcinoma, affecting fewer than 8% of cases.[31]

Pre-operative US identifies involved cervical lymph nodes undetected by physical examination, thereby altering surgical management in 39% of patients.[32] In a series of 550 patients with PTC who underwent neck dissection, patients with ultrasonically diagnosed nodal metastases had a higher rate of disease recurrence than those with sonographically occult but pathologically proven metastases.[33] Involved nodes may be abnormal in shape (round), echotexture or size, or exhibit abnormal patterns of vascularity such as exaggerated hilar, capsular or mixed patterns. Size alone is a poor indicator of metastatic nodal involvement and, whilst US findings may be highly suspicious of involvement, there is some overlap in the appearance of reactive and malignant lymph nodes.

Metastatic nodes lying adjacent to the gland may mimic extensions of the primary tumour. Manifestations of metastatic PTC include echogenic cortical foci and punctuate calcification (see Fig. 4.6). Notably, up to 70% of metastatic PTC nodes have a cystic component. Lymph nodes may be entirely cystic or contain colloid regardless of the appearance of the thyroid tumour.[34] The presentation of palpable metastatic PCT nodes and an occult primary tumour is well recognized. Metastatic medullary carcinoma nodes may contain areas of coarse calcification.[17] Lymphomatous nodes may exhibit a subtle reticular cortical pattern.

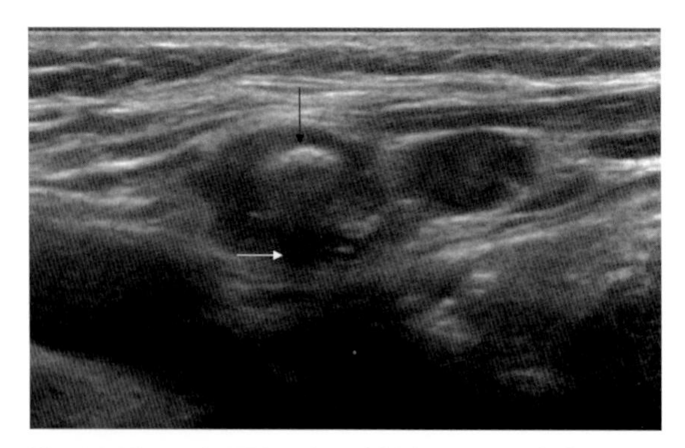

Fig. 4.6 Metastatic PTC nodes exhibiting coarse calcification (black arrow) with posterior acoustic shadowing (white arrow).

Local extent of malignant tumours

US is reliable for diagnosing vascular involvement. The real-time nature of the study allows assessment of independent mobility of the carotid artery.[35] Extracapsular tumour extension may be apparent, manifesting as invasion of adjacent structures. However, US is not generally accurate in the assessment of the local tumour extension. A study of 220 patients with well-differentiated PCT demonstrated that the most accurate US predictor of extracapsular spread is when more than 25% of the tumour circumference is in contact with the thyroid capsule[38] (Fig. 4.4A). When tumour is not surrounded by a cuff of normal thyroid tissue, assessment with magnetic resonance imaging (MRI) is probably warranted.[36,37]

THE ROLE OF CROSS-SECTIONAL IMAGING IN THYROID DISEASE

Non-contrast CT is frequently used in patients with a multinodular goitre to assess the calibre of the airway in patients with compressive symptoms or retrosternal extension. In thyroid malignancy cross-sectional imaging is useful to assess the local extent of tumour, usually with MRI. Distant metastases are best assessed with CT. Iodinated contrast, used in CT but not MRI, is contraindicated in patients with suspected well-differentiated thyroid cancer.

Local extent of the tumour

MRI is probably the most accurate modality for assessing invasion of adjacent structures. A few studies have assessed the MRI features of local tumour extension in the context of known malignancy but this modality should be used with caution if the diagnosis is not established.[39] Assessment is based on the degree of contact with adjacent structures. The optimal thresholds for tumour invasion of laryngeal cartilage and oesophagus are >90° contact. For the trachea it is >135° contact and for the carotid artery it is >225° contact (accuracy of 86–94%), although some authorities suggest that >270° contact with the carotid artery is the best indicator of

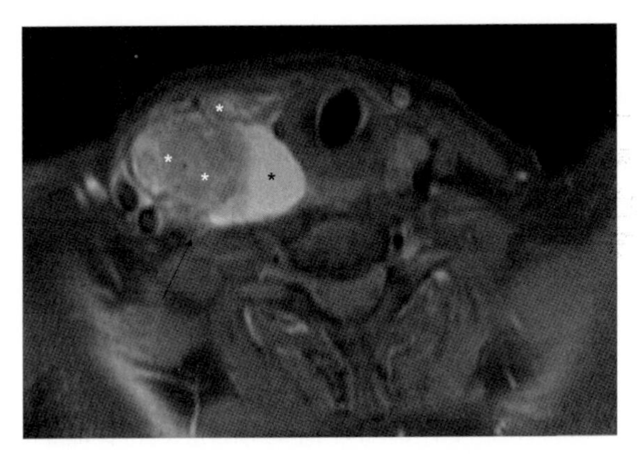

Fig. 4.7 Axial fat-saturated post-gadolinium MRI in a patient with PTC. The enhancing tumour (white asterisks) is ill defined posteriorly (arrow) consitent with extracapsular spread. There is a haemorrhagic cyst (black asterisk) medially.

malignant invasion.[39,40] An intraluminal tracheal mass indicates deep invasion but does not necessarily suggest tracheal cartilage involvement because tumour can penetrate between tracheal rings.[41] Extracapsular spread to the adjacent fat (without organ invasion) manifests as ill definition on MRI[39] (Fig. 4.7). Effacement of fat in the tracheo-oesophageal groove on one or more images is the best predictor of malignant invasion of the recurrent laryngeal nerve, with an accuracy of 88%.[42]

Lymph node metastasis

Cross-sectional imaging has a poor sensitivity for nodal involvement (59%) compared with US (92%).[43] The best indicators of metastasis are the presence of cystic foci, enlargement (on CT and MRI) or the presence of coarse calcification (on CT)[43] (see Fig. 4.8). Haemorrhagic and colloid-containing nodes may be hyperintense on T1-weighted MRI sequences.

Distant metastasis

Haematogenous spread to the lungs, bones and central nervous system occurs in 5% of PTC.[31] Pulmonary metastases are best assessed on CT and characteristically manifest as multiple tiny soft tissue nodules which are more numerous in the lung bases. Anaplastic tumours have a high predilection for vascular invasion and distant metastases. Coarse calcification within metastatic deposits may be seen as papillary, anaplastic and medullary tumours.

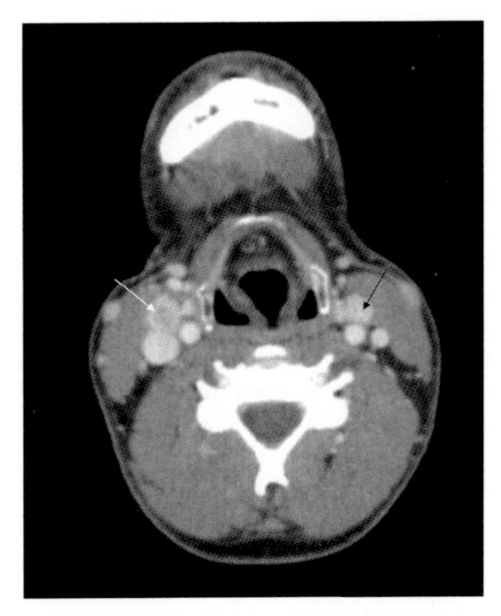

Fig. 4.8 Axial contrast-enhanced CT showing enlarged rounded nodes due to metastatic medullary carcinoma. Note the low density necrotic centre in the right-sided node.

Emerging MRI techniques

There is increasing evidence that restriction of diffusion on diffusion-weighted MRI may be a useful non-invasive method of differentiating malignant and benign tumours. The technique involves quantitative analysis of the apparent diffusion coefficient value in specific regions of interest. It has been widely used to assess lymphoma and is under investigation in a variety of head and neck tumours. There are currently limited data about this investigation in thyroid malignancy, although a prospective study of 67 patients with solitary nodules demonstrated an accuracy of nearly 99%.[44]

FOLLOW-UP IMAGING

Disease recurrence is observed in 15–30% of patients with PTC, and 8% of patients with local recurrence eventually die from their disease. Conventional post-operative surveillance involves serum thyroglobulin measurements and ^{131}I whole-body scans (WBS). The latter is performed following thyroxine withdrawal or after administration of human recombinant thyroid-stimulating hormone.[45] However, 25% of recurrent differentiated thyroid cancer does not accumulate iodine.[45] More recently, US surveillance of the thyroid bed and cervical lymph nodes has become the main modality for assessment of locoregional recurrence. The overall accuracy of this modality approaches 94%.[30]

FDG-PET and PET-CT co-registration are mainly used in non-iodine-avid or de-differentiated tumours. FDG avidity tends to be inversely related to iodine uptake on the WBS. It is associated with a poor response to radioiodine treatment and therefore a worse prognosis.[46] PET is used in patients with previously treated differentiated thyroid cancers who have a persistently raised thyroglobulin, despite a negative ^{131}I WBS. In this group, PET and PET-CT are reported to alter the surgical management in 14–38% of patients, although these studies do not take into account the US neck findings.[46] Although it has not been demonstrated in the literature, the major application of PET and PET-CT is probably in patients with non-iodine-avid distant metastatic disease not demonstrated on ^{131}I WBS.

The reported sensitivity and specificity of FDG-PET for the detection of recurrent disease ranges widely. In part, this variation reflects differences in study design. A multicentre trial of 222 patients with differentiated thyroid cancer suggests that the sensitivity of this modality is 75%. It rises to 85% in the subset of patients with negative ^{131}I WBS.[47] The sensitivity of PET is improved with increasing levels of thyroglobulin. Giammarile *et al.* reported sensitivities of 50, 62 and 83% in patients with unstimulated thyroglobulin levels <1.0, 1.0–10.0 and >10.0 mg/dl, respectively.[48]

The major advantage of PET-CT co-registration is enhanced anatomical localization which allows more accurate localization of involved lymph nodes. It improves specificity by reducing the number of false-positive results which arise due to physiological uptake by brown fat, vocal cords, muscular activity and uptake by inflammatory post-operative tissue.[46]

EVIDENCE APPRAISAL

Aspects of this review chapter reflect the opinion of the author and should be considered low level evidence; Oxford Centre Evidence Based Medicine (EBM) Level V.

Due to a lack of high level evidence, the articles quoted in this section are at best EBM Levels III and IV.

There is wide variation in the methodology used in most radiological studies involving thyroid disease which limits any direct comparison of the results of these studies.

REFERENCES

1. Frates MC, Benson CB, Charboneau JW, *et al.* Society of Radiologists in Ultrasound. Management of thyroid nodules detected at US: Society of Radiologists in Ultrasound consensus conference statement. Radiology 2005;237:794–800.
2. Cochand-Priollet B, Guillausseau PJ, Chagnon S, *et al.* The diagnostic value of fine-needle aspiration biopsy under ultrasonography in nonfunctional thyroid nodules: a prospective study comparing cytologic and histologic findings. Am J Med 1994;97:152–7.
3. Nam-Goong IS, Kim HY, Gong G, *et al.* Ultrasonography-guided fine-needle aspiration of thyroid incidentaloma: correlation with pathological findings. Clin Endocrinol 2004;60:21–8.
4. Frates MC, Benson CB, Doubilet PM, *et al.* Prevalence and distribution of carcinoma in patients with solitary and multiple thyroid nodules on sonography. J Clin Endocrinol Metab 2006;91:3411–7.
5. Izquierdo R, Arekat MR, Knudson PE, *et al.* Comparison of palpation-guided versus ultrasound-guided fine-needle aspiration biopsies of thyroid nodules in an outpatient endocrinology practice. Endocr Pract 2006;12:609–14.
6. Kang HW, No JH, Chung JH, Min YK, *et al.* Prevalence, clinical and ultrasonographic characteristics of thyroid incidentalomas. Thyroid 2004;14:29–33.
7. Kim DL, Song KH, Kim SK. High prevalence of carcinoma in ultrasonography-guided fine needle aspiration cytology of thyroid nodules. Endocr J 2008;55:135–42.
8. Are C, Hsu JF, Schoder H, *et al.* FDG-PET detected thyroid incidentalomas: need for further investigation? Ann Surg Oncol 2007;14:239–47.
9. Hay ID, Grant CS, van Heerden JA, *et al.* Papillary thyroid microcarcinoma: a study of 535 cases observed in a 50-year period. Surgery 1992;112:1139–46.
10. Cappelli C, Castellano M, Braga M, *et al.* Aggressiveness and outcome of papillary thyroid carcinoma (PTC) versus microcarcinoma (PMC): a mono-institutional experience. J Surg Oncol 2007;95:555–60.
11. Berker D, Aydin Y, Ustun I, *et al.* The value of fine-needle aspiration biopsy in subcentimeter thyroid nodules. Thyroid 2008;18:603–8.
12. Moon WJ, Jung SL, Lee JH, *et al.* Benign and malignant thyroid nodules: US differentiation—multicenter retrospective study. Radiology 2008;247:762.
13. Mazzaferri EL, Sipos J. Should all patients with subcentimeter thyroid nodules undergo fine-needle aspiration biopsy and preoperative neck ultrasonography to define the extent of tumor invasion? Thyroid 2008;18:597–602.
14. Gharib H, Papini E, Paschke R. Thyroid nodules: a review of current guidelines, practices, and prospects. Eur J Endocrinol 2008;159:493–505.
15. Gharib H,. Goellner JR. Fine-needle aspiration biopsy of the thyroid: an appraisal. Ann Intern Med 1993;118:282–9.
16. Khoo ML, Asa SL, Witterick IJ, *et al.* Thyroid calcification and its association with thyroid carcinoma. Head Neck 2002;24:651–5.
17. Gorman B, Charboneau JW, James EM, *et al.* Medullary thyroid carcinoma: role of high-resolution US. Radiology 1987;162:147–50.

18. Taki S, Terahata S, Yamashita R, *et al.* Thyroid calcifications sonographic patterns and incidence of cancer. Clin Imaging 2004;28:368–71.
19. Ellison E, Lapuerta P, Martin SE. Psammoma bodies in fine-needle aspirates of the thyroid: predictive value for papillary carcinoma. Cancer 1998;84:169–75.
20. Kim BM, Kim MJ, Kim EK, *et al.* Sonographic differentiation of thyroid nodules with eggshell calcifications. J Ultrasound Med 2008;27:1425–30.
21. Wienke JR, Chong WK, Fielding JR, *et al.* Sonographic features of benign thyroid nodules: interobserver reliability and overlap with malignancy. J Ultrasound Med 2003;22: 1027–31.
22. Chan BK, Desser TS, McDougall IR, *et al.* Common and uncommon sonographic features of papillary thyroid carcinoma. J Ultrasound Med 2003;22:1083–90.
23. Papini E, Guglielmi R, Bianchini A, *et al.* Risk of malignancy in nonpalpable thyroid nodules: predictive value of ultrasound and color-Doppler features. J Clin Endocrinol Metab 2002;87:1941–6.
24. Ahuja AT. The thyroid and parathyroids. In: Ahuja AT, Evans RM, eds. Practical head and neck ultrasound. New York: Cambridge University Press, 2006:35–64.
25. Yuan WH, Chiou HJ, Chou YH, *et al.* Gray-scale and color Doppler ultrasonographic manifestations of papillary thyroid carcinoma: analysis of 51 cases. Clin Imaging 2006; 30:394–401.
26. Lu C, Chang TC, Hsiao YL, *et al.* Ultrasonographic findings of papillary thyroid carcinoma and their relation to pathologic changes. J Formos Med Assoc 1994;93:933–8.
27. Frates MC, Benson CB, Doubilet PM, *et al.* Can color Doppler sonography aid in the prediction of malignancy of thyroid nodules? J Ultrasound Med 2003;22:127–31.
28. Sippel RS, Elaraj DM, Khanafshar E, *et al.* Does the presence of additional thyroid nodules on ultrasound alter the risk of malignancy in patients with a follicular neoplasm of the thyroid? Surgery 2007;142:851–7.
29. Takashima S, Sone S, Nomura N, *et al.* Nonpalpable lymph nodes of the neck: assessment with US and US-guided fine-needle aspiration biopsy. J Clin Ultrasound 1997;25: 283–92.
30. Stulak JM, Grant CS, Farley DR, *et al.* Value of preoperative ultrasonography in the surgical management of initial and reoperative papillary thyroid cancer. Arch Surg 2006;141: 489–94.
31. Loevner L. Thyroid and parathyroid glands. In: Som. PM, Curtin HD, eds. Head and neck imaging, 4th edn. St Louis: Mosby, 2003:2134–72.
32. Kouvaraki MA, Shapiro SE, Fornage BD, *et al.* Role of preoperative ultrasonography in the surgical management of patients with thyroid cancer. Surgery 2003;134:946–54.
33. Ito Y, Tomoda C, Uruno T, *et al.* Ultrasonographically and anatomopathologically detectable node metastases in the lateral compartment as indicators of worse relapse-free survival in patients with papillary thyroid carcinoma. World J Surg 2005;29:917–20.
34. Kessler A, Rappaport Y, Blank A, *et al.* Cystic appearance of cervical lymph nodes is characteristic of metastatic papillary thyroid carcinoma. J Clin Ultrasound 2003;31:21–5.
35. Mann WJ, Beck A, Schreiber J, *et al.* Ultrasonography for evaluation of the carotid artery in head and neck cancer. Laryngoscope 1994;104:885–8.
36. King AD, Ahuja AT, To EW, *et al.* Staging papillary carcinoma of the thyroid: magnetic resonance imaging vs ultrasound of the neck. Clin Radiol 2000;55:222–6.
37. Takashima S, Nomura N, Noguchi Y, *et al.* Primary thyroid lymphoma: evaluation with US, CT, and MRI. J Comput Assist Tomogr 1995;19:282–8.
38. Kwak JW, Kim EK, Youk JH, *et al.* Extrathyroid extension of well-differentiated papillary thyroid microcarcinoma on ultrasound. Thyroid 2008;18:609–14.
39. Takashima S, Takayama F, Wang Q, *et al.* Differentiated thyroid carcinomas. Prediction of tumor invasion with MR imaging. Acta Radiol 2000;41:377–83.
40. Yousem DM, Hatabu H, Hurst RW, *et al.* Carotid artery invasion by head and neck masses: prediction with MR imaging. Radiology 1995;195:715–20.
41. Wang JC, Takashima S, Takayama F, *et al.* Tracheal invasion by thyroid carcinoma: prediction using MR imaging. AJR Am J Radiol 2001;177:929–36.
42. Takashima S, Takayama F, Wang J, *et al.* Using MR imaging to predict invasion of the recurrent laryngeal nerve by thyroid carcinoma. AJR Am J Radiol 2003;180:837–42.
43. Takashima S, Sone S, Takayama F, Wang Q, *et al.* Papillary thyroid carcinoma: MR diagnosis of lymph node metastasis. AJNR Am J Neuroradiol 1998;19:509–13.
44. Razek AA, Sadek AG, Kombar OR, *et al.* Role of apparent diffusion coefficient values in differentiation between malignant and benign solitary thyroid nodules. AJNR Am J Neuroradiol 2008;29:563–8.
45. Lee JH, Lee HK, Lee DH, *et al.* Ultrasonographic findings of a newly detected nodule on the thyroid bed in postoperative patients for thyroid carcinoma: correlation with the results of ultrasonography-guided fine-needle aspiration biopsy. Clin Imaging 2007;31:109–13.
46. Johnson NA, Tublin ME. Postoperative surveillance of differentiated thyroid carcinoma: rationale, techniques, and controversies. Radiology 2008;249:429–44.
47. Grünwald F, Kälicke T, Feine U, *et al.* Fluorine-18 fluorodeoxyglucose positron emission tomography in thyroid cancer: results of a multicentre study. Eur J Nucl Med. 1999;26:1547–52.
48. Giammarile F, Hafdi Z, Bournaud C, *et al.* Is [18F]-2-fluoro-2-deoxy-d-glucose (FDG) scintigraphy with non-dedicated positron emission tomography useful in the diagnostic management of suspected metastatic thyroid carcinoma in patients with no detectable radioiodine uptake? Eur J Endocrinol 2003;149:293–300.

MULTIPLE CHOICE QUESTIONS

Select more than one option where appropriate.

1. Regarding the ultrasound features of malignant thyroid tumours
A. The majority of malignant tumours are hyperechoic
B. Metastases to the thyroid gland are hypoechoic
C. A spongiform appearance is suggestive of necrosis in a malignant tumour
D. Ill-defined hypoechoic nodules should undergo FNAC

2. Regarding US features of thyroid nodules
A. Calcification within a multinodular goitre is a sinister sign
B. Peripheral calcification usually indicates a malignant nodule
C. Microcalcification may occasionally be observed in benign conditions but warrants FNAC
D. A solid nodule with intranodular vascularity raises the suspicion of a follicular tumour

3. Metastatic PTC lymph nodes
A. Should be primarily assessed with cross-sectional imaging
B. Invariably mimic the US appearances of the primary tumour
C. Are rarely cystic
D. May be the presenting feature of the disease

4. MRI of the neck
A. Is the best modality for the assessment of pulmonary metastases
B. Is the best modality for assessment of the local extent of tumour
C. In the presence of known malignancy an ill-defined margin is suggestive of extracapsular spread
D. 90° or greater contact with the carotid artery is suspicious of invasion

5. CT-PET
A. Sensitivity for detection of recurrent tumour increases with high levels of serum thyroglobulin
B. Has a higher false-positive rate than PET due to misregistration artefact
C. Is most useful in iodine-avid recurrent disease
D. Negates the need for post-operative US surveillance of the neck

Answers

1. B, D
2. C, D
3. D
4. B, C
5. A

5 The role of nuclear medicine

Ravinder K. Grewal, Steven M. Larson & Jorge A. Carrasquillo
Department of Radiology, Memorial Sloan-Kettering Cancer Center, New York, NY, USA

KEY POINTS

- Radioactive iodine imaging is often used to differentiate between the various aetiologies of hyperthyroidism
- The main use of radioactive iodine scanning in a solitary thyroid nodule is when the TSH is decreased to determine if it is 'hot' as this is rarely malignant
- ^{131}I therapy plays an important role in management of hyperthyroidism and thyroid cancer
- Patients undergoing radioactive iodine imaging and/or therapy for thyroid cancer require a low iodine diet. TSH stimulation may be obtained by inducing hypothyroidism or using recombinant human TSH (rhTSH)
- Focal uptake in a thyroid gland on FDG-PET scan represents malignancy in 27–50% of patients and warrants further management.

Benign and malignant thyroid disorders are frequently encountered in medical practice. Thyroid scintigraphy plays an important role in guiding clinical and surgical management of patients with thyroid disorders, and ^{131}I continues to play an important role in the therapy of thyroid cancer and hyperthyroidism.

RADIOPHARMACEUTICALS IN THYROID IMAGING AND THERAPY

Procedure guidelines for scintigraphy of benign conditions[1] and differentiated thyroid cancer (DTC) have been developed.[2] Thyroid scintigraphy relies heavily on the radioisotopes of iodine such as ^{131}I, ^{123}I and more recently ^{124}I.[3]

^{131}I has been used for diagnostic and therapeutic purposes in both benign and malignant thyroid disorders. ^{131}I has an 8.02 day half-life, γ emissions (364 keV) that can be imaged and β particles that are useful for therapy. In patients with thyroid cancer being assessed for tumour recurrence or metastatic disease, ^{131}I is frequently used for imaging. The amount of ^{131}I usually varies, with many centres using less than 185 MBq to prevent the possibility of stunning. This is defined as decreased fractional uptake of ^{131}I induced by a pre-therapy diagnostic dose.[4] For diagnostic imaging, ^{123}I is an alternative to ^{131}I. The advantages of ^{123}I over ^{131}I are its short half-life (13 hours) lower energy γ emissions (159 keV) and lack of β emission. This results in improved imaging characteristics and dosimetry. The diagnostic accuracy of ^{123}I and ^{131}I in the initial post-thyroidectomy scan is similar, although the success rate of radioablation therapy appears to be better following the ^{123}I scan. In contrast, ^{131}I appears to be more sensitive than ^{123}I for post-ablation follow-up imaging, although there is a risk of stunning.[5,6] A comparison of post-therapy ^{123}I and ^{131}I scans showed that approximately 85% (228 out of 263) of patients with a positive ^{123}I whole-body scan had concordant post-treatment ^{131}I images. There were 44 additional abnormal foci detected on the post-treatment ^{131}I scans although these findings did not impact on therapeutic management. In conclusion, ^{123}I appears to be a reasonable alternative to ^{131}I.

Tc-99m (administered as Tc-99m pertechnetate) is another ideal isotope for thyroid imaging. It gives off 140 keV γ emissions, has a half-life of 6 hours, a low radiation dose and is rapidly taken up by thyroid tissue. However, a proportion of non-functioning 'cold' nodules demonstrated on an ^{123}I scan will misleadingly appear warm or hot on a Tc-99m scan.[7] Tc-99m is therefore not adequate for detecting metastatic thyroid disease because of the unacceptably high number of false-negative results.[8]

IMAGING AND UPTAKE MEASUREMENTS OF THE THYROID

Planar imaging of the thyroid with ^{123}I, ^{131}I or Tc-99m is performed with a γ camera equipped with a parallel hole or a pinhole collimator. Single photon emission computed tomography (SPECT) is increasingly used due to the improved contrast afforded with this modality. Machines that combine SPECT and CT allow even more precise localization of disease.[9]

A Practical Manual of Thyroid and Parathyroid Disease, 1st Edition.
Edited by Asit Arora, Neil Tolley & R. Michael Tuttle.

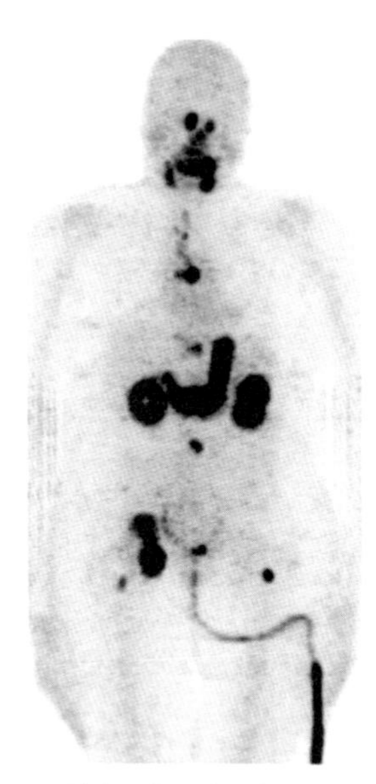

Fig. 5.1 A 56-year-old female with a history of papillary thyroid carcinoma. ^{124}I SPECT images were obtained 48 hours after oral administration of 222 MBq. A maximum intensity projection image of the PET scan (MIP) demonstrates metastatic lesions in the thoracolumbar spine, right hemipelvis, bilateral femora, kidneys and mediastinum. Activity is also seen around an indwelling urinary catheter.

Recently, ^{124}I has been used in positron emission tomography (PET) imaging (Fig. 5.1). The isotope has a half-life of 4 days which enables extended imaging with higher resolution compared with ^{123}I and ^{131}I. It is quantitative and, when used with PET-CT, can be accurately co-registered to a corresponding anatomic structure.

Thyroid uptake determination is the measurement of the fraction of administered radioactive iodine (RAI) which accumulates in the thyroid gland or thyroid bed. It is used to calculate the activity needed for therapy of hyperthyroidism or remnant ablation.

Guidelines for performing thyroid uptake have been developed.[10] The usual indications are to differentiate subacute or painless thyroiditis and factitious hyperthyroidism from Graves' disease and other forms of hyperthyroidism.

Non-radioiodine radiopharmaceuticals

Alternative radiopharmaceuticals can also be used to detect thyroid tumour. They have varied mechanisms of localization. [^{18}F]Fluorodeoxyglucose (FDG) utilizes glucose metabolism, ^{201}Tl relies on blood flow, Tc-99m Sestamibi uses blood flow and mitochondrial potential,[11,12] and radiolabelled somatostatin analogues use somatostatin receptor binding.[13]

ROLE OF IMAGING AND THERAPY IN HYPERTHYROIDISM

Hyperthyroidism is a clinical syndrome caused by either acute or chronic excess production and/or release of thyroid hormones. It is caused by Graves' disease, toxic adenomas, thyroiditis, toxic multinodular goitre, iodine-induced hyperthyroidism, excessive pituitary thyroid-stimulating hormone (TSH) or trophoblastic disease, and excessive ingestion of thyroid hormone. The thyroid scan and uptake are invaluable in differentiating between the various aetiologies of hyperthyroidism. High uptake is usually associated with Graves' disease, autonomous toxic nodules or multinodular goitres. In contrast, hyperthyroidism due to thyroiditis or factitious hyperthyroidism is associated with decreased thyroid uptake.

Treatment of hyperthyroidism due to Graves, multinodular goitre or autonomous hyperfunctioning nodules (AFTNs) often involves ^{131}I therapy.[14] In patients with multinodular goitre, treatment with ^{131}I is also used, although surgery is usually preferable with large goitres to relieve compressive symptoms.[15] Numerous methods have been proposed to select the correct radioiodine treatment dose.[16,17] These methods use either fixed doses of ^{131}I (generally 185–555 MBq) or dosimetric estimates adjusted for gland size, percentage uptake and the desired radiation dose (e.g. 2.96–7.4 MBq/g deposited at 24 hours or a desired absorbed dose ranging from 5000 to 15 000 cGy). There is no evidence that patient-specific methods have an advantage over fixed dose methods.[18,19] A recent study by Grosso *et al.* showed similar control of hyperthyroidism at doses of 150, 300 or >300 Gy to the thyroid. Following initial treatment, 5–10% of patients may require further therapy to control hyperthyroidism adequately.[20] Hypothyroidism may develop in up to 90% of patients.[21,22]

Patient preparation

Patient preparation prior to radioiodine imaging or therapy is important. It is recommended that patients start a low iodine diet (LID) for 1–2 weeks (<50 mg of iodine/day) prior to ablation or surveillance scanning. It is essential to decrease total body iodine[23] because non-radioactive iodine competes with RAI and decreases uptake of the latter. Therefore, substances containing high levels of iodine, such as contrast media, certain foodstuffs and drugs, are contraindicated. Studies utilizing LID demonstrate reduced urinary iodine excretion, up to 2.3-fold increased iodine uptake and an increased remnant ablation rate.[24,25]

Female patients must not be pregnant or breastfeeding since iodine accumulates in the fetal thyroid.[26] To minimize the breast radiation dose, breastfeeding should be stopped 6–8 weeks prior to RAI[23] because the lactating breast accumulates iodine.[27]

TSH stimulation is necessary for thyroid uptake of iodine. Elevated TSH activates various thyroid-specific proteins and is required for remnant ablation, subsequent monitoring and treatment of residual/recurrent disease with radioiodine. Increased TSH levels are achieved by thyroid hormone withdrawal[28–30] or recombinant human TSH (rhTSH) injections which exogenously stimulate thyroid/thyroid cancer tissue. One frequently utilized approach involves substituting T3 for l-T4 for 4–6 weeks and discontinuing T3 2 weeks prior to administration of radioiodine.[29] This results in TSH levels >30 mU/l in the majority of patients,[31,32] which is generally accepted as the target level associated with increased radioiodine uptake in thyroid cancers.[33]

Significant morbidity and inconvenience are induced by the hypothyroid state.[34] Furthermore, withdrawal is not always effective in patients with hypopituitarism and TSH deficiency or functional metastases. Therefore, the use of rhTSH has been explored. The pharmacokinetics and clinical use of rhTSH have been reviewed elsewhere.[35] The recommended regimen when rhTSH is used in conjunction with whole-body scintigraphy (WBS) consists of 0.9 mg/day for 2 days with RAI administered 24 hours after the second dose. The rapid effect of rhTSH permits greater flexibility in treatment planning and a shorter duration of TSH stimulation (3–4 days) compared with hypothyroidism induced by hormone withdrawal.[36] A comparison of thyroid scanning under rhTSH or hypothyroid stimulation demonstrates some differences in the pharmacokinetics of iodine distribution,[32] although findings are concordant in 89% of cases.[37]

THYROID NODULES

Thyroid nodules are discrete lesions that are recognized as separate from the surrounding thyroid by palpation or imaging. The vast majority are benign.[38] Thus, the clinical goal is to identify nodules that require surgical excision. At the time of diagnosis the risk factors for malignancy should be assessed by history and physical examination, focusing on the thyroid and nodal structures.[39]

The most commonly used imaging procedure for the evaluation of a thyroid nodule is thyroid ultrasonography (US).[40] Fine needle aspiration cytology (FNAC), often guided by US, has become the accepted method for screening a solitary nodule for malignancy.[41] If FNAC reveals a follicular neoplasm (which occurs in >15% of cases), a radionuclide scan may be performed. If a functioning nodule is identified, surgery can be avoided.[42]

Nodules smaller than 1 cm are less likely to harbour clinically significant cancers and therefore current guidelines recommend evaluation of nodules >1 cm.[23] Nevertheless, smaller nodules associated with other high risk factors may also warrant further investigation with serial US and physical exam. Patients presenting with a 1–1.5 cm solitary thyroid nodule should have their TSH level checked. When the TSH is suppressed, a thyroid uptake scan is recommended to determine if the nodule is functional. Functional nodules only account for 5% of cases and do not generally require histological confirmation as they are typically benign. Patients with normal or elevated TSH and those with cold nodules on scintigraphy should proceed to US evaluation.

Multinodular goitres have an incidence of 1–2%.[43] The risk of thyroid cancer in multinodular goitres is similar to that in patients with solitary nodules.[44,45] The decision to perform FNAC is usually made on US characteristics of the nodules since it is not always the largest nodule that is malignant[45] (see Chapter 3). As in the setting of the solitary nodule, thyroid scintigraphy may be useful in identifying functional nodules which rarely harbour malignancy.

Retrospective studies utilizing FDG imaging have found incidental focal accumulation in the thyroid gland in 1– 4% of patients.[46–49] Such uptake warrants further evaluation, since 27–50% of these lesions are malignant. The amount of uptake does not differentiate benign from malignant lesions.[46–49] Diffuse FDG accumulation in the thyroid has also been reported in 3.4% of patients. These cases are often found to represent thyroiditis, although patients with Graves' disease can also demonstrate diffuse uptake.[50]

Few prospective studies have been performed in patients with thyroid nodules to assess adequately the role of FDG in their management. Nonetheless some studies suggest there may be some utility in the management of cold nodules.[51,52]

SCINTIGRAPHY IN THE FOLLOW-UP OF PATIENTS WITH THYROID CANCER

Although the prognosis is generally excellent for most patients with DTC, recurrent disease does occur in some patients. This may arise many years after initial presentation, which is why long-term surveillance is vital. Early detection of local or metastatic disease leads to long-term survival when the disease is removed surgically and/or treated with RAI. Therefore, the optimal management is to identify and treat recurrence early in order to facilitate cure and reduce morbidity. Patients at low risk include those without distant or locoregional metastasis, no evidence of local tumour invasion, size <1 cm in diameter and favourable histology.[53,54] These patients usually do not require routine follow-up RAI imaging. They are monitored for disease recurrence with thyroglobulin (Tg) and US. RAI imaging is indicated if the Tg is elevated or when the physical exam or US findings are abnormal[55,56] (see Chapters 11 and 12). Intermediate risk patients are those with microscopic invasion of tumour into the peri-thyroidal soft tissues at the time of initial surgery, tumours with aggressive histology or vascular invasion. These may require follow-up diagnostic RAI WBS.[57,58] High risk patients are those with tumours >4 cm in diameter, macroscopic tumour invasion, incomplete tumour resection, distant metastases or post-ablation uptake beyond the thyroid bed on RAI WBS.[59,60] These patients will typically need routine follow-up every 6–12 months with diagnostic RAI WBS. This is followed by RAI therapy if lesions are detected. Studies have shown that diagnostic RAI WBS is less sensitive for detecting residual or recurrent disease compared with measurement of Tg.[37,61]

^{131}I THERAPY FOR METASTATIC THYROID CANCER

Patient preparation and dose determination

As with remnant ablation, patients with metastatic disease must be made hypothyroid or administered rhTSH prior to treatment with ^{131}I. Although there is growing evidence that rhTSH may be used effectively in these patients, well controlled randomized trials have not been performed.[62,63] In selected patients, when induction of hypothyroidism is undesirable, this represents an alternative.

The amount of ^{131}I used to treat metastatic disease is variable and either consists of a fixed, empirically selected dose or is based on dosimetric methods.[64–66] The goal of dosimetry in the treatment of cancer is to estimate the maximum dose of RAI that can be administered safely. Dosimetric estimates are performed to restrict the dose to blood, as a surrogate for bone marrow, to <2 Gy as originally described by Benua *et al.*[65] Furthermore, in order to avoid pulmonary fibrosis in patients with metastatic lung disease, a whole-body retention of 2.96 GBq at 48 hours should not be exceeded[65] (see Chapter 12).

Who should receive ^{131}I treatment for metastatic thyroid cancer?

RAI therapy may improve survival in patients with metastatic disease, although patients are not usually cured by ^{131}I alone.[67–69] Therefore, in patients with potentially curable locoregional disease, the preferred mode of treatment is surgery often followed by RAI therapy. In these patients, pre-operative diagnostic RAI WBS should still be performed as it may reveal additional sites of disease which alter management. Patients treated with RAI should routinely undergo follow-up post-therapy scans as these frequently detect further sites of disease (Fig. 5.2).[70,71]

Lung metastases are not generally amenable to surgery. One strategy is to treat these patients every 6–12 months with RAI for as long as they continue to respond. Rather than using an empirical fixed dose therapy (ranging from 3.7 to 11.1 GBq) many centres administer doses based on individualized dosimetry. The intention is to deliver a maximally tolerated dose and avoid lung toxicity.[64,65]

Bone metastases may be diagnosed on a bone scan, but ^{131}I WBS is usually a more sensitive way to detect bone lesions in thyroid disease.[72] When bone metastases are present it is crucial to determine if there is a risk of neurological deficit or pathological fracture. If this is determined to be the case, emergent care including surgery and external beam radiation must be considered.[68] Typically, patients with bone metastases are not cured by RAI therapy, although it may improve survival.[68,73]

Brain metastases are usually associated with poor prognosis.[74] The mainstay of treatment is surgery and external beam radiation therapy.[74,75] There is little evidence supporting the efficacy of ^{131}I therapy, but it is often used because of the high likelihood of metastases elsewhere.

Approach to the patient with suspected metastatic disease and negative RAI

Management of patients with iodine-negative WBS and elevated Tg requires other investigation (CT, US, FDG

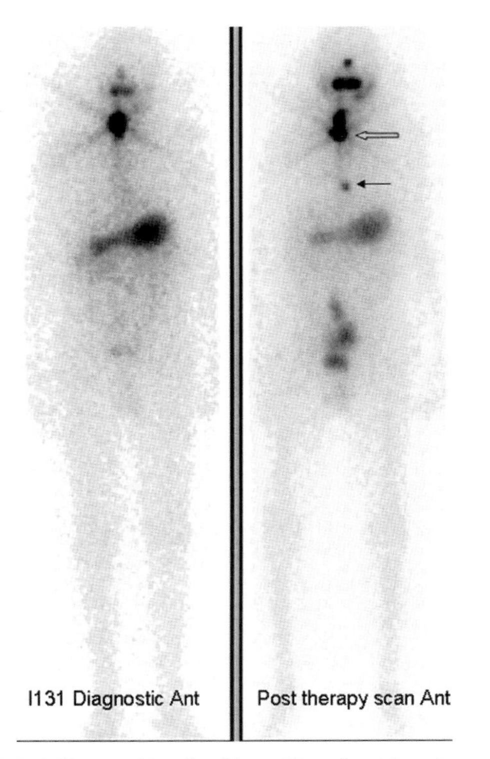

Fig. 5.2 A 78-year-old male with papillary thyroid carcinoma. A diagnostic whole-body scan was obtained 72 hours after oral ingestion of 185 MBq of ^{131}I and shows uptake in the thyroid bed and physiological uptake in the nasopharynx, mouth and stomach. A post-therapy scan obtained 5 days after 7.4 GBq of ^{131}I, in addition to targeting of the thyroid bed, showed focal uptake in an anterior mediastinal node (block arrow) which was confirmed on SPECT-CT (data not shown). Although the lesion was not clearly visualized on the diagnostic scan, a metastatic focus was identified corresponding to a para-aortic node at the level of the manubrium (arrow).

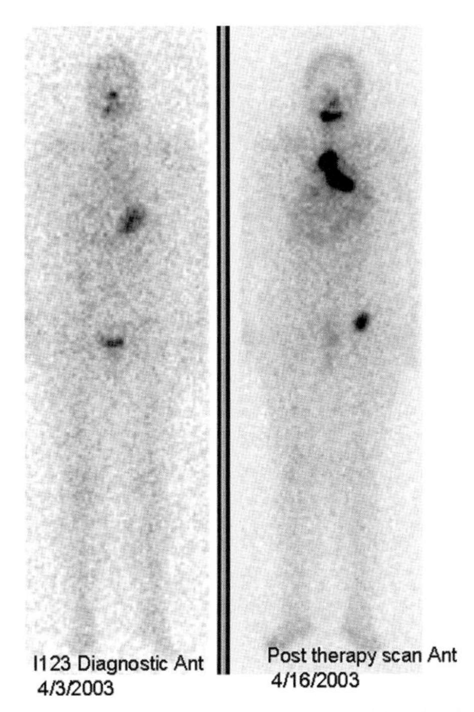

Fig. 5.3 A 55-year-old female with metastatic follicular thyroid cancer. A ^{123}I diagnostic scan showed no evidence of iodine-avid disease. Because of elevated thyroglobulin levels she was treated with 12.95 GBq ^{131}I. The post-therapy scan showed a large area of iodine-avid metastatic disease in the superior mediastinum extending to the left hilar region which was not seen on the diagnostic scan. In addition, focal metastatic disease was detected in the left femur.

and other radionuclide tests) to determine the location and extent of disease. When additional diagnostic imaging fails to localize the site of disease, an empiric therapeutic RAI dose[76–78] is administered if the Tg remains elevated. In this setting the post-therapy WBS localizes disease in 50% of patients[79,80] (Fig. 5.3). A significant proportion of WBS-negative patients will demonstrate a drop in Tg levels, suggesting a clinical response.[76–78] If an empiric dose of RAI fails to localize disease then it is considered 'iodine negative' and other modalities should be sought (see Chapters 8, 11 and 12). FDG-PET may be particularly useful as it tends to be positive in patients with thyroid disease which is no longer iodine avid (Fig. 5.4). In these patients, the extent of disease on FDG is the strongest predictor of survival[81] (see Chapter 4).

Imaging and RAI therapy in pregnancy

Radioiodine is contraindicated in pregnancy because ^{131}I concentrates in the fetal thyroid and results in a high radiation dose. Thus, monitoring local disease is best done by US. Female patients who receive ^{131}I therapy should avoid conception for a minimum of 6 months and men for a period of 4 months following treatment.[23] A slightly higher risk of miscarriage has been observed in the first year following RAI therapy.[82,83]

Thyroid cancer in childhood

Although thyroid cancer is rare in children it is not uncommon in individuals who have been exposed to

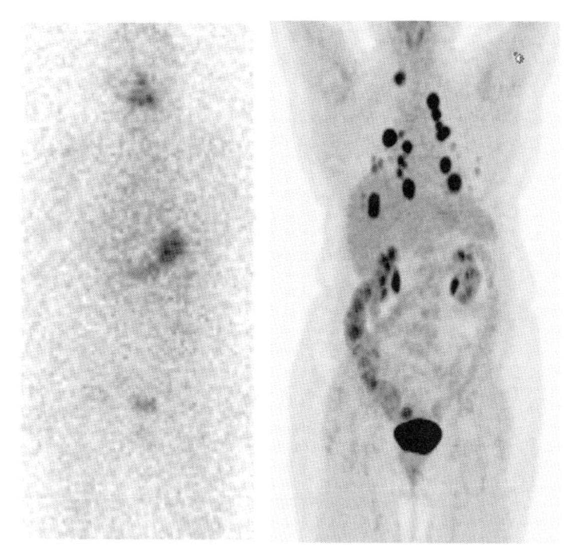

Fig. 5.4 A 68-year-old female with metastatic Hurthle cell carcinoma. A diagnostic scan performed 72 hours after 185 MBq of ^{131}I was negative. MIP images of FDG-PET show multiple hypermetabolic pulmonary nodules consistent with metastatic disease.

radiotherapy of the head and neck. The presence of a thyroid nodule in a child is more likely to be malignant than in an adult. The management of thyroid nodules and thyroid cancer in children is similar to that in adults, although the potential long-term side effects of radiation in children must be considered. Post-thyroidectomy ablation is often performed in children less than 10 years of age.[84]

Anaplastic thyroid cancer

Radioiodine scans are seldom of value in pre-operative imaging or therapy because anaplastic cancer does not take up RAI. Anaplastic thyroid cancer is highly metabolic and therefore FDG-PET may be useful in the evaluation of distant metastases.[85]

Medullary thyroid cancer

Medullary thyroid cancer (MTC) represents 5–10% of thyroid cancer.[86] These tumours arise from C cells that are derived from neuroectodermal cells. Due to this embryological derivation, these tumours do not concentrate iodine and thus a variety of alternative radiopharmaceuticals have been used. FDG-PET has a sensitivity of 70–75% for localizing metastatic disease in medullary thyroid cancer patients with an elevated calcitonin level post-thyroidectomy.[87] Radiolabelled metaiodobenzylguanidine (MIBG) scintigraphy may have a role in the imaging of MTC although it has a low sensitivity.

Side effects of RAI

Following RAI therapy, patients may complain of symptoms of sialadenitis such as mild discomfort, mouth dryness and abnormal taste.[88] Chronic persistent sialadenitis results in a dry oral cavity and intermittent swelling of the salivary gland, especially after high doses. Nausea following therapy may be reduced by using anti-emetics. Radiation pneumonitis can occur in patients with diffuse lung disease, although the use of dosimetry in treatment planning has reduced its incidence. A small increase in the risk of leukaemia and second malignancies has also been reported.[89–92]

CONCLUSION

Radionuclide scintigraphy continues to play an important role in the imaging, therapy and management of thyroid disorders. Isotopes of iodine are important for performing a functional assessment of the thyroid gland and for the optimal treatment of thyroid cancer. While ^{123}I and ^{131}I are important imaging isotopes, the advent of ^{124}I and FDG with PET provides important new tools for the evaluation of thyroid disorders.

EVIDENCE APPRAISAL

The Society of Nuclear Medicine (SNM) has written and approved guidelines for imaging the thyroid and for thyroid uptake. This serves as an educational tool designed to promote cost-effective use of high quality nuclear medicine procedures. SNM guidelines also assist with the conduct of research. Data are based on literature review and expert opinion, and therefore constitute Level IV evidence.[1,2,10]

Selection of the most appropriate amount of ^{131}I for therapy in hyperthyroidism is controversial. Most references are Level III or IV evidence, although Leslie *et al.*[18] present Level II evidence (a prospective study looking at low or high fixed/adjusted doses based on thyroid uptake).

A low iodine diet is recommended by the American Cancer Association. Studies evaluating the effect of low iodine diet have generally been retrospective[24,25] and represent Level IV evidence.

For hypothyroidism versus rhTSH: most studies are Level III. Haugen *et al.*[37] performed a large prospective study providing Level II evidence.

For the role of RAI on patient survival: there are a number of studies all providing Level III or IV evidence.

For the role of FDG-PET in management of thyroid cancer: there is mainly Level II–IV evidence.

REFERENCES

1. Becker DV, Charkes ND, Hurley JR, *et al.* Society of Nuclear Medicine procedure guideline for thyroid scintigraphy version 2.0. http://interactivesnmorg/docs/pg_ch05_0403pdf. 1999.
2. Silberstein EB, Alavi A, Balon HR, *et al.* Society of Nuclear Medicine procedure guideline for scintigraphy for differentiated papillary and follicular thyroid cancer. http://interactivesnmorg/docs/Scintigraphy%20for%20Differentiated%20 Thyroid%20Cancer%20V3%200%20(9-25-06)pdf. 2006.
3. Eschmann SM, Reischl G, Bilger K, *et al.* Evaluation of dosimetry of radioiodine therapy in benign and malignant thyroid disorders by means of iodine-124 and PET. Eur J Nucl Med Mol Imaging 2002;29:760–7.
4. Sisson JC, Avram AM, Lawson SA, *et al.* The so-called stunning of thyroid tissue. J Nucl Med 2006;47:1406–12.
5. Park HM, Park YH, Zhou XH. Detection of thyroid remnant/metastasis without stunning: an ongoing dilemma. Thyroid 1997;7:277–80.
6. Mandel SJ, Shankar LK, Benard F, *et al.* Superiority of iodine-123 compared with iodine-131 scanning for thyroid remnants in patients with differentiated thyroid cancer. Clin Nucl Med 2001;26:6–9.
7. Ryo UY, Vaidya PV, Schneider AB, *et al.* Thyroid imaging agents—a comparison of I-123 and Tc-99m pertechnetate. Radiology 1983;148:819–22.
8. Khammash NF, Halkar RK, Abdeldayem HM. The use of technetium-99m pertechnetate in postoperative thyroid-carcinoma—a comparative-study with I-131. Clin Nucl Med 1988;13:17–22.
9. Tharp K, Israel O, Hausmann J, *et al.* Impact of I-131-SPECT/CT images obtained with an integrated system in the follow-up of patients with thyroid carcinoma. Eur J Nucl Med Mol Imaging 2004;31:1435–42.
10. Balon HR, Silberstein EB, Meier DA, *et al.* Society of Nuclear Medicine procedure guideline for thyroid uptake measurement version 3. http://interactivesnmorg/docs/Thyroid%20 Uptake%20Measure%20v3%200pdf. 2006.
11. Mallin WH, Elgazzar AH, Maxon HR. Imaging modalities in the follow-up of non-iodine avid thyroid carcinoma. Am J Otolaryngol 1994;15:417–22.
12. Spanu A, Schillaci O, Madeddu G. Tc-99m labelled cationic lipophilic complexes in malignant and benign tumors: the role of SPET and pinhole-SPET in breast cancer, differentiated thyroid carcinoma and hyperparathyroidism. Q J Nucl Med Mol Imaging 2005;49:145–69.
13. Baudin E, Schlumberger M, Lumbroso J, *et al.* Octreotide scintigraphy in patients with differentiated thyroid carcinoma: contribution for patients with negative radioiodine scan. J Clin Endocrinol Metab 1996;81:2541–4.
14. Weetman AP. Radioiodine treatment for benign thyroid diseases. Clin Endocrinol 2007;66:757–64.
15. Hurley DL, Gharib H. Evaluation and management of multinodular goiter. Otolaryngol Clin North Am 1996;29: 527–40.
16. Clarke SEM. Radionuclide therapy of the thyroid. Eur J Nucl Med 1991;18:984–91.
17. Howarth D, Epstein M, Lan L, *et al.* Determination of the optimal minimum radioiodine dose in patients with Graves' disease: a clinical outcome study. Eur J Nucl Med 2001;28: 1489–95.
18. Leslie WD, Ward L, Salamon EA, *et al.* A randomized comparison of radioiodine doses in Graves' hyperthyroidism. J Clin Endocrinol Metab 2003;88:978–83.
19. Jarlov AE, Hegedus L, Kristensen LO, *et al.* Is calculation of the dose in radioiodine therapy of hyperthyroidism worth while. Clin Endocrinol 1995;43:325–9.
20. Alexander EK, Larsen PR. High dose I-131 therapy for the treatment of hyperthyroidism caused by Graves' disease. J Clin Endocrinol Metab 2002;87:1073–7.
21. Graham GD, Burman KD. Radioiodine treatment of Graves-disease—an assessment of its potential risks. Ann Intern Med 1986;105:900–5.
22. Cunnien AJ, Hay ID, Gorman CA, *et al.* Radio-iodine-induced hypothyroidism in Graves-disease—factors associated with the increasing incidence. J Nucl Med 1982;23: 978–83.
23. Smith BR, Cooper DS, Doherty GM, *et al.* Management guidelines for patients with thyroid nodules and differentiated thyroid cancer. Thyroid 2006;16:109.
24. Lakshmanan M, Schaffer A, Robbins J, *et al.* A simplified low iodine diet in I-131 scanning and therapy of thyroid cancer. Clin Nucl Med 1988;13:866–8.
25. Pluijmen M, Eustatia-Rutten C, Goslings BM, *et al.* Effects of low-iodide diet on postsurgical radioiodide ablation therapy in patients with differentiated thyroid carcinoma. Clin Endocrinol 2003;58:428–35.
26. Gorman CA. Radioiodine and pregnancy. Thyroid 1999;9: 721–6.
27. Robinson PS, Barker P, Campbell A, *et al.* I-131 in breast-milk following therapy for thyroid carcinoma. J Nucl Med 1994;35:1797–801.
28. Hilts SV, Hellman D, Anderson J, *et al.* Serial TSH determination after T3 withdrawal or thyroidectomy in the therapy of thyroid carcinoma. J Nucl Med 1979;20:928–32.
29. Goldman JM, Line BR, Aamodt RL, *et al.* Influence of triiodothyronine withdrawal time on I-131 uptake post-thyroidectomy for thyroid cancer. J Clin Endocrinol Metab 1980;50:734–9.

30. Grigsby PW, Siegel BA, Bekker S, *et al.* Preparation of patients with thyroid cancer for I-131 scintigraphy or therapy by 1–3 weeks of thyroxine discontinuation. J Nucl Med 2004;45:567–70.
31. Sanchez R, Espinosa-de-los-Monteros A, Mendoza V, *et al.* Adequate thyroid-stimulating hormone levels after levothyroxine discontinuation in the follow-up of patients with well-differentiated thyroid carcinoma. Arch Med Res 2002;33:478–81.
32. Meier CA, Braverman LE, Ebner SA, *et al.* Diagnostic use of recombinant human thyrotropin in patients with thyroid carcinoma (phase I/II study). J Clin Endocrinol Metab 1994;78:188–96.
33. Edmonds CJ, Kermode JC, Hayes S, *et al.* Measurement of serum TSH and thyroid hormones in management of treatment of thyroid carcinoma with radioiodine. Br J Radiol 1977;50:799–807.
34. Rosario PWS, Fagundes TA, Rezende LL, *et al.* Assessing hypothyroidism in the preparation of patients with thyroid cancer—cardiovascular risk, renal function, drug metabolism, persistence of elevated thyroid-stimulating hormone, and absence from work. Endocrinologist 2006;16:25–9.
35. Luster M, Lippi F, Jarzab B, *et al.* rhTSH-aided radioiodine ablation and treatment of differentiated thyroid carcinoma: a comprehensive review. Endocr Relat Cancer 2005;12: 49–64.
36. Robbins RJ, Tuttle RM, Sharaf RN, *et al.* Preparation by recombinant human thyrotropin or thyroid hormone withdrawal are comparable for the detection of residual differentiated thyroid carcinoma. J Clin Endocrinol Metab 2001;86:619–25.
37. Haugen BR, Pacini F, Reiners C, *et al.* A comparison of recombinant human thyrotropin and thyroid hormone withdrawal for the detection of thyroid remnant or cancer. J Clin Endocrinol Metab 1999;84:3877–85.
38. Mortensen JD, Woolner LB, Bennett WA. Gross and microscopic findings in clinically normal thyroid glands. J Clin Endocrinol Metab 1955;15:1270–80.
39. Hegedus L, Bonnema SJ, Bennedbaek FN. Management of simple nodular goiter: current status and future perspectives. Endocr Rev 2003;24:102–32.
40. Frates MC, Benson CB, Charboneau JW, *et al.* Management of thyroid nodules detected at us: Society of Radiologists in Ultrasound consensus conference statement. Radiology 2006;238:794–800.
41. Gharib H, Goellner JR. Fine-needle aspiration biopsy of the thyroid—an appraisal. Ann Intern Med 1993;118:282–9.
42. Hegedus L. The thyroid nodule. N Engl J Med 2004;351: 1764–71.
43. Baldwin DB, Rowett D. Incidence of thyroid disorders in connecticut. JAMA 1978;239:742–4.
44. Frates MC, Benson CB, Doubilet PM, *et al.* Prevalence and distribution of carcinoma in patients with solitary and multiple thyroid nodules on sonography. J Clin Endocrinol Metab 2006;91:3411–7.
45. Marqusee E, Benson CB, Frates MC, *et al.* Usefulness of ultrasonography in the management of nodular thyroid disease. Ann Intern Med 2000;133:696–700.
46. Cohen MS, Arslan N, Dehdashti F, *et al.* Risk of malignancy in thyroid incidentalomas identified by fluorodeoxyglucose-positron emission tomography. Surgery 2001;130:941–6.
47. Are C, Hsu JF, Schoder H, *et al.* FDG-PET detected thyroid incidentalomas: need for further investigation? Ann Surg Oncol 2007;14:239–47.
48. Kim TY, Kim WB, Ryu JS, *et al.* F-18-fluorodeoxyglucose uptake in thyroid from positron emission tomogram (PET) for evaluation in cancer patients: high prevalence of malignancy. Laryngoscope 2005;115:1074–8.
49. Choi JY, Lee KS, Kim HJ, *et al.* Focal thyroid lesions incidentally identified by integrated 18F-FDG PET/CT: clinical significance and improved characterization. J Nucl Med 2006;47:609–15.
50. Chen YK, Chen YL, Cheng RH, *et al.* The significance of FDG uptake in bilateral thyroid glands. Nucl Med Commun 2007;28:117–22.
51. de Geus-Oei LF, Pieters G, Bonenkamp JJ, *et al.* 18F-FDG PET reduces unnecessary hemithyroidectomies for thyroid nodules with inconclusive cytologic results. J Nucl Med 2006;47:770–5.
52. Kresnik E, Gallowitsch HJ, Mikosch P, *et al.* Fluorine-18-fluorodeoxyglucose positron emission tomography in the preoperative assessment of thyroid nodules in an endemic goiter area. Surgery 2003;133:294–9.
53. Schlumberger M, Berg G, Cohen O, *et al.* Follow-up of low-risk patients with differentiated thyroid carcinoma: a European perspective. Eur J Endocrinol 2004;150:105–12.
54. Rouxel A, Hejblum G, Bernier MO, *et al.* Prognostic factors associated with the survival of patients developing loco-regional recurrences of differentiated thyroid carcinomas. J Clin Endocrinol Metab 2004;89:5362–8.
55. Mazzaferri EL, Robbins RJ, Spencer CA, *et al.* A consensus report of the role of serum thyroglobulin as a monitoring method for low-risk patients with papillary thyroid carcinoma. J Clin Endocrinol Metab 2003;88:1433–41.
56. Pacini F, Capezzone M, Elisei R, *et al.* Diagnostic 131-iodine whole-body scan may be avoided in thyroid cancer patients who have undetectable stimulated serum Tg levels after initial treatment. J Clin Endocrinol Metab 2002;87:1499–501.
57. Akslen LA, LiVolsi VA. Prognostic significance of histologic grading compared with subclassification of papillary thyroid carcinoma. Cancer 2000;88:1902–8.
58. Prendiville S, Burman KD, Ringel MD, *et al.* Tall cell variant: an aggressive form of papillary thyroid carcinoma. Otolaryngol Head Neck Surg 2000;122:352–7.
59. Cailleux AF, Baudin E, Travagli JP, *et al.* Is diagnostic iodine-131 scanning useful after total thyroid ablation for differentiated thyroid cancer? J Clin Endocrinol Metab 2000;85: 175–8.
60. Bachelot A, Cailleux AF, Klain M, *et al.* Relationship between tumor burden and serum thyroglobulin level in patients

with papillary and follicular thyroid carcinoma. Thyroid 2002;12:707–11.
61. Pacini F, Molinaro E, Castagna MG, *et al.* Recombinant human thyrotropin-stimulated serum thyroglobulin combined with neck ultrasonography has the highest sensitivity in monitoring differentiated thyroid carcinoma. J Clin Endocrinol Metab 2003;88:3668–73.
62. Rudavsky AZ, Freeman LM. Treatment of scan-negative, thyroglobulin-positive metastatic thyroid cancer using radioiodine I-131 and recombinant human thyroid stimulating hormone—authors' response. J Clin Endocrinol Metab 1997;82:4277–8.
63. Lippi F, Capezzone M, Angelini F, *et al.* Radioiodine treatment of metastatic differentiated thyroid cancer in patients on l-thyroxine, using recombinant human TSH. Eur J Endocrinol 2001;144:5–11.
64. Van Nostrand D, Atkins F, Yeganeh F, *et al.* Dosimetrically determined doses of radioiodine for the treatment of metastatic thyroid carcinoma. Thyroid 2002;12:121–34.
65. Benua RS, Rawson RW, Sonenberg M, *et al.* Relation of radioiodine dosimetry to results and complications in treatment of metastatic thyroid cancer. Am J Roentgenol Radium Ther Nucl Med 1962;87:171–82.
66. Maxon HR, Smith HS. Radioiodine-131 in the diagnosis and treatment of metastatic well differentiated thyroid cancer. Endocrinol Metab Clin North Am 1990;19:685–718.
67. Leeper RD. Effect of I-131 therapy on survival of patients with metastatic papillary or follicular thyroid carcinoma. J Clin Endocrinol Metab 1973;36:1143–52.
68. Bernier MO, Leenhardt L, Hoang C, *et al.* Survival and therapeutic modalities in patients with bone metastases of differentiated thyroid carcinomas. J Clin Endocrinol Metab 2001;86:1568–73.
69. Beierwaltes WH, Nishiyama RH, Thompson NW, *et al.* Survival-time and cure in papillary and follicular thyroid carcinoma with distant metastases—statistics following University of Michigan therapy. J Nucl Med 1982;23:561–8.
70. Do Rosario PWS, Barroso AL, Rezende LL, *et al.* Post I-131 therapy scanning in patients with thyroid carcinoma metastases: an unnecessary cost or a relevant contribution? Clin Nucl Med 2004;29:795–8.
71. Fatourechi V, Hay ID, Mullan BP, *et al.* Are posttherapy radioiodine scans informative and do they influence subsequent therapy of patients with differentiated thyroid cancer? Thyroid 2000;10:573–7.
72. Castillo LA, Yeh SDJ, Leeper RD, *et al.* Bone scans in bone metastases from functioning thyroid carcinoma. Clin Nucl Med 1980;5:200–9.
73. Schlumberger M, Challeton C, DeVathaire F, *et al.* Radioactive iodine treatment and external radiotherapy for lung and bone metastases from thyroid carcinoma. J Nucl Med 1996;37:598–605.
74. Chiu AC, Delpassand ES, Sherman SI. Prognosis and treatment of brain metastases in thyroid carcinoma. J Clin Endocrinol Metab 1997;82:3637–42.
75. McWilliams RR, Giannini C, Hay ID, *et al.* Management of brain metastases from thyroid carcinoma—a study of 16 pathologically confirmed cases over 25 years. Cancer 2003;98:356–62.
76. Schlumberger M, Arcangioli O, Piekarski JD, *et al.* Detection and treatment of lung metastases of differentiated thyroid-carcinoma in patients with normal chest x-rays. J Nucl Med 1988;29:1790–4.
77. Pacini F, Lippi F, Formica N, *et al.* Therapeutic doses of I-131 reveal undiagnosed metastases in thyroid cancer patients with detectable serum thyroglobulin levels. J Nucl Med 198;28:1888–91.
78. Pineda JD, Lee T, Ain K, Reynolds JC, Robbins J. I-131 therapy for thyroid cancer patients with elevated thyroglobulin and negative diagnostic scan. J Clin Endocrinol Metab 1995;80:1488–92.
79. Ma C, Xie JW, Kuang A. Is empiric I-131 therapy justified for patients with positive thyroglobulin and negative I-131 whole-body scanning results? J Nucl Med 2005;46:1164–70.
80. Schlumberger M, Mancusi F, Baudin E, *et al.* I-131 therapy for elevated thyroglobulin levels. Thyroid 1997;7:273–6.
81. Wang W, Larson SM, Fazzari M, *et al.* Prognostic value of [18F]fluorodeoxyglucose positron emission tomographic scanning in patients with thyroid cancer. J Clin Endocrinol Metab 2000;85:1107–13.
82. Chow SM, Yau S, Lee SH, *et al.* Pregnancy outcome after diagnosis of differentiated thyroid carcinoma: no deleterious effect after radioactive iodine treatment. Int J Radiat Oncol Biol Phys 2004;59:992–1000.
83. Schlumberger M, DeVathaire F, Ceccarelli C, *et al.* Exposure to radioactive iodine-131 for scintigraphy or therapy does not preclude pregnancy in thyroid cancer patients. J Nucl Med 1996;37:606–12.
84. Dottorini ME, Vignati A, Mazzucchelli L, *et al.* Differentiated thyroid carcinoma in children and adolescents: a 37-year experience in 85 patients. J Nucl Med 1997;38:669–75.
85. Poppe K, Lahoutte T, Everaert H, *et al.* The utility of multimodality imaging in anaplastic thyroid carcinoma. Thyroid 2004;14:981–2.
86. Roman S, Lin R, Sosa JA. Prognosis of medullary thyroid carcinoma—demographic, clinical, and pathologic predictors of survival in 1252 cases. Cancer 2006;107:2134–42.
87. Schoder H, Yeung HWD. Positron emission imaging of head and neck cancer, including thyroid carcinoma. Semin Nucl Med 2004;34:180–97.
88. Mandel SJ, Mandel L. Radioactive iodine and the salivary glands. Thyroid 2003;13:265–71.
89. Bhattacharyya N, Chien W. Risk of second primary malignancy after radioactive iodine treatment for differentiated thyroid carcinoma. Ann Otol Rhinol Laryngol 2006;115:607–10.
90. Sandeep TC, Strachan MWJ, Reynolds RM, *et al.* Second primary cancers in thyroid cancer patients: a multinational

record linkage study. J Clin Endocrinol Metab 2006;91: 1819–25.
91. Rubino C, de Vathaire F, Dottorini ME, *et al.* Second primary malignancies in thyroid cancer patients. Br J Cancer 2003;89:1638–44.
92. Verkooijen RBT, Smit JWA, Romijn JA, *et al.* The incidence of second primary tumors in thyroid cancer patients is increased, but not related to treatment of thyroid cancer. Eur J Endocrinol 2006;155:801–6.

MULTIPLE CHOICE QUESTIONS

Select more than one option where appropriate.

1. Except for low-risk patient groups, ^{131}I ablation:
A. Permits subsequent identification by whole-body scanning of any residual or metastatic carcinoma
B. Increases the sensitivity of Tg measurement for follow-up
C. Decreases tumour recurrence
E. Increases cause-specific survival

2. Prior to ablation or therapeutic ^{131}I, the TSH level should be greater than:
A. 15 mU/l
B. 20 mU/l
C. 30 mU/l
D. 40 mU/l
E. 50 mU/l

3. In patients with recurrent lymph node disease in the neck, ^{131}I scanning will reveal uptake in:
A. 0–20%
B. 20–40%
C. 40–60%
D. 60–80%

4. A 45-year-old male with a palpable nodule undergoes a ^{123}I thyroid scan that shows 40% radioactive iodine uptake and a hot nodule. The patient most probably has:
A. An autonomous functioning thyroid nodule
B. A lesion at high risk for cancer
C. A lesion at low risk for cancer
D. Both A and C

5. The following is true regarding patients who undergo radioiodine treatment:
A. A low iodine diet is necessary for 4 weeks prior to therapy
B. Women should avoid breast feeding for 6–8 weeks prior to therapy
C. Women should avoid pregnancy for 1 year following treatment
D. Dosimetric estimates are performed to restrict the dose to <1 Gy

Answers

1. A, B, C, D, E
2. C
3. D
4. D
5. B

6 Endocrine disorders: medical management

Nick Oliver & Stephen Robinson
St Mary's Hospital, Imperial Healthcare NHS Trust, London, UK

KEY POINTS

- Hyperthyroidism is biochemically confirmed by a low thyroid-stimulating hormone (TSH) and elevated free thyroid hormones (thyroxine and tri-iodothyronine)
- Technetium uptake scanning is useful to diagnose the cause of hyperthyroidism. The aetiology of hyperthyroidism may be divided into low and high uptake causes
- Thionamide drugs are the ideal first-line therapy for hyperthyroidism. Surgery is an important treatment modality for goitre and thyroid eye disease. Radioiodine therapy is used in primary or relapsing autoimmune hyperthyroidism, toxic multinodular goitre and single toxic adenomata
- Primary hypothyroidism is biochemically confirmed by an elevated TSH and low free thyroxine. Treatment is with thyroxine to normalize the TSH regardless of aetiology
- An acutely unwell patient with a non-thyroidal illness may exhibit temporary derangement of thyroid function

HYPERTHYROIDISM

Introduction

Hyperthyroidism is an endocrine condition characterized by hypermetabolism. The causes of hyperthyroidism may be divided into those which show increased uptake on technetium scanning and those with low uptake Table 6.1).

Hyperthyroidism has an annual incidence of 0.5 cases per 1000 people, and the majority of cases (60–80%) are due to Graves' disease. Toxic multinodular goitre accounts for 15–20% of cases and is prevalent in areas of iodine deficiency. Single toxic adenomata account for 3–5% of annual cases, while rarer causes include thyroiditis and drug-induced hyperthyroidism.

Autoimmune hyperthyroidism (Graves' disease) has a peak incidence between the ages of 20 and 40 years, and is much more common in women than men (between 5:1 and 10:1). Toxic multinodular goitre occurs in individuals with long-standing multinodular disease and therefore tends to present over the age of 50 years. Single toxic adenomata may present at an earlier age than toxic multinodular goitre. Both toxic multinodular goitre and single toxic adenomata are more common in women than men, with a ratio of 2:1–4:1. Autoimmune hyperthyroidism occurs with the same frequency in Caucasian, Hispanic and Asian populations, but is less common in Black populations. It is associated with type 1 diabetes mellitus, Addison's disease, vitiligo, pernicious anaemia, alopecia areata, myasthenia gravis, coeliac disease and other autoimmune diseases associated with the human leucocyte antigen (HLA)-DR3 haplotype. The Royal College of Physicians suggest that all cases of hyperthyroidism should be reviewed by a specialist endocrinologist.

Clinical features

The presenting features of hyperthyroidism are variable and do not correlate with the degree of biochemical hyperthyroidism (Table 6.2).

Patients develop symptoms of sympathetic overstimulation, including tachycardia, anxiety, tremor, diarrhoea and hyperactivity. Tachyarrhythmias may occur particularly in elderly patients. The incidence of atrial fibrillation associated with hyperthyroidism increases with age, as does the risk of stroke and associated mortality. Hypermetabolism leads to weight loss despite increased appetite and increased food intake (hyperphagia). Heat intolerance and increased sweating are common due to increased metabolic thermogenesis. When myopathy occurs, patients often complain of difficulty climbing stairs or doing physical work. Women with hyperthyroidism report oligomenorrhoea or amenorrhoea, and fertility can be adversely affected.

A smoking history should be sought as this exacerbates autoimmune hyperthyroidism. It may also exacerbate

A Practical Manual of Thyroid and Parathyroid Disease, 1st Edition. Edited by Asit Arora, Neil Tolley & R. Michael Tuttle.

Table 6.1 The aetiology of hyperthyroidism by technetium uptake (common causes in bold)

High uptake	Low uptake
Autoimmune hyperthyroidism	**Subacute thyroiditis**
Toxic multinodular goitre	**Post-partum thyroiditis**
Single toxic adenoma	**Amiodarone-induced hyperthyroidism***
Thyroid hormone resistance	Excess thyroid hormone ingestion
TSH-secreting pituitary adenoma	Hashimoto's thyroiditis

* Amiodarone-induced hyperthyroidism shows low uptake on technetium uptake scanning. Iodine uptake scanning may be low but detectable in type 1 disease.

thyroid ophthalmopathy particularly in patients receiving radioactive iodine treatment. Susceptibility to autoimmune thyroid disease (both hypo- and hyperthyroid) is linked to haplotype. It is therefore important to enquire about family history of thyroid disease. Forty to 50% of patients with autoimmune thyroid disease have another family member with a thyroid disorder. Population studies have shown associations with HLA loci, and other candidate genes such as those encoding CTLA-4 (cytotoxic T cell antigen 4), CD40 and tyrosine phosphatase-22 have also been identified.

Clinical examination of a thyrotoxic patient will confirm the signs of hyperthyroidism and may also indicate the aetiology. General features common to all causes of hyperthyroidism include tremor, palmar erythema, tachycardia, warm or moist skin, hair loss, hyper-reflexia, myopathy and lid lag. Less common manifestations include high output cardiac failure, chorea, periodic paralysis (primarily seen in Asian men) and psychosis.

Autoimmune hyperthyroidism

Autoimmune hyperthyroidism is commonly known as Graves' disease (Graves' disease was described by Robert Graves, a Dublin physician, in 1835 as a triad of goitre, palpitations and exophthalmos observed in three patients. However, the first description was by Caleb Parry, a physician working in Bath, UK, who noted exophthalmos and thyrotoxic symptoms in a patient and published 10 years before Graves. In 1840, Karl Basedow, a German physician, described the Merseburger triad of exophthalmos, diffuse goitre and hyperthyroidism in Berlin.) Features specific to Graves' disease include thyroid-associated dermopathy and ophthalmopathy. Thyroid-associated dermopathy includes acropachy (finger-clubbing and subperiosteal new bone formation) and pre-tibial myxoedema. The soft tissue swelling seen in both conditions is due to glycosaminoglycan deposition. Pre-tibial myxoedema typically appears as raised, discoloured and indurated lesions over the tibia (Fig. 6.1). Lesions have also been described on the foot and hand. They are usually asymptomatic but can become painful or pruritic.

Thyroid-associated ophthalmopathy is caused by cross-reactivity between the anti-thyroid antibodies and

Table 6.2 Clinical features of hyperthyroidism and hypothyroidism

System	Hyperthyroidism	Hypothyroidism
General	Weight loss* Heat intolerance Tremor Sweating Pruritis Myopathy/weakness Hyperactivity	Weight gain Cold intolerance Dry skin Fatigue Muscle weakness Hoarseness Hair loss
Cardiovascular	Palpitations Arrhythmia Dyspnoea Cardiac failure Exacerbation of ischaemic heart disease	Bradycardia Hypertension Pericardial effusion Cardiac failure
Gastrointestinal	Diarrhoea Hyperphagia	Constipation
Endocrine	Oligomenorrhoea Subfertility Osteoporosis Loss of libido Gynaecomastia	Oligomenorrhoea Subfertility Galactorrhoea
Autoimmune hyperthyroidism	Gritty/uncomfortable eyes Exophthalmos Diplopia Chemosis Optic neuropathy Thyroid-associated dermopathy	
Central nervous system	Irritability Insomnia Psychosis	Depression Poor memory Ataxia

* Rarely, paradoxical weight gain can be seen in hyperthyroidism, presumably as a consequence of hyperphagia overcoming the hypermetabolism.

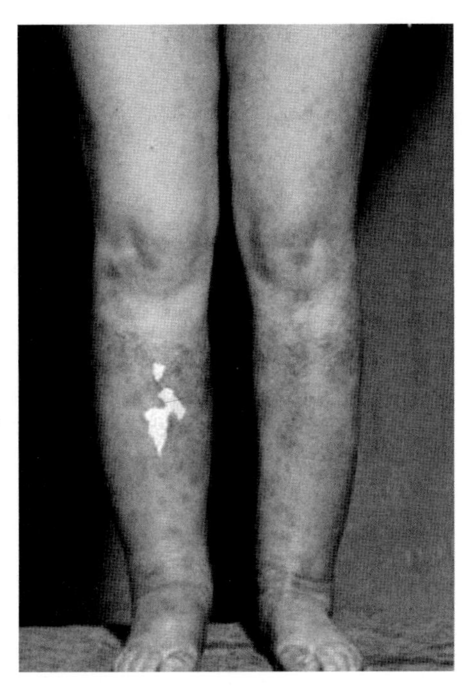

Fig. 6.1 A patient with pre-tibial myxoedema.

TSH receptors (TSHRs) found in extraocular muscles (the role of TSHRs in extraocular muscle is unclear). This causes inflammation, lymphocytic infiltration and proliferation of orbital soft tissue. The patient may complain of grittiness in the eyes, red eyes, diplopia or deteriorating vision. It is important to identify and monitor thyroid-associated ophthalmopathy to ensure that ocular emergencies such as corneal ulceration and optic neuropathy do not develop.

The clinical features of thyroid-associated ophthalmopathy include peri-orbital oedema, proptosis, lid retraction, chemosis, scleral injection, ophthalmoplegia and optic neuropathy. Lid lag is a feature of increased sympathetic autonomic tone and may be seen in all forms of hyperthyroidism. Although the terms proptosis and exophthalmos are used interchangeably, conventionally exophthalmos is reserved for cases of endocrine-mediated ocular protrusion. Other clinical features which guide the diagnosis are the presence of a palpable multinodular goitre or a single palpable nodule.

Thyroiditis

Thyroiditis refers to inflammation of the thyroid and may be infectious, autoimmune or drug related. It is typified by destruction of thyroid follicular cells and rapid release of intrathyroid hormone stores. The histopathological changes which occur in various forms of thyroiditis are outlined in Chapter 2.

Biochemical hyperthyroidism, with inhibition of pituitary TSH secretion, results from rapid release of stored hormone and does not represent an increase in the rate of thyroid hormone production. The thyrotoxic phase of thyroiditis is often followed by a hypothyroid phase as the follicular cells recover function slowly. Subacute (also known as De Quervain's or post-viral) thyroiditis commonly follows a viral illness, and the aetiology is thought to be directly related to viral infection although the specific causative virus has not been identified. The diagnosis is suggested by a painful thyroid gland, fever and malaise. Clinical examination differs from other differential diagnoses in the finding of a tender, firm thyroid which may be asymmetrical. There may also be associated cervical lymphadenopathy.

Post-partum thyroiditis (also known as silent or lymphocytic thyroiditis) occurs in 1–17% of women depending on geographical location and genetic susceptibility. It is most common in women with pre-existing anti-thyroid antibodies, which suggests that an autoimmune aetiology is likely. Some patients follow the classic 'triphasic' thyroiditis course (hyperthyroid, hypothyroid, recovery to normal), but presentation is varied. Patients may experience hyperthyroidism which recovers back to normal without a hypothyroid phase, while others become hypothyroid without a toxic phase. Around 25% of women develop permanent hypothyroidism, and the recurrence rate is 80%. It usually occurs following delivery at term, but can also arise following miscarriage. Silent thyroiditis usually arises following pregnancy, but also occurs outside of this context in women and rarely in men.

Amiodarone-induced hyperthyroidism

Amiodarone is an iodinated anti-arrhythmic drug in common use. It contains 37.3% iodine by weight and causes hyperthyroidism by two possible mechanisms. Type 1 amiodarone-induced hyperthyroidism is caused by release of iodine during the metabolism of amiodarone and tends to occur in patients with a pre-existing multinodular goitre. Type 2 amiodarone-induced hyperthyroidism is a thyroiditis caused by a direct toxic effect of the drug on the thyroid gland. In the USA, 3% of patients taking amiodarone develop hyperthyroidism. Differentiating between type 1 and type 2 can be difficult since technetium and iodine uptake are poor in both conditions. Iodine uptake may be low but detectable in type 1 disease. Colour-flow Doppler ultrasound scanning is useful because it detects blood flow, which is reduced in thyroiditis. Type 1 disease may be treated with anti-thyroid medication. Patients who do not respond to thionamides or radioiodine therapy require surgery. Type 2 disease follows the natural history of a typical thyroiditis.

Laboratory testing

The diagnosis of hyperthyroidism is dependent upon the finding of a suppressed serum TSH concentration in conjunction with elevated free hormone levels. Suppression of TSH below the reference range alone is not specific for hyperthyroidism as this occurs in non-thyroidal illness and pituitary disease, and may also be drug induced. Confirmation of hyperthyroidism therefore requires elevated free circulating thyroid hormone levels in addition to suppression of TSH. In most cases of hyperthyroidism, the TSH will be undetectable, with elevated free thyroxine (FT4) and free tri-iodothyronine (FT3) (Table 6.3).

Thyroid function testing may be affected by medications such as amiodarone, lithium and carbamazepine.

In early autoimmune hyperthyroidism and single toxic adenoma, T3 toxicosis has been described (TSH is suppressed with a normal FT4 and an elevated FT3). It is therefore important to measure FT3 in cases where the TSH is suppressed with a normal FT4. Biochemical hyperthyroidism is often more severe in autoimmune disease.

Table 6.3 Interpretation of thyroid function testing

TSH	Free thyroid hormones	Differential diagnosis
Normal	Normal	Normal thyroid function
↓	↑	Hyperthyroidism
↓	Normal	Non-thyroidal illness Subclinical hyperthyroidism Pregnancy
↓	↓	Non-thyroidal illness Pituitary disease
Normal	↑	Non-thyroidal illness Thyroid hormone resistance TSH-secreting tumour
Normal	↓	Non-thyroidal illness
↑	↓	Primary hypothyroidism
↑	Normal	Subclinical hypothyroidism
↑	↑	Thyroid hormone resistance TSH-secreting tumour

Subclinical hyperthyroidism is defined as a suppressed TSH with normal free thyroid hormones in the absence of concurrent illness. Clinical features in subclinical hyperthyroidism are mild or absent, but it is important to identify this condition because it can progress to frank hyperthyroidism. It also contributes to subfertility, osteoporosis and increases the risk of atrial fibrillation. Survival from cardiovascular disease in the older age group is significantly reduced when the TSH is less than 0.5 mU/l.[1] However, the evidence base for treatment of subclinical hyperthyroidism is not substantial at present.[2]

Euthyroid hyperthyroxinaemia is a common finding in acutely unwell patients and reflects changes in binding protein concentrations, thyroid hormone peripheral conversion and the pituitary–thyroid axis. It is characterized by a normal TSH with elevated free thyroid hormones. It is not an uncommon finding in hospital inpatients and it is important to check thyroid function when the patient has recovered from the acute illness. If a normal TSH persists in the presence of elevated free thyroid hormones, rarer differential diagnoses should be considered such as thyroid hormone resistance and TSH-secreting pituitary adenoma. Thyroid hormone resistance syndrome is an inherited defect of the thyroid hormone receptor. It may present with goitre and should not be treated with surgery. TSH-secreting pituitary adenomas are confirmed by pituitary investigation.

Persistently abnormal thyroid function in patients with no clinical features of thyroid dysfunction suggests the presence of circulating antibodies which interfere with the assay of thyroid function tests. Antibodies may be confirmed by dilution test, heterophilic antibody removal or by using an alternative assay methodology.

Once biochemical hyperthyroidism has been confirmed, other laboratory tests may assist the diagnosis. Clinical features may indicate a likely aetiology, and measurement of autoantibodies is useful. Thyroid peroxidase (TPO) antibodies and TSHR antibodies may be seen in Graves' disease. TPO antibodies are positive in around 75% of patients with Graves' disease. TSHR antibody is a more specific indicator of disease but is not measured routinely as there is no evidence to suggest this alters management. TSHR antibodies are positive in over 80% of patients with autoimmune hyperthyroidism and are of particular importance in pregnancy because they cross the placenta and may cause neonatal autoimmune hyperthyroidism. Measurement of TSHR antibody may also be useful in patients who are biochemically euthyroid but have clinical signs suggestive of Graves' disease such as ophthalmopathy.

Other biochemical abnormalities occur in the context of hyperthyroidism. Deranged liver function tests may be observed, with a rise in transaminases. Anti-thyroid medication is also associated with elevated transaminase levels and, in order to establish the correct aetiology in the thyrotoxic patient, it is important to assess liver function prior to treatment. Similarly, a full blood count should ideally be assessed prior to the commencement of treatment.

Thionamide drugs rarely cause agranulocytosis, leading to neutropenia and thrombocytopenia which may result in sepsis and bleeding complications. In view of this, all patients prescribed thionamides must be clearly warned of the associated risks, which are further outlined later in this chapter. Erythrocyte sedimentation rate (ESR) is a useful test when viral thyroiditis is suspected. It is often elevated, and very high levels are typical in the thyrotoxic phase.

In pregnancy, serum human chorionic gonadotrophin (HCG) is present in high concentrations. It shares a similar chemical morphology to TSH. In high concentrations it binds to and activates the thyroid TSHR, increasing thyroxine secretion. This may cause suppression of TSH particularly in the first trimester when HCG concentrations are at their highest. The compensatory suppression of TSH prevents free thyroid hormones becoming significantly elevated.

Radiology in hyperthyroidism

Once biochemical hyperthyroidism has been confirmed, ideally all patients should have a radionuclide uptake scan (see Chapter 5). This quantifies the uptake of labelled technetium or iodine by the thyroid gland. It should be undertaken prior to treatment with anti-thyroid medication because the latter reduces marker uptake. Causes of hyperthyroidism can be divided radiologically into high and low uptake (see Table 6.1).

Uptake scanning also demonstrates the pattern of uptake, which provides useful functional and anatomical information. Single toxic adenomas are identifiable as a 'hot' area within the gland and there is reduced activity in the thyroid tissue surrounding the nodule. Diffuse increased uptake is consistent with autoimmune hyperthyroidism and toxic multinodular goitre. A dominant nodule with asymmetrical uptake may also be seen in multinodular goitre. Clinical examination and antibody status is required to differentiate further autoimmune disease from multinodular goitre.

In the presence of a clinically palpable nodule, an ultrasound (US) scan is useful to assess its size, vascularity and calcification status. However, this is not a substitute for functional assessment with an uptake scan as US only provides anatomical information. Depending on the US findings, fine needle aspiration may be undertaken for cytological assessment. Full guidelines on the management of thyroid nodules are published by the American Thyroid Association and the role of fine needle aspiration cytology is outlined in Chapter 3.[3] It is worth noting that 'hot' nodules very rarely represent thyroid carcinoma.

Hyperthyroid patients with clinical evidence of a retrosternal goitre require further imaging such as plain chest radiograph and computed tomography (CT) scanning to assess the full extent of the thyroid gland. This is important when considering future definitive therapies such as surgery or radioiodine treatment.

Hyperthyroidism is rarely due to ectopic thyroxine secretion. Struma ovarii is an ovarian teratoma containing thyroid tissue which may be autonomously functioning. Metastatic follicular thyroid carcinoma may also cause ectopic hyperthyroidism, and wider radionuclide scans are employed in these cases.

Management of hyperthyroidism

Anti-thyroid medication

Medical treatment of hyperthyroidism is dependent upon its aetiology and should be individually tailored to the patient. Treatment modalities include symptomatic management, management of complications, anti-thyroid medication and radioisotope treatment.

Hyperthyroidism causes symptoms of increased sympathetic tone such as palpitations, anxiety and tremor. These symptoms can be managed with β-adrenergic blockade if the patient does not have asthma or significant peripheral vascular disease. β-Blockade also reduces the risk of atrial fibrillation. Propranolol 40 mg twice or three times daily is frequently used, but all β-blockers are effective and the dose should be titrated to symptoms. When the patient is biochemically euthyroid, β-blockade should be titrated down and then completely stopped. Sometimes the patient is unable to tolerate oral agents, e.g. during the peri-operative period, if the patient has severe vomiting or during a thyroid storm. In these situations, intravenous esmolol or metoprolol can be used. Long-acting β-blockers should be used pre-operatively to ensure adequate intra-operative blockade. Patients who do not tolerate β-blockers may be treated with calcium channel blockers such as diltiazem or verapamil.

Autoimmune hyperthyroidism, toxic multinodular goitre and single toxic adenoma can all be treated with thionamides. These include carbimazole (UK), methimazole (USA/Europe) and propylthiouracil. Methimazole is an active metabolite of carbimazole. The thionamides inhibit thyroid peroxidase and thus thyroid hormone synthesis. Propylthiouracil also inhibits peripheral conversion of T4 to T3, thus reducing the peripheral circulating concentration of FT3 rapidly. This additional property of propylthiouracil is particularly useful in the management of thyroid storm. Carbimazole and methimazole are both once-daily drugs compared with the twice-daily propylthiouracil regime. The latter achieves control of hyperthyroidism more rapidly. Once euthyroid, the thionamides may be titrated down to a maintenance dose. Regular thyroid function testing is essential so that further management may be planned. In the case of toxic multinodular goitre and single toxic adenoma, pre-existing hyperthyroidism will relapse if drug treatment is discontinued. Once the patient is rendered euthyroid, definitive management should be planned such as radioiodine treatment or surgery.

Autoimmune hyperthyroidism does remit spontaneously. Thionamides may be given for 12–18 months following achievement of biochemical euthyroid status and then stopped. Approximately 50% of patients will relapse at some point, although this may occur years later. When relapse does occur, thionamide treatment should be restarted and, once euthyroid status has been re-established, definitive treatment is planned. Thirty to 40% of patients with autoimmune hyperthyroidism treated with an anti-thyroid drug remain euthyroid 10 years later. Retrospective and prospective data have shown that at diagnosis, the presence of a large goitre, severe biochemical hyperthyroidism, an increased FT3:FT4 serum ratio, repeated relapse and high antibody titres are all associated with a greater probability of relapse. During treatment, a persistent large goitre, high FT3:FT4 ratio, requirement for high dose anti-thyroid medication to maintain euthyroid status, persistently positive antibodies and suppressed TSH all predict relapse. However, these features are not sufficiently predictive to direct early definitive treatment with radioiodine or surgery in individual cases.

Some endocrinologists prefer a 'block and replace' regime when prescribing thionamides. Instead of titrating the dose of thionamide downwards according to frequent thyroid function test results, thyroxine is added to a suppressive dose of thionamide and the thyroxine dose is titrated to achieve normal thyroid function. This has the advantage of fewer clinic visits and blood tests, and reduces the risk of fluctuations in thyroid hormone levels. Avoiding high concentrations of TSH by ensuring constant exogenous thyroxine also prevents release of thyroid antigens which may play a role in promoting remission of autoimmune hyperthyroidism. Avoiding release of excess thyroid antigen may also reduce the severity of thyroid-associated ophthalmopathy. A low relapse rate of hyperthyroidism with a block and replace regime has been reported, but has not been widely reproduced in further studies.[4]

Thionamide drugs can potentially cause agranulocytosis which occurs in <3 cases per 10000 patient years (although some estimates are higher).[5] The incidence is very low but the consequences may be serious. Therefore, all patients started on thionamides should be warned that if they develop a sore throat, fever, arthralgia, mouth ulcers (refer plate 6.1) or rash, the drug should be discontinued immediately. In such cases, a full blood count is required to assess the white cell count. Routine monitoring of the full blood count is not required provided that the patient is adequately counselled regarding this risk. Treatment of agranulocytosis requires hospitalization, barrier care, broad-spectrum antibiotic cover and discontinuation of the drug.

Another serious side effect is hepatotoxicity. Small rises in transaminase concentrations are common with anti-thyroid drugs. Rarely, hepatitis occurs which necessitates discontinuation of the drug. Hepatitis is more common with propylthiouracil than with carbimazole or methimazole.

Patients requiring rapid control of hyperthyroidism prior to surgery or during thyroid storm can be treated with Lugol's iodine which is a solution of 5% molecular iodine (I_2) and 10% potassium iodide (KI). It was first manufactured by Jean Lugol, a French physician, in 1829 and has several dose-dependent effects on the thyroid gland. In high doses, it inhibits organification and hormone release, and decreases the size and vascularity of the gland. Lugol's iodine may also be used in patients intolerant of other anti-thyroid agents.

Thyroid hormone resistance syndrome and TSH-secreting adenomas should be investigated and managed in specialist endocrine centres.

Radioactive iodine therapy

Once the patient is biochemically euthyroid, definitive treatment can be planned to cure hyperthyroidism and prevent relapse of autoimmune hyperthyroidism. Definitive treatment involves either radioiodine ablation with ^{131}I or surgery.

Radioiodine is a safe treatment with no evidence from longitudinal studies to suggest that fertility, intrathyroid or extrathyroid malignancy risks are adversely affected. Local guidelines should be followed for counselling, consent and administration. The dose given in benign thyroid disease is lower than that used in the management of thyroid carcinoma. It should ideally be given to euthyroid patients and caution should be exercised in patients with thyroid ophthalmopathy as radioiodine may exacerbate eye disease, especially in smokers. Thyroid ophthalmopathy may be further exacerbated following radioiodine treatment if the patient becomes hypothyroid. If radioiodine is given to patients prior to achieving euthyroid status, worsening hyperthyroidism may be precipitated and cases of thyroid storm have been reported. Patients being consented for radioiodine should be made aware that it is an ablative treatment which may cause life-long hypothyroidism. In a retrospective study of patients with Graves' disease treated with a standard dose of 555 MBq, 64% were hypothyroid at 1 year.[6] Radioiodine treatment may be dose adjusted to aim for euthyroid status. The annual incidence of hypothyroidism in Graves' disease treated with radioiodine is 2–3%, even when the patient is initially euthyroid.[7]

Radioiodine is given orally in capsule or solution form and is taken up primarily by the thyroid gland. Radioiodine not absorbed by the thyroid is excreted by the kidneys and the rest is lost in sweat, faeces, saliva and breath. Radioiodine is contraindicated in pregnant and breastfeeding women. ^{131}I decays to stable xenon, emitting β particles which ablate the thyroid with little effect on surrounding tissue. Decay of radioiodine also emits γ rays which are detectable in the external environment. For this reason, patients receiving radioiodine should have restricted contact with others, particularly pregnant women and children, following treatment.

Concomitant use of anti-thyroid drugs during radioiodine therapy varies and while anti-thyroid drugs reduce radioiodine uptake, there is no change in outcome for patients on anti-thyroid medication providing a dose of >370 MBq is administered. Depending on the severity of hyperthyroidism and concomitant risk factors such as cardiovascular disease and previous arrhythmias, anti-thyroid medication may be continued after radioiodine treatment. Patients with large goitres or severe hyperthyroidism may require repeat doses of radioiodine.

Radioiodine is a safe treatment, but some patients may experience a transient radiation thyroiditis following treatment. There may be a small rise in thyroid hormones associated with some discomfort, but this is transient and self-limiting.

Thyroid surgery for hyperthyroidism

Surgery in the form of hemi- or complete thyroidectomy is the alternative definitive treatment for hyperthyroidism. This is ideally performed in the euthyroid patient, and surgery may be covered with β-blockade and Lugol's iodine. Surgery is preferable to radioiodine in patients with large goitres or nodules with compressive symptoms, refractory recurrent autoimmune hyperthyroidism or in patients in whom there is a contraindication to radioiodine treatment. The decision to proceed with definitive treatment for benign thyroid disease is based upon informed patient choice.

Management of thyroid-associated ophthalmopathy

Thyroid ophthalmopathy should be referred to an ophthalmologist for specialist review. Symptoms of gritty eyes may be managed with synthetic tear eye drops such as hypermellose, and patients should be given smoking cessation advice. It is important to ensure that the patient remains biochemically euthyroid.

More severe ophthalmopathy with pronounced exophthalmos may prevent the patient from closing their eyes and presents a risk of corneal ulceration. Eye patches and prism visual aids can be used to improve diplopia. Other treatments used in ophthalmopathy include glucocorticoids, azathioprine, local radiotherapy and surgical intervention.

HYPOTHYROIDISM

Introduction

Hypothyroidism is the most common endocrine condition. It is characterized by reduced secretion of thyroid hormone from the thyroid gland and has an annual incidence of 4.1 cases per 1000 people.[8] The probability of developing hypothyroidism increases with age and it is more common in women than men, with a female to male ratio between 2:1 and 8:1. The prevalence of an abnormally elevated TSH in the US population is 4.6%.[9]

Hypothyroidism is classified as primary or secondary (central). Primary hypothyroidism describes intrinsic thyroid disease leading to hyposecretion of T4. Secondary (or central disease) is far less common and refers to reduced TSH secretion from the anterior pituitary gland leading to reduced T4 secretion.

Worldwide, the most common cause of primary hypothyroidism is iodine deficiency, but in areas with sufficient iodine intake, the most common cause is autoimmune thyroiditis (Hashimoto's thyroiditis). In contrast to autoimmune hyperthyroidism, there is destruction of the thyroid by non-stimulating autoantibodies, leading to reduced thyroid gland activity. Autoimmune hypothyroidism is associated with other autoimmune disorders including type 1 diabetes, vitiligo, atrophic gastritis, pernicious anaemia, systemic sclerosis and Sjögren's syndrome. It may also occur as part of a polyglandular autoimmune syndrome. Type 1 polyglandular autoimmune syndrome comprises autoimmune hypothyroidism, hypoparathyroidism, adrenal insufficiency and chronic mucocutaneous candidiasis. Type 2 polyglandular autoimmune syndrome comprises hypothyroidism, adrenal insufficiency, type 1 diabetes and primary ovarian failure.

Other causes of primary hypothyroidism are iatrogenic (drugs including amiodarone and lithium, radiotherapy and surgery), the hypothyroid phase of thyroiditis and congenital hypothyroidism.

Clinical features

Patients with hypothyroidism present with a variety of symptoms and signs reflecting the reduced action of thyroid hormone. It often has an indolent onset. Common presenting symptoms include cold intolerance, weight gain, constipation, dry skin and depression. Patients with mild disease may be asymptomatic, whilst severe disease, particularly in elderly patients, may present as myxoedema coma which is a life-threatening illness. This is a late and unusual presentation of hypothyroidism.

Drugs which impair thyroid function include lithium, amiodarone, interferon α and stavudine. As seen in hyperthyroidism, a strong family history of autoimmune thyroid disease is common.

On clinical examination, patients may be bradycardic, and slow relaxing deep tendon reflexes may be present. A goitre may be palpable, reflecting sustained exposure to abnormally elevated TSH concentrations. More unusual clinical signs include pericardial or pleural effusion, jaundice, peri-orbital oedema, peripheral oedema (myxoedema) and cerebellar ataxia.

Laboratory testing

The first-line diagnostic test is serum TSH. In the presence of normal pituitary function TSH is elevated in primary hypothyroidism. This reflects the reduced negative feedback on pituitary TSH secretion. In mild (subclinical) hypothyroidism the FT4 may be at the lower end of the normal range, but in overt hypothyroidism it is low. FT3 measurement is not helpful in the assessment of hypothyroidism. A low FT4 with a normal TSH should prompt further investigation as this may represent an inadequate pituitary response to reduced thyroxine production. Non-thyroidal illness may affect thyroid function test results causing a low FT4 and altering the TSH level. This reflects physiological changes in the hypothalamo-pituitary–thyroid axis and is termed 'sick euthyroid' state. Therefore, thyroid function should not be assessed in patients with acute illness.

Differentiating the aetiology of primary hypothyroidism is primarily by careful history taking to exclude features of subacute or silent thyroiditis. A careful drug history is also important. Circulating TPO antibodies are found in up to 95% of patients with autoimmune hypothyroidism and may be useful in confirming the diagnosis. Antibody status is also useful in patients with subclinical hypothyroidism for predicting disease progression to overt hypothyroidism. However, measurement of TPO antibodies to predict primary hypothyroidism has no utility in the general population.

Other biochemical abnormalities seen in hypothyroidism are hypercholesterolaemia, hyponatraemia, hyperprolactinaemia, hypoglycaemia and an elevated creatine kinase (predominantly the MM isozyme).

The reference range of TSH (typically 0.35–5.5 mU/l) is distributed logarithmically, with its mean in the lower half of this range. Some investigators recommend that TSH values in the upper half of the reference range represent true thyroid dysfunction and that the upper limit of the reference range warrants re-assessment. At present, there is no evidence to suggest that patients with a TSH level within the reference range benefit from early treatment.

Subclinical hypothyroidism

Subclinical hypothyroidism is defined as an elevated TSH above the upper limit of the reference with a normal FT4. The prevalence may be as high as 15% in patients over 65 years of age, although few are symptomatic. It may be a transient phenomenon or progress to overt hypothyroidism. A high percentage of patients with subclinical hypothyroidism and positive antibody status eventually progress to overt hypothyroidism.

There is controversy surrounding the treatment of subclinical disease. No evidence exists to suggest that treating patients with TSH levels below 10 mU/l has any benefit (upper limit of normal is 5.5 mU/l) although, anecdotally, some patients feel better with thyroxine therapy. There is also no evidence to suggest that symptoms described by patients with subclinical hypothyroidism are attributable to thyroid disease. However, given the frequency of progression to overt hypothyroidism, all patients with subclinical disease should have their thyroid function assessed annually. Recent recommendations published in 2004, suggest that treatment be considered if the TSH is greater than 10 mU/l.[2]

Routine radiological assessment is not required in hypothyroidism unless there is a palpable thyroid nodule. If this is the case, investigation should proceed as for a thyroid nodule in the euthyroid patient.

Management

The principal management is treatment with levothyroxine (thyroxine). This is a direct hormone replacement treatment which has an identical structure and function to endogenous thyroxine. When given in appropriate doses it therefore has no adverse effects. The dose required varies between patients, depending on individual pharmacokinetics and the amount of residual endogenous thyroid function remaining. Doses vary from around 50 to 300 μg once daily. Patients are conventionally started on 50 μg once daily and the dose is titrated to TSH measurements. The elderly and patients with ischaemic heart disease are started on a lower dose (25 μg) with slower titration. This avoids exacerbation of cardiac disease which occurs due to hyperthyroxinaemia or when there is a rapid return to euthyroidism. TSH should be measured at 4- to 6-week intervals until the level is within the lower half of the normal range (approximately 1.0 mU/l).

The treatment of primary hypothyroidism is the same regardless of aetiology. However, in the treatment of hypothyroidism following surgery for differentiated thyroid carcinoma, the thyroxine dose is suppressive to ensure an undetectable TSH.

There is anecdotal evidence that some hypothyroid patients have neuropsychological symptoms which persist despite a normalized TSH. Some of these patients appear to benefit from a combination of T3 replacement in addition to T4 replacement therapy. However, a recent meta-analysis study showed that combined T4 and T3 therapy has no clear advantage over T4 monotherapy for improving thyroid function, quality of life, mood and psychometric parameters.[10]

T3 monotherapy is well established in the management of thyroid cancer to minimize the period of hypothyroidism prior to therapeutic radioiodine treatment. There is no evidence for its use in the treatment of primary hypothyroidism. It is associated with fluctuations in thyroid hormone levels due to its short half-life, and is associated with a greater frequency of iatrogenic hyperthyroidism. Biological and synthetic combined thyroid hormone preparations are available (e.g. from desiccated pig thyroid) although these are not recommended because they frequently lead to fluctuating and elevated free thyroid hormone concentrations.

EVIDENCE APPRAISAL

The majority of the evidence cited is Level II or III with systematic reviews or individual case–control studies. The epidemiological studies[7,8] are Level II, as are references 3 and 6.

REFERENCES

1. Parle J, Maisonneuve P, Sheppard M, *et al.* A single low serum thyrotrophin (TSH) concentration predicts increased all cause and cardiovascular mortality in older persons in the community: a 10-year cohort study. Lancet 2001;358:861–5.
2. Surks MI, Ortiz E, Daniels GH, *et al.* Subclinical thyroid disease scientific review and guidelines for diagnosis and management. JAMA 2004;291:228–38.
3. Cooper DS, Doherty GM, Haugen BR, *et al.* Management guidelines for patients with thyroid nodules and differentiated thyroid cancer: the American Thyroid Association Guidelines Taskforce. Thyroid 2006;16:109–42.
4. Hashizume K, Ichikawa K, Sakurai A, *et al.* Administration of thyroxine in treated Graves' disease: effects on the level of antibodies to thyroid-stimulating hormone receptors and on the risk of recurrence of hyperthyroidism. N Engl J Med 1991;324:947–53.
5. International Agranulocytosis and Aplastic Anaemia Study. Risk of agranulocytois and aplastic anaemia in relation to the use of antithyroid drugs. BMJ 1988;297:262–5.
6. Kendall-Taylor P, Keir MJ, Ross WM. Ablative radioiodine therapy for hyperthyroidism: longterm follow up study. BMJ 1984;289:361–3.
7. Franklyn JA, Daykin J, Drolc Z, *et al.* Longterm follow up of treatment of hyperthyroidism by three different methods. Clin Endocrinol 1991;34:71–6.

8. Vanderpump MPJ, Tunbridge WMG, French JM, *et al.* The incidence of thyroid disorders in the community: a twenty year follow up of the Whickham survey. Clin Endocrinol 1995;43:55–68.
9. Hollowell JG, Staehling NW, Flanders WD, *et al.* Serum TSH, T4 and thyroid antibodies in the United States Population (1988–1994): National Health and Nutrition Examination Survey (NHANES III). J Clin Endocrinol Metab 2002;87:489–99.
10. Escobar-Morreale HF, Botella-Carretero JI, Escobar del Rey F, *et al.* Review: treatment of hypothyroidism with combinations of levothyroxine plus liothyronine. J Clin Endocrinol Metab 2005;90:4946–54.

MULTIPLE CHOICE QUESTIONS

Select the single most appropriate option.

1. Which of the following biochemical abnormalities confirms primary hypothyroidism?
A. Low free thyroxine and low free tri-iodothyronine
B. Low thyroid-stimulating hormone
C. Positive thyroid peroxidase antibodies
D. Raised thyroid-stimulating hormone and low free thyroxine
E. Hypercholesterolaemia

2. Which of the following is a cause of high technetium uptake thyrotoxicosis?
A. Post-partum thyroiditis
B. Type 1 amiodarone-induced thyrotoxicosis
C. Toxic multinodular goitre
D. Type 2 amiodarone-induced thyrotoxicosis
E. Hashimoto's thyroiditis

3. Combination treatment with thyroxine (T4) and tri-iodothyronine (T3) has an evidence base for use in which scenario?
A. Secondary hypothyroidism
B. Block and replace regime
C. Thyroid-associated ophthalmopathy
D. Primary hypothyroidism
E. None of the above

4. The presence of anti-thyroid peroxidase antibodies in a euthyroid patient may be predictive of:
A. Thyroid malignancy
B. Primary hyperparathyroidism
C. Silent thyroiditis
D. Thyroid-associated ophthalmopathy
E. Primary hypothyroidism

5. A patient with pneumonia ventilated on the Intensive Care Unit has a thyroid-stimulating hormone of <0.01 mU/l and a free thyroxine of 9.0 pmol/l (Normal range 10–22 pmol/l). What is the diagnosis and management?
A. Hypothyroid, urgent thyroxine therapy
B. Hyperthyroid, urgent thionamide
C. Primary hypothyroidism, no treatment required
D. Sick euthyroid, no action required
E. None of the above

Answers

1. D
2. C
3. E
4. E
5. D

7 Clinical anatomy and developmental aberrations

Vishy Mahadevan

The Royal College of Surgeons of England, Lincoln's Inn Fields, London, UK

KEY POINTS

- The entire thyroid gland is enveloped within a single layer of deep cervical fascia termed the pre-tracheal fascia. The latter is firmly attached to the cartilage of the anterior wall of the upper trachea behind the thyroid isthmus. On either side it is attached to the lateral aspects of the cricoid and thyroid cartilages, medial to the corresponding thyroid lobe. The intimate attachment of this fascial envelope to the larynx and trachea ensures that the thyroid moves upwards with these structures during deglutition
- The follicular and stromal elements within the thyroid develop from the thyroglossal duct—a midline, ventrally directed diverticulum which migrates caudally from the floor of the primitive pharynx. The parafollicular C cells are derived from the ultimobranchial body
- Two arterial pedicles (superior thyroid artery and inferior thyroid artery) on either side of the midline supply the thyroid gland, forming a rich anastomosis with each other
- In the vicinity of the thyroid, each of the two arteries are closely related to an important nerve: the superior thyroid artery to the external laryngeal nerve and the inferior thyroid artery to the recurrent laryngeal nerve. Appreciation of these inter-relationships is crucial to avoid major complications during surgery
- The lymphatic drainage of the thyroid gland is principally to the middle and lower groups of jugular lymph nodes (Levels III and IV) on either side and to the pre-laryngeal/pre-tracheal lymph nodes

INTRODUCTION

A thorough appreciation of the topographical arrangement of the fascial and muscular planes in the anterior aspect of the neck is fundamental to understanding the clinical anatomy of the thyroid and parathyroid glands. Furthermore, it is an essential prerequisite to safety and precision in thyroid and parathyroid surgery.

A Practical Manual of Thyroid and Parathyroid Disease, 1st Edition. Edited by Asit Arora, Neil Tolley & R. Michael Tuttle.

This chapter begins with a detailed description of the tissue planes in the anterior cervical region, followed by a detailed account of the normal surgical anatomy of the thyroid. This description will also include the anatomical hazards and pitfalls which arise during thyroid surgery with which the surgeon should be thoroughly familiar.

Finally, it is important for the surgeon to appreciate the embryological development of the thyroid gland. Developmental aberrations of the thyroid are not uncommon and may manifest themselves in anomalies of form, number, location or function of the gland. The understanding of these developmental abnormalities is considerably facilitated by a knowledge of the basic principles underlying its embryological development. The final section of this chapter will therefore describe the embryological derivation of the thyroid followed by an account of its common developmental abnormalities.

TISSUE PLANES AND FASCIAL LAYERS IN THE ANTERIOR PART OF NECK (FIG. 7.1)

Deep to the skin of the neck is the superficial fascia or panniculus adiposus. This is a layer of subcutaneous fat which is more or less homogeneous. The degree of adiposity in this layer varies between individuals, and also, to some extent, between the anterior and posterior aspects of the neck in the same individual. Generally it is somewhat thinner in the front of the neck than in the back. Lying immediately deep to the subcutaneous fat on either side of the anterior midline is the platysma. This is a relatively thin but wide sheet of muscle. The platysma is a feature of the anterolateral part of the neck and does not extend to the back of the neck. Superiorly, platysma crosses superficial to the lower border of the mandible to blend with the SMAS (superficial musculo-aponeurotic system) layer of the face. Inferiorly, it crosses superficial to the clavicle, blending with the fascia overlying the pectoralis major approximately 1–2 cm below the level of the clavicle. Above the level of the hyoid, the medial borders

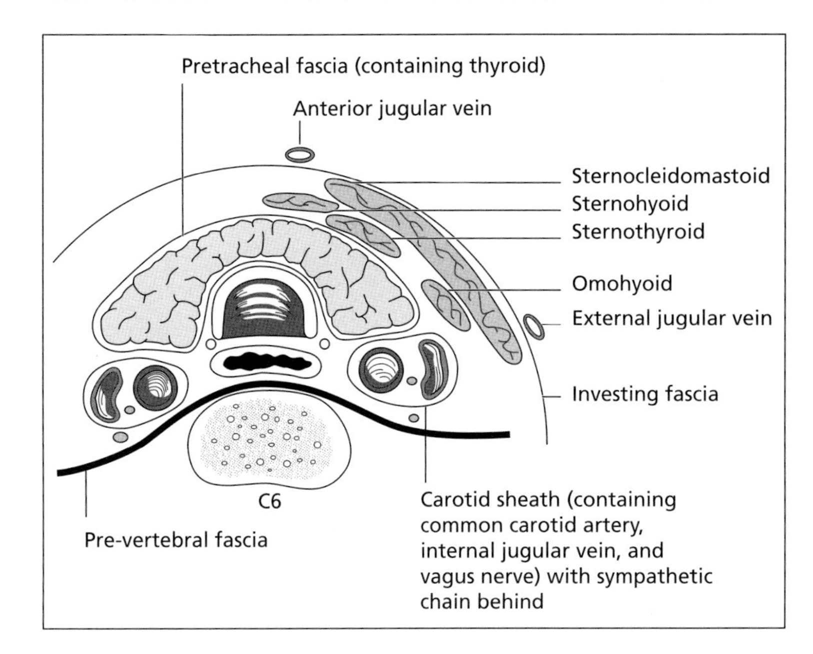

Fig. 7.1 Schematic cross-sectional representation of the neck showing the fascial and muscular planes. Reproduced from Ellis, H. Clinical Anatomy, 11th edn. with permission from Blackwell Publishing.

of the right and left platysma muscles are contiguous, whereas below this level they are separated from each other by an interval of 2–3 cm. Subjacent to the platysma is the investing layer of deep cervical fascia which forms the most superficial of the multiple layers of deep cervical fascia. It invests the neck like a collar. Superiorly, its attachment may be traced circumferentially along the entire length of the lower border of the mandible, the mastoid processes and superior nuchal lines on either side, and to the external occipital protuberance in the posterior midline. In the interval between the angle of the mandible and the mastoid process, the investing layer of deep cervical fascia encloses the parotid salivary gland as the parotid fascia.

Inferiorly on each side, the investing layer of deep cervical fascia circumferentially attaches to the sternal notch (i.e. the notched, thick upper border of the manubrium sterni), the upper surface of the clavicle, the acromion and corresponding spine of the scapula (and thus to the posterior midline). Traced laterally from the anterior midline, between its upper and lower attachments on each side, the investing layer meets the medial border of the corresponding sternocleidomastoid muscle. It splits to enclose the muscle and thereafter continues posterolaterally as the fascial roof of the ipsilateral posterior triangle of the neck. Upon reaching the anterior edge of the trapezius muscle it splits to enclose this muscle (Fig. 7.1).

In its descent from the lower border of the mandible, the investing layer of deep cervical fascia is firmly adherent to the front of the hyoid body and to the lateral aspects of the greater horns of the hyoid. Thus all the cervical viscera, major blood vessels and nerves of the neck and all the cervical muscles (with the sole exception of the platysma) lie within the sweep of this investing fascial layer.[1–4]

Immediately deep to the investing layer of deep cervical fascia and running longitudinally on either side of the anterior midline of the neck are the infrahyoid anterior cervical muscles or 'strap' muscles (Figs 7.1 and 7.2). On each side of the vertical midline the strap muscles are disposed in two planes. The superficial plane consists of the sternohyoid and omohyoid muscles lying side by side, with sternohyoid medial to omohyoid. The deep plane consists of the sternothyroid muscle which extends vertically from the posterior surface of the manubrium sterni to the oblique line of the thyroid cartilage. Extending upwards from the oblique line of the thyroid cartilage to the greater horn of the hyoid is the thyrohyoid muscle. This muscle is generally regarded as the upward continuation of sternothyroid.

The deepest layer of the deep cervical fascia is the prevertebral fascia. This is a relatively dense layer which covers the anterior aspects of the pre-vertebral musculature and the cervical vertebral column (Fig. 7.1).

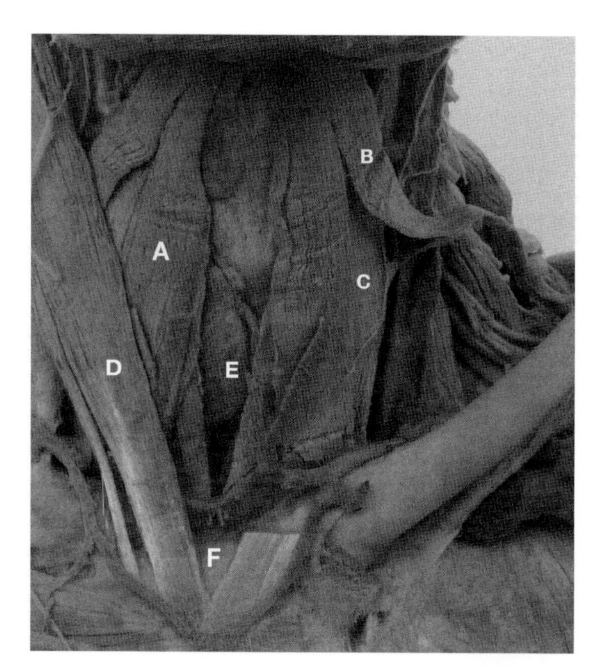

Fig. 7.2 Dissection of the anterior part of the neck showing strap muscles and related structures. A = sternohyoid; B = omohyoid; C = sternothyroid; D = sternocleidomastoid; E = thyroid isthmus; F = sternal notch.

Deep to the strap muscles and anterior to the pre-vertebral fascial layer is the centrally located visceral compartment of the neck. Lying lateral to the cervical visceral column in front of the pre-vertebral fascia are the right and left carotid sheaths. Situated posteromedial to the carotid sheath (outside from it) and anterior to the pre-vertebral fascia is the ipsilateral, ganglionated cervical sympathetic chain.

The cervical visceral compartment is flanked by the right and left carotid sheaths. Posteriorly, it comprises the pharynx and its distal continuation with the oesophagus. The pharyngo-oesophageal junction is typically at the level of the lower border of the cricoid cartilage which also corresponds to the level of the lower border of the sixth cervical vertebra. Situated in front of the pharynx and oesophagus are the larynx and trachea, respectively. The laryngo-tracheal junction arises at the same horizontal level as the pharyngo-oesophageal junction. Lying astride the anterior aspect of the upper trachea is the thyroid isthmus, which is confluent with the corresponding thyroid lobe either side of the midline. The entire thyroid gland is enveloped in a further layer of deep cervical fascia termed the pre-tracheal fascia. The pre-tracheal fascia is firmly adherent to the front of the upper trachea behind the isthmus and to the sides of the cricoid and thyroid cartilages (Figs 7.1 and 7.2). This encasement of the thyroid gland by pre-tracheal fascia (with its attachment to the trachea and laryngeal cartilages) is the anatomical basis to the clinical observation that all thyroid swellings move upwards during the second phase of swallowing. As the larynx and trachea ascend so does the thyroid gland contained within the pre-tracheal fascia.[1,2,4]

The cervical lymph nodes may be broadly categorized into two groups:

1. Superficial cervical lymph nodes: those superficial to the investing layer of deep cervical fascia.
2. Deep cervical lymph nodes: those deep to the investing layer of deep cervical fascia.

Each of these categories is further divided into subgroups on the basis of location and territory of drainage. The lymphatic drainage of the thyroid is discussed in further detail later in the chapter.

THE THYROID GLAND (FIGS 7.3 AND 7.4)

The normal thyroid gland is a firm, richly vascularized, reddish-brown organ located in the anterior aspect of the lower part of the neck. It weighs 17 g in an average adult and consists of a right and left lobe, one on either side of the larynx and trachea. Each lobe is approximately 5 cm in length and is roughly pyramidal in shape. The apex of the pyramid corresponds to the relatively narrow upper pole, while the lower pole of the lobe constitutes its broad base. The thyroid lobe lies in a bed which is made up medially of the trachea, oesophagus and tracheo-oesophageal groove.[1–3] Posteriorly is the carotid sheath and anterolaterally are the strap muscles and overlying sternocleidomastoid. Thus, in cross-section, each lobe of the thyroid appears triangular, presenting a superficial or anterolateral surface (related to the strap muscles), a posterior surface (related to the carotid sheath) and a medial surface (related to the tracheo-oesophageal groove, trachea and oesophagus). The anteromedial aspect of the lower part of one thyroid lobe is joined to the corresponding part of the other lobe by the isthmus which is a flattened bridge of thyroid tissue. This lies transversely across the front of the upper trachea usually overlying the second and third (and sometimes fourth) tracheal rings. The isthmus is approximately 1.5 cm in width and height. A superiorly directed, conical projection of thyroid tissue from the isthmus, somewhat to the left of the midline, is

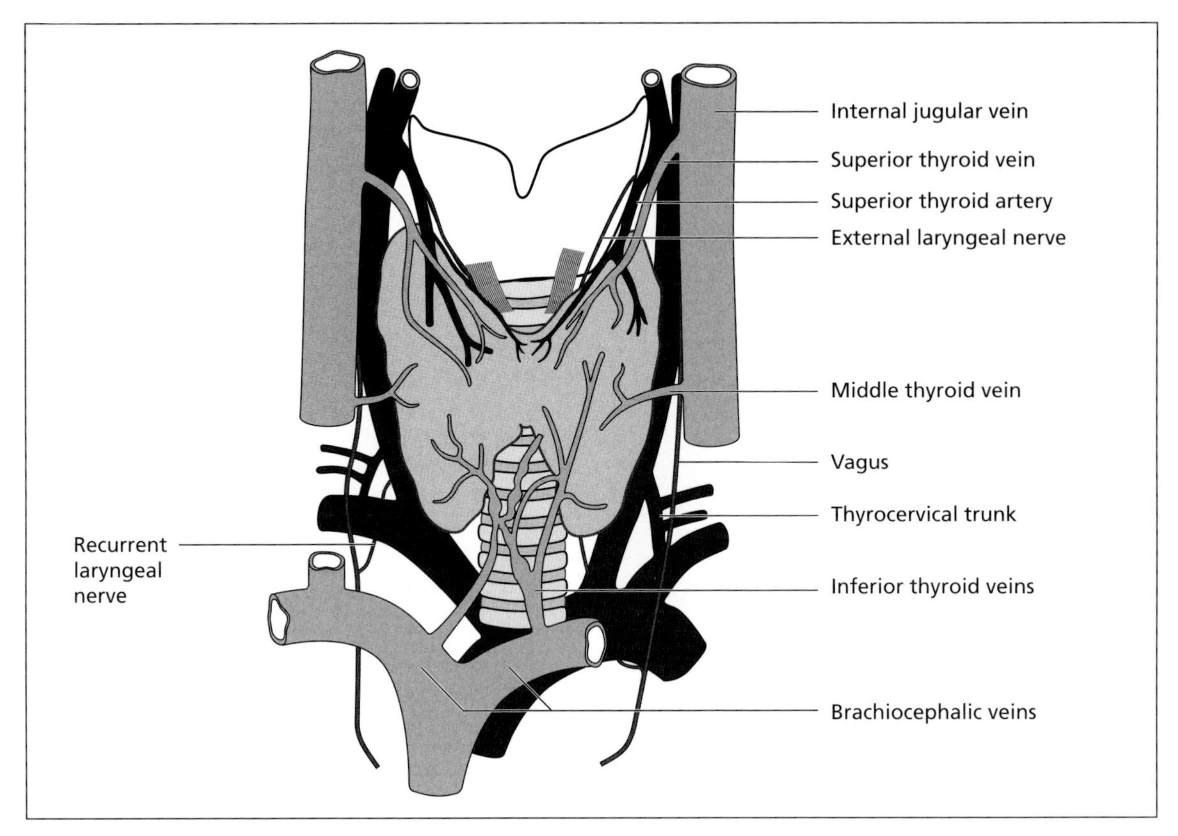

Fig. 7.3 Anterior view of the thyroid and related structures.

a frequent feature. Termed the pyramidal lobe, it is thought to occur in 40–50% of individuals. It is an important consideration in surgery for thyrotoxicosis as failure to remove the pyramidal lobe may result in recurrence of thyrotoxicosis. Occasionally a fibrous or fibromuscular band extends from the upper pole of the pyramidal lobe to the inferior margin of the hyoid body. It denotes the route of embryological migratory descent of the thyroid and is termed levator glandulae thyroid.

The thyroid gland possesses a thin capsule beyond which lies the pre-tracheal fascia. This fascial layer has been already been described in detail with respect to its attachment to the trachea and larynx. It develops a distinct thickening between the medial aspect of the thyroid lobe and cricoid cartilage. This fascial band is termed the lateral ligament of the thyroid or the ligament of Berry (Fig. 7.4).

An element of controversy prevails as to whether the pre-tracheal fascia encloses the thyroid completely or merely covers its anterior and anterolateral surfaces. Histological studies favour the view that the thyroid is completely enclosed by pre-tracheal fascia. At the microscopic level, the pre-tracheal fascial envelope is an important landmark in the histopathological staging of differentiated and medullary thyroid cancer.

TOPOGRAPHICAL RELATIONS OF THE THYROID

Anterolateral relations

Each thyroid lobe is overlapped antero-laterally by the ipsilateral strap muscles. The sternothyroid forms the immediate relation with the sternohyoid and superior belly of the omohyoid overlapping the sternothyroid (Figs 7.1 and 7.2). The upper pole of each thyroid lobe is limited by the attachment of the sternothyroid muscle to the oblique ridge (oblique line) on the lateral aspect of the thyroid lamina. To facilitate optimal exposure of the superior pole of the thyroid lobe, or when mobilizing a

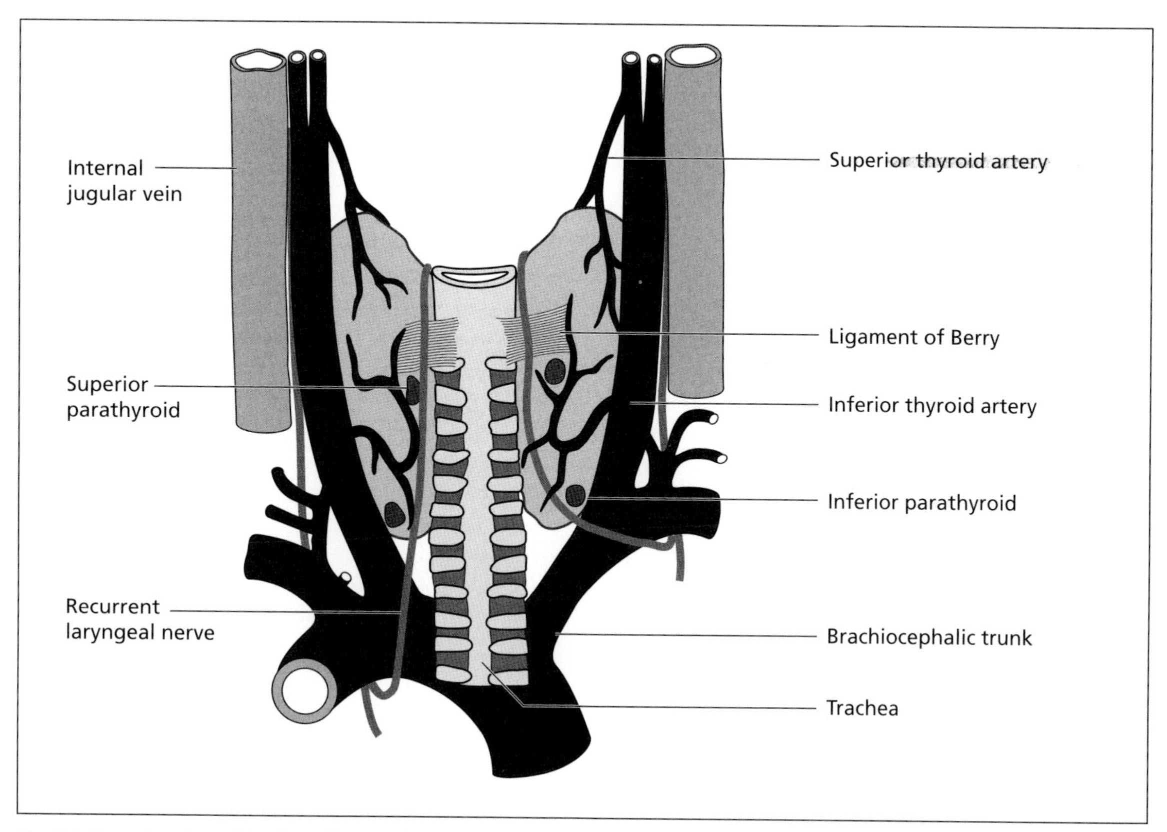

Fig. 7.4 Posterior view of the thyroid and related structures.

large goitre, it may be necessary for the surgeon to divide the strap muscles (sternohyoid and sternothyroid). In these circumstances, it is advisable to divide the strap muscle transversely near their upper attachments and to re-approximate the divided muscles following thyroidectomy. The rationale for high division of the strap muscles is that the nerves supplying the strap muscles (branches of the ansa cervicalis) enter the muscles near their lower ends and course upwards within the muscles.

Posterior relations

Posterior to each thyroid lobe is the common carotid artery lying within the carotid sheath. Lateral to the artery within the carotid sheath is the internal jugular vein, and interposed between the two is the vagus nerve.

More immediately related to the posterior aspect of the thyroid lobe are the two ipsilateral parathyroids. Their embryological derivation and anatomical location are outlined in detail in Chapter 16. They may be located within the pre-tracheal fascial covering of the thyroid or outside this fascia. Rarely, they are embedded within the thyroid substance. The inferior parathyroid is usually located behind the lower pole of the thyroid lobe. The approximate location of the superior parathyroid is a third of the way up from the lower pole of the thyroid lobe (Fig. 7.4).

Medial relations

Medially, the thyroid lobe is related to the lateral aspects of the larynx, trachea and the tracheo-oesophageal groove. On either side, running upwards in the tracheo-oesophageal groove before entering the larynx, is the corresponding recurrent laryngeal nerve (RLN); see Fig. 7.4.

Depending on their direction of growth, expanding neoplasms of the thyroid may compress any of the related structures mentioned above.

(Note: the term inferior laryngeal nerve which is sometimes used in surgical literature is synonymous with recurrent laryngeal nerve.)

BLOOD SUPPLY OF THE THYROID (FIGS 7.3 AND 7.4)

In common with all endocrine organs, the thyroid possesses a very generous arterial blood supply which it derives from two complementary pairs of arteries: the right and left superior and inferior thyroid arteries. These four arteries form a rich anastomosis with each other within the gland and also on its surface.[1–3]

Typically, the superior thyroid artery arises from the anterior or anteromedial aspect of the external carotid artery at the level of the greater horn of the hyoid, a short distance above the level of the upper border of the thyroid cartilage. It is usually the first branch arising from the anterior aspect of the external carotid artery. The vessel descends obliquely in an anteromedial direction on the surface of the inferior pharyngeal constrictor but deep to sternothyroid muscle to reach the superior pole of the ipsilateral thyroid lobe. In approximately 5–7% of individuals, the superior thyroid artery arises from the terminal part of the common carotid artery. This variant origin may be unilateral or bilateral.

On reaching the upper pole of the thyroid lobe, the superior thyroid artery typically divides into an anterior and posterior branch. The posterior branch descends along the posterior surface of the thyroid lobe and eventually anastomoses with a branch of the inferior thyroid artery. The anterior branch, typically larger than its posterior counterpart, descends on the medial aspect of the lobe and then along the upper border of the isthmus to anastomose with its fellow from the other side.

The inferior thyroid artery typically arises from the thyrocervical artery (trunk) which in turn arises in the root of the neck from the superior aspect of the first part of the subclavian artery, immediately distal to the origin of the vertebral artery.

From its origin, the inferior thyroid artery courses superomedially behind the carotid sheath, anterior to the scalenus anterior muscle and its covering of pre-vertebral fascia. Approximately at the level of the lower border of the cricoid cartilage it loops inferomedially towards the lower pole of the thyroid lobe and gives off a branch called the ascending cervical artery. As it approaches the lower pole of the thyroid lobe, the inferior thyroid artery crosses anterior to the cervical sympathetic chain. The inferior thyroid artery may be absent in 5% of individuals.

Rarely, a fifth artery termed the thyroidea ima artery may also be present. It only occurs in 1–3% of individuals. Its origin, in descending order of frequency, is from the brachiocephalic artery, right common carotid artery or aortic arch. An aberrant artery arising from either subclavian artery which supplies the thyroid is usually regarded as an anomalous inferior thyroid artery rather than a thyroidea ima artery.

The inferior thyroid artery, as it approaches the posterior surface of the thyroid lobe, runs close to the recurrent laryngeal nerve. Accompanying the superior thyroid artery towards the upper pole of the thyroid is the external branch of the superior laryngeal nerve. Also known as the external laryngeal nerve, this is a terminal branch of the superior laryngeal nerve which in turn is a branch of the vagus nerve. The artery is typically somewhat posterolateral to the nerve. The external laryngeal nerve is an exclusively motor nerve which innervates the cricothyroid muscle. The proximity of the recurrent and external laryngeal nerves to the thyroid vessels puts these nerves at risk of inadvertent injury during thyroid surgery. Injury to the external laryngeal nerve and consequent paralysis of the cricothyroid muscle results in laxity of the vocal fold which causes impairment of voice projection and loss of high-pitched phonation. Invasive thyroid neoplasms may, on occasion, invade the recurrent laryngeal nerve causing dysphonia and/or inspiratory stridor.

VENOUS DRAINAGE OF THE THYROID (FIG. 7.3)

The pattern of venous drainage is subject to greater variation than its arterial supply. The venous drainage of the thyroid gland is initially into a capsular venous plexus which surrounds the thyroid gland. This is situated, for the most part, in the interval between the capsule of the thyroid and the pre-tracheal fascial envelope. The plexus is made up of thin-walled, freely intercommunicating venous channels. Three principal channels emerge from this capsular plexus on either side of the midline. The superior thyroid vein emerges from the upper part of the thyroid lobe and accompanies the superior thyroid artery (usually running postero-lateral to the artery) before draining directly into the ipsilateral internal jugular vein. Not uncommonly, the superior thyroid vein drains into the terminal part of the ipsilateral facial vein (usually at the level of the common carotid artery bifurcation). The facial vein in turn drains into the internal jugular vein. The middle thyroid vein is present in 50%

of individuals. It emerges from the anterolateral aspect of the thyroid lobe somewhat nearer the lower than the upper pole. It runs laterally, anterior to the common carotid artery, before draining into the internal jugular vein. During thyroidectomy, gentle lateral retraction of the carotid sheath facilitates identification (and thus ligation) of the middle thyroid vein. Each inferior thyroid vein emerges from the lower part of the corresponding thyroid lobe. The right vein runs inferolaterally and crosses anterior to the brachiocephalic artery before draining into the right brachiocephalic vein. The left inferior thyroid vein runs down in front of the trachea to drain into the left brachiocephalic vein.[1–3] It is not uncommon for the right and left inferior thyroid veins to anastomose in front of the trachea via multiple venous channels. The surgeon should be mindful of this feature when dissecting the pre-tracheal region during thyroidectomy or when performing a tracheostomy. Large retrosternal goitres can compress the brachiocephalic veins and the resulting venous obstruction may cause considerable engorgement of the inferior thyroid veins in the pre-tracheal region.

LYMPHATIC DRAINAGE OF THE THYROID

A sound understanding of the lymphatic drainage of the thyroid gland is essential for the effective clinical management of thyroid malignancy, particularly those with a tendency for lymph node metastasis. Papillary thyroid carcinoma has a propensity to spread to lymph nodes, as does medullary thyroid carcinoma.

The thyroid has a rich lymphatic drainage which may flow in multiple directions. At the histological level, intrathyroid lymphatic channels are numerous and surround the thyroid follicles. They form an extensive network within the gland and enable lymph flow from one lobe to the other. The lymphatic drainage of the thyroid gland is principally to the pre-laryngeal and pre-tracheal lymph nodes which lie in front of the thyrohyoid membrane and upper trachea, respectively. Drainage also occurs to the tracheo-oesophageal lymph nodes which are situated alongside the tracheo-oesophageal grooves bilaterally. These sets of lymph nodes all belong to the anterior cervical group of deep cervical lymph nodes and therefore are situated deep to the investing layer of deep cervical fascia. Lymphatics from the thyroid also drain to the middle and lower jugular groups of lymph nodes which lie alongside the internal jugular vein.

ANATOMICAL HAZARDS IN THYROID SURGERY

On either side of the midline two functionally important nerves are closely related to the corresponding lobe of the thyroid: the recurrent laryngeal nerve and the external laryngeal nerve. No account of the surgical anatomy of the thyroid gland would be complete without a detailed consideration of the proximity of these nerves to the thyroid and their consequent susceptibility to inadvertent damage during surgery.

The recurrent laryngeal nerve is a direct branch of the vagus, while the external laryngeal nerve is a branch of the superior laryngeal nerve (which in turn is a direct branch of the vagus).

A further anatomical hazard in relation to thyroid surgery is inadvertent parathyroid devascularization with resultant post-operative hypocalcaemia.

Recurrent laryngeal nerve

Most medico-legal claims relating to thyroid surgery involve the recurrent laryngeal nerve. A thorough understanding of the anatomy of this nerve (including its anatomical variations) and meticulous surgical technique, facilitated by optimal illumination and magnification, are of paramount importance in avoiding iatrogenic nerve injury.[5–9]

The right recurrent laryngeal nerve arises from the right vagus in the root of the neck anterior to the first part of the right subclavian artery. It winds around the subclavian artery passing from front to back, and ascends in the neck behind the common carotid artery. It then curves medially to ascend in the right tracheo-oesophageal groove. The left recurrent laryngeal nerve, a branch of the left vagus, has a significantly longer course. It originates lateral to the aortic arch and winds around this, passing from lateral to medial below the arch before ascending in the left tracheo-oesophageal groove. Once in the vicinity of the tracheo-oesophageal groove, both recurrent laryngeal nerves pursue a similar course on their respective sides. Each nerve runs behind the ipsilateral inferior cornu of the thyroid cartilage, either behind or through the ligament of Berry, before running deep to the cricothyroid muscle to enter the larynx.

Awareness of the following anatomical points in relation to the recurrent laryngeal nerve are of great practical usefulness in reducing the incidence of operative nerve injury.

The right recurrent laryngeal nerve may have an aberrant (non-recurrent) course in 0.5–0.7% of individuals. In these individuals, the nerve branches off from the vagus at the level of the cricoid cartilage or even higher. It runs medially behind the common carotid artery to reach the larynx (Plate 7.1). Very rarely the left recurrent laryngeal nerve may have a non-recurrent course (incidence 0.04%). This anomaly is associated with malformations of the aortic arch.

Another important anatomical feature of practical significance concerns the relative positions of the right and left recurrent laryngeal nerves in relation to the tracheo-oesophageal groove. The nerve on the left side is more predictably situated in the groove (~80% of individuals) compared with the nerve on the right side (65% of individuals). In the remainder, the nerve is situated somewhat more anteriorly and lies lateral to the trachea. Exceptionally, either nerve may be situated posterior to the tracheo-oesophageal groove and lie beside the oesophagus.

The recurrent laryngeal nerve and inferior thyroid artery are closely related to each other, but a specific and consistent anatomical relationship between the two does not exist. Thus the artery is not a useful landmark in identifying and locating the nerve. In contrast, the inferior cornu of the thyroid cartilage is a more useful landmark. The nerve typically lies immediately behind the inferior cornu.

A further anatomical variation of the recurrent laryngeal nerve of practical significance is the occasional tendency for the nerve, in its extra-laryngeal ascent, to run as a duplicated structure. When this occurs, the anterior branch carries the motor fibres to the intrinsic laryngeal muscles while the posterior branch carries sensory fibres for distribution to the trachea and oesophagus.

Idiopathic, unilateral vocal cord paralysis is believed to occur in approximately 1% of the population and is usually asymptomatic. For this reason and as a defence against potential litigation, it is essential to perform pre-operative fibreoptic nasoendoscopy to document vocal cord function prior to thyroid surgery. The an uthors also advocate routine use of an intra-operative laryngeal nerve stimulator and post-operative vocal cord examination.

External laryngeal nerve (see Fig. 7.3)

The external laryngeal nerve is vulnerable when ligating the superior thyroid vascular pedicle.[10,11] The nerve is rather slender and runs in close proximity to the superior thyroid artery, typically lying anteromedial to it. In a significant number of individuals (15–20%) the nerve is intimately related or intertwined with the artery at the level of the upper pole of the thyroid. In order to avoid accidental injury to the nerve, it is important to display the upper pole of the thyroid adequately. If necessary, the sternothyroid muscle should be divided to facilitate this manouevre. Regrettably the external laryngeal nerve is often not identified during thyroid surgery. The laryngeal nerve stimulator facilitates this process intra-operatively.

Compromise of parathyroid blood supply and consequent hypocalcaemia

A serious concern when performing thyroid surgery, particularly during total thyroidectomy, is the potential for accidentally devascularizing the parathyroids and rendering the patient hypocalcaemic. In over 80% of individuals the blood supply to the four parathyroids is derived largely, if not exclusively, from the two inferior thyroid arteries.[12] In order to avoid the serious metabolic complication of post-operative hypocalcaemia it is advisable to avoid ligating the main trunk of the inferior thyroid artery. The very terminal branches of the vessel should be ligated as near as possible to the thyroid capsule to preserve the parathyroid blood supply. However, one study demonstrated that ligating the main trunk of the artery during subtotal thyroidectomy did not result in a higher incidence of post-operative hypocalcaemia (ascertained clinically and biochemically) compared with matched patients who underwent ligation of tertiary branches of the inferior thyroid artery just outside the thyroid capsule.[13]

EMBRYOLOGY OF THE THYROID GLAND (FIG. 7.5)

Understanding the development of the thyroid and parathyroid glands is greatly facilitated by a preliminary consideration of the development of the neck and pharynx. In all mammalian embryos the primitive mouth (stomodeum) is bound cranially by the forebrain projection and caudally by the cardiac prominence. The intervening area—the primitive pharynx—gives rise to the mandibular region, lower face and the neck. Embryological development of these parts is characterized and greatly influenced by the appearance of the pharyngeal (branchial) arches. These appear during the fourth and fifth weeks of intrauterine development. The mesoderm of the primitive pharynx is reinforced by a large number of migratory

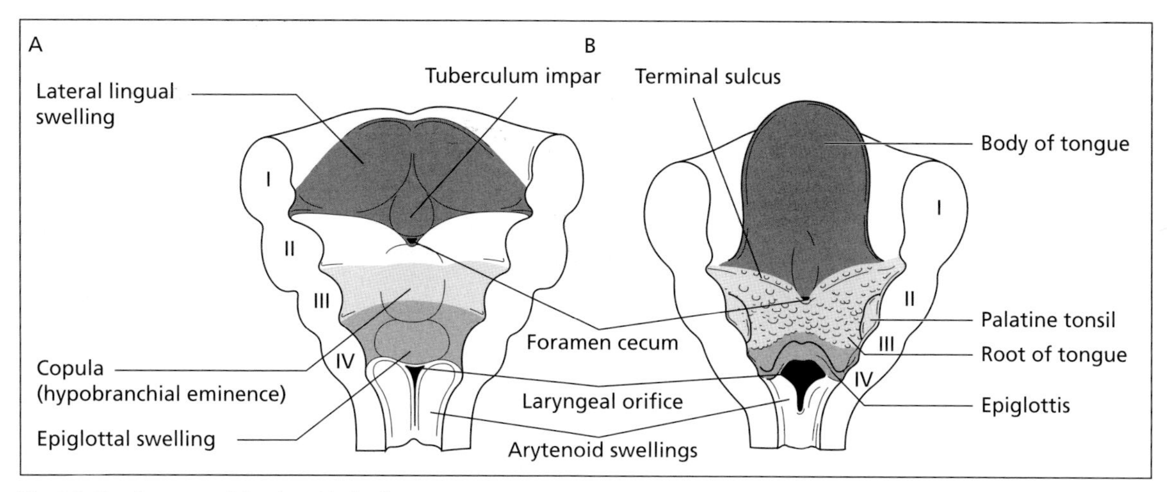

Fig. 7.5 Development of the thyroid gland.

neural crest cells. The resulting mesenchyme gives rise to six curved (arched) cylindroid thickenings, termed pharyngeal arches, in the pharyngeal wall on either side. Each pharyngeal arch commences lateral to the hindbrain and grows ventrally through the lateral wall of the pharynx to meet its fellow on the contralateral side in the ventral midline. As the ventral ends of the arches approach the midline there is a progressive separation of the cardiac region from the stomodeum. In all, six such arches appear in a cranio-caudal sequence, with the first one being the most cranial. In the human embryo, the fifth arch has a very transient existence and does not give rise to any definitive structures. Each arch comprises a core of mesenchyme covered externally by ectoderm and internally by endoderm. Ventrally, successive arches are virtually contiguous one with another. Laterally on either side, adjacent pharyngeal arches are separated on the external aspect by ectodermal depressions termed pharyngeal clefts (branchial grooves). On the corresponding internal aspect, adjacent arches are separated by endodermal outpouchings termed pharyngeal pouches.[14]

Embryologically, the thyroid gland is essentially an endodermal derivative which appears initially as a midline cellular proliferation in the floor of the primitive pharynx between the first and second pharyngeal arches. The site of origin of this bud is marked in later life by the midline foramen caecum on the dorsum of the tongue (see Fig. 7.6). The thyroid bud descends in the ventral midline as the thyroglossal duct (thyroglossal tract) in front of the pharyngeal gut. It successively crosses the anterior aspect of the developing hyoid and larynx before reaching its definitive position in front of the trachea. In its descent, after crossing in front of the hyoid, the thyroglossal duct loops upwards behind the body of the hyoid before recommencing its midline descent (see Fig. 7.6). The distal end of the thyroid bud bifurcates, and subsequent proliferation of this bifurcation gives rise to the thyroid isthmus and bilateral lobes. A further contribution to the developing thyroid comes from the ultimobranchial body (a derivative of the fourth pharyngeal pouch). This gives rise to the parafollicular C cells which secrete calcitonin.[14] The tubercle of Zuckerkandl represents a remnant of the ultimobranchial body. It is a small visible elevation on the posterolateral aspect of the thyroid lobe located halfway between the upper and lower poles.

During descent, the thyroid remains connected to its site of pharyngeal origin via the thyroglossal duct. With further development, this duct disintegrates completely.

DEVELOPMENTAL ABERRATIONS OF THE THYROID

Aberrant location of the thyroid gland may be explained on the basis of incomplete or exaggerated descent of the developing thyroid bud.

Rarely (1 in 3500 individuals) there may be a total failure of thyroglossal duct (tract) descent. The condition presents as a lingual thyroid located at the base of the tongue.

Incomplete embryological descent of the thyroglossal duct may result in the thyroid being situated superior to

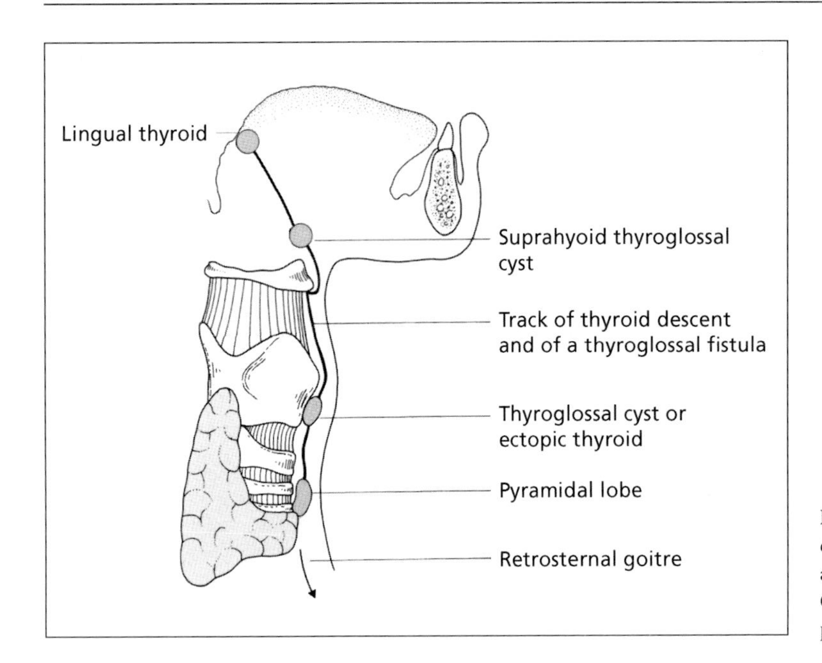

Fig. 7.6 Schematic diagram of embryological descent of the thyroid anlagen. Reproduced from Ellis, H. Clinical Anatomy, 11th edn. with permission from Blackwell Publishing.

its normal position. Thus the thyroid gland may be found at the level of the hyoid bone or in an infrahyoid position.

Conversely, the thyroglossal duct may show excessive descent, resulting in the thyroid being located at the level of the root of the neck or in the superior mediastinum (intrathoracic thyroid).

Another class of developmental abnormalities is attributable to persistence of part (or all) of the thyroglossal duct. The most common example of this is the presence of the pyramidal lobe and levator glandulae thyroidea. This occurs when the lower end of the thyroglossal duct fails to obliterate. This is such a common occurrence that it is regarded as an anatomical variation rather than an anomaly. Persistence of the thyroglossal duct also predisposes to thyroglossal cyst formation, which typically occurs in the midline (or just off it) in the anterior neck, corresponding to the line of descent of the thyroglossal duct. The majority of thyroglossal cysts are found in the vicinity of the hyoid. Thyroglossal cysts are the most common of all congenital, midline cystic lesions, accounting for nearly 70% of such lesions (see Fig. 7.6 and Plate 7.2). A diagnostic clinical sign is the distinct 'tug' felt by the examiner's palpating fingers when holding the cyst while the patient protrudes their tongue (Plate 7.3). Thyroglossal cysts are prone to infection and fistulation, so it is advisable to excise these lesions. When doing so, it is important to define the cyst and thyroglossal duct and to remove them along with the body of the hyoid. This is the principle of the Sistrunk operation. Failure to remove the hyoid is likely to result in recurrence within remnants of the thyroglossal duct lodged behind the body of the hyoid.

Other developmental anomalies of the thyroid are the result of partial agenesis of the thyroid anlagen. Thus in 0.1–0.2% of individuals the isthmus or one or other lobe fails to develop.

EVIDENCE APPRAISAL

This chapter is intended, largely, as a comprehensive and contemporary description and review of the surgical anatomy and embryology of the thyroid. The anatomical descriptions and variations mentioned in the cited papers are based, without exception, on substantial studies and elaborate observations, and thus have a considerable evidence base.

The inferences drawn in Reference 13 are at variance with general experience and traditional opinion. However, as they are based on a well-designed and well-executed study involving a significant number of patients, the observations are worthy of serious consideration and further study.

REFERENCES

1. Bailey BJ, Calhoun KH, Friedman NR. Thyroid and parathyroid. In: Bailey BJ, Calhoun KH, eds. Atlas of head and neck surgery—otolaryngology, 2nd edn. Philadelphia, PA: Lippincott Williams and Wilkins, 2001:228–34.
2. Bliss RD, Gauger PC, Delbridge LW. Surgeon's approach to the thyroid gland: surgical anatomy and the importance of technique. World J Surg 2000;24:891–7.
3. Hunt PS. A reappraisal of the surgical anatomy of the thyroid and parathyroid glands. Br J Surg 1968;55:63–6.
4. Wang C. The anatomic basis of thyroid surgery. Ann Surg 1976;3:271–5.
5. Farrar WB. Complications of thyroidectomy. Surg Clin North Am 1983;6:1353–61.
6. Gavilan J, Gavilan C. Recurrent laryngeal nerve: identification during thyroid and parathyroid surgery. Arch Otolaryngol Head Neck Surg 1986;112:1286–8.
7. Medina JE, Boyd EM Jr. Complications of thyroid and parathyroid surgery. In: Weissler MC, Pillsbury HC, eds. Complications of head and neck surgery. New York: Thieme Medical Publishers, 1995.
8. Randolph GW. Surgical anatomy of the recurrent laryngeal nerve. In: Randolph GW, ed. Surgery of the thyroid and parathyroid glands. Philadelphia, PA: Saunders, 2003.
9. Wang D. The use of the inferior cornu of the thyroid cartilage in identifying the recurrent laryngeal nerve. Surg Gynecol Obstet 1975;140: 91–4.
10. Mooseman DA, DeWeese MS. The external laryngeal nerve as related to thyroidectomy. Surg Gynecol Obstet 1968; 126:1011–6.
11. Shemen L, Strong EW. Complications after total thyroidectomy. Otolaryngol Head Neck Surg 1989;101:472–5.
12. Flament JB, Delattre JF, Pluot M. Arterial blood supply to the parathyroid glands: implications for thyroid surgery. Anat Clin 1982;3:279–87.
13. Nies C, Sitter H, Zielke A, *et al.* Parathyroid function following ligation of the inferior thyroid arteries during bilateral subtotal thyroidectomy. Br J Surg 1994;81:1757–9.
14. Sadler TW. Langman's medical embryology. Philadelphia, PA: Lippincott Williams and Wilkins, 2006.

MULTIPLE CHOICE QUESTIONS

Select the single most appropriate option.

1. The inferior thyroid artery is a direct branch of:
A. External carotid artery
B. Thyrocervical artery
C. Subclavian artery
D. Vertebral artery
E. Internal carotid artery

2. The fascial sheath which envelops the thyroid gland is derived from which of the following layers?
A. Pre-tracheal fascia
B. Pre-vertebral fascia
C. Investing layer of deep cervical fascia
D. Carotid sheath
E. Buccopharyngeal fascia

3. In the context of neurovascular structures related to the thyroid:
A. The recurrent laryngeal nerve is most vulnerable to injury during surgical dissection in the vicinity of the upper pole of the thyroid
B. The cervical sympathetic chain is embedded in the anterior wall of the carotid sheath
C. The recurrent laryngeal nerve is more deeply situated in the tracheo-oesophageal groove on the right side than on the left
D. The incidence of a non-recurrent laryngeal nerve is approximately 5%
E. The external laryngeal nerve is motor to the cricothyroid muscle

4. Regarding the developmental anatomy and embryological aberrations of the thyroid gland:
A. The thyroid lobes are developed from the second pharyngeal pouch
B. The parafollicular cells are derived from the third pharyngeal pouch
C. In its descent, the thyroglossal tract courses posterior to the body of the hyoid bone
D. The pyramidal lobe is typically situated to the right of the midline
E. A thyroglossal cyst is commonly located at the level of the cricothyroid interval

5. Which one of the following topographical relationships of the thyroid gland is incorrect?
A. The thyroid isthmus overlaps the second, third and fourth tracheal rings
B. The strap muscles overlap the anterolateral surface of the thyroid lobe
C. The posterior surface of the thyroid lobe overlaps the carotid sheath
D. The medial surface of the thyroid lobe is related to the recurrent laryngeal nerve
E. The superior parathyroid is usually located adjacent to the posterior aspect of the upper pole of the thyroid lobe

Answers

1. B
2. A
3. E
4. C
5. E

8 Surgical management of benign thyroid disease

David J. Lesnik[1], Miriam A. O'Leary[2], J. Pieter Noordzij[2] & Gregory W. Randolph[1]

[1] Division of Thyroid and Parathyroid Surgery, Department of Laryngology and Otology, Harvard Medical School, Massachusetts Eye and Ear Infirmary, Boston, MA, USA
[2] Department of Otolaryngology, Boston Medical Center, Boston, MA, USA

KEY POINTS

- Ultrasound and autopsy studies demonstrate that thyroid nodules occur in 30–50% of the population, yet only 5% of these are malignant
- Treatment options for non-toxic multinodular goitre include suppression with thyroid hormone, radioactive iodine ablation and surgery
- CT imaging is particularly useful for the evaluation of retrosternal thyroid extension. Iodinated contrast will result in a short delay in post-operative radioiodine therapy and should not be used unless a normal TSH is confirmed
- Adequate pre-operative evaluation includes laryngoscopy in all patients undergoing thyroid surgery. Intra-operative neural monitoring is an invaluable adjunct when performing thyroid surgery.
- The majority of retrosternal goitres can be removed via a cervical incision without the need for sternotomy. In patients with a large retrosternal goitre it is advisable to identify the recurrent laryngeal nerve superiorly near its laryngeal entry point once the superior pedicle has been ligated.

COMMON BENIGN THYROID DISORDERS

It is important for the thyroid surgeon to have a thorough understanding of the range of benign disorders which affect the thyroid gland because they occur frequently in the Western population. Approximately 3–7% of adults have palpable thyroid nodules.[1] Furthermore, ultrasound and autopsy studies have detected thyroid nodules in 30–50% of the population.[2] A mere 5% of these nodules are malignant.[3] Many benign thyroid masses are resected each year in order to exclude carcinoma. The majority of goitres are excised because of their large size or potential growth in size, associated pressure symptoms and toxic function.

Benign disorders are categorized as non-toxic, toxic and inflammatory. Non-toxic thyroid lesions include diffuse and multinodular goitre. Toxic lesions include diffuse toxic goitre (Graves' disease), toxic multinodular goitre (Plummer's disease) and solitary toxic adenoma. Inflammatory disorders are further subdivided into acute, subacute and chronic thyroiditis. The most common benign thyroid neoplasm is follicular adenoma, which occurs as a solitary nodule, a dominant nodule within a thyroid goitre (non-toxic or toxic) or in the setting of thyroiditis. Less common benign thyroid neoplasms include atypical follicular adenoma, hyalinizing trabecular neoplasm and signet-ring follicular adenoma.[4]

NATURAL HISTORY

When left untreated, most goitres grow slowly and steadily over years, gradually causing compressive symptoms. Sometimes goitres undergo a rapid increase in size with associated acute compressive symptoms. Precipitants include pregnancy, iodine deficiency, ingestion of goitrogens (foods that affect iodine uptake) and haemorrhage within a nodule.[5]

TREATMENT

Treatment options for non-toxic multinodular goitre include suppression with thyroid hormone, radioactive iodine ablation and surgery. Treatment of toxic thyroid lesions has been outlined in Chapters 5 and 6, and will be reiterated briefly below.

Thyroid suppression is an effective treatment modality for non-toxic goitre in some patients. However, not all patients respond, and those who do demonstrate a

A Practical Manual of Thyroid and Parathyroid Disease, 1st Edition. Edited by Asit Arora, Neil Tolley & R. Michael Tuttle.

Table 8.1 Retrosternal goitre classification

Type	Location	Anatomy	Prevalence	Approach—Comments
I	Anterior mediastinum	Anterior to great vessels, trachea, RLN	85%	Transcervical (sternotomy only if intrathoracic goitre diameter >thoracic inlet diameter
II	Posterior mediastinum	Posterior to great vessels, trachea, RLN	15%	As above. Also consider sternotomy or right posterolateral thoracotomy if type IIB
IIA	Ipsilateral extension			
IIB	Contralateral extension			
B1	Extension posterior to both trachea and oesophagus			
B2	Extension between trachea and oesophagus			
III	Isolated mediastinal goitre	No connection to orthotopic gland; may have mediastinal blood supply	<1%	Transcervical or sternotomy

RLN, recurrent laryngeal nerve.
From Randolph GW. Surgery of the thyroid and parathyroid glands. Philadelphia, PA: Saunders, 2003.

variable reduction in goitre size. Furthermore, re-growth often occurs following cessation of suppressive doses of thyroxine.[6] Suppressive therapy increases the risk of atrial fibrillation in elderly patients and worsens osteoporosis. It cannot be used if the patient's thyroid-stimulating hormone (TSH) is already suppressed, which is common in patients with chronic multinodular goitre.

With radioiodine therapy, relatively high doses may be required to treat Graves' disease. This reflects the decreased iodine avidity of thyroid epithelium in multinodular goitre and the large thyroid volume which requires treatment. Nevertheless, this is an effective strategy for appropriate patients. The evidence suggests 33–66% volume reduction in the vast majority (80%) of patients, with symptomatic improvement achieved in a similar majority. The radioiodine dose needed to treat benign multinodular goitre may be associated with significant patient morbidity. Radiation thyroiditis occurs in 5% of patients with an acute worsening of airway obstruction. Radiation-induced Graves' disease occurs in up to 10% of patients, and radioiodine may also carry an increased risk of developing secondary malignancies beyond the thyroid gland. Sixty percent of patients will be rendered hypothyroid, and up to 1 in 5 patients require a further therapeutic dose.[6]

Surgery is a good option available for the treatment of progressive multinodular non-toxic goitre. It provides a direct and expeditious way of controlling regional aerodigestive tract compression and is associated with low operative morbidity when performed by experienced surgical teams. It also allows histological assessment and achieves complete resolution of hyperthyroidism. Patients with obvious compressive symptoms or who have significant cosmetic concerns related to the size of a thyroid goitre are best treated with surgery. In our experience, thyroid masses >5 cm frequently cause troublesome symptoms. Subsequently, we have a very low threshold for offering surgery in this group of patients. The same applies for patients with radiographic evidence of tracheal or oesophageal obstruction (i.e. significant deviation or compression) and retrosternal goitre extension. Surgery is mandatory for all patients in whom the preoperative work-up suggests malignancy. This includes patients with hard or fixed masses, vocal cord paralysis, cervical lymphadenopathy and suspicious or positive fine needle aspiration cytology (FNAC).

Surgery is a good management option for retrosternal goitre as this is very likely to cause regional (oesophageal and vascular) compressive symptoms and airway obstruction. We have developed a classification system which reflects the surgical considerations involved when contemplating resection of these lesions (Table 8.1). This information, obtained by axial computed tomography (CT) scanning, allows the surgeon to anticipate the various anatomical locations of a retrosternal goitre. This facilitates appropriate surgical preparation for safe removal of the goitre which can occasionally involve the assistance of a thoracic surgeon.

TOXIC GOITRE

The majority of patients with a toxic benign thyroid lesion (most commonly Graves' disease) are initially managed with anti-thyroid medications (e.g. propylthiouracil, methimazole or carbimazole) in the USA. This achieves lasting remission in only one-third of patients,[10] and therefore is usually followed by radioactive iodine.[7] Medical management is least successful (<30% remission rate) when patients require high doses of maintenance thionamide, e.g. >400 mg/day of propylthiouracil. Other factors which predict poor outcome include high titres of TSH receptor antibodies and goitre size >3 cm.[11]

A significant issue, implicit with use of anti-thyroid medications, is the 0.5% risk of agranulocytosis.[8] This rare, but potentially life-threatening risk generally limits anti-thyroid medications to short-term use. In the USA, radioactive iodine (RAI) is the most common definitive treatment for Graves' disease (see Chapter 5). Surgery is considered when there is allergy to anti-thyroid agents, a suspicious nodule, a compressive goitre or a goitre which needs expedient definite management.[9] In Japan, surgery is performed much more extensively to treat Graves' disease than in the USA. The UK approach is outlined in Chapter 6.

Thyroidectomy is very effective in treating hyperthyroidism, with a recurrence rate of only 5%.[12] Surgery for Graves' disease does appear to be associated with a greater risk of surgical complications including post-operative haemorrhage, recurrent laryngeal nerve (RLN) injury and hypoparathyroidism.[6] Nevertheless, in skilled hands, total thyroidectomy remains an excellent treatment choice.

PRE-OPERATIVE CONSIDERATIONS

Suppressive doses of thyroxine may decrease the size of a non-toxic nodular goitre particularly in cases with underlying Hashimoto's thyroiditis.[13] However, it is unlikely to have a significant impact on the vascularity of the gland. The pre-operative use of anti-thyroid medications in toxic nodules and Graves' disease diminishes hormone stores within the thyroid gland and re-establishes a normal metabolic state.[14] Surgery should not be performed until a normal euthyroid state has been established. Anti-thyroid agents do not, however, decrease the size or vascularity of the gland. Potassium iodide salts are used to achieve this. SSKI (potassium iodide; 50–250 mg three times a day) is usually administered for 10–14 days pre-operatively for this purpose.[15] Dexamethasone is sometimes used as an adjunctive treatment. It blocks glandular hormone secretion and inhibits peripheral conversion of T4 to T3. Propranolol may be helpful in the peri-operative period, but is usually not sufficient by itself to prevent thyroid storm.[16]

Table 8.2 Work-up for benign goitre

History and physical examination (see Plate 8.1)
Symptomatic*
Massive goitre*
Bilateral circumferential goitre*
Suspect retrosternal goitre*
Suspect cancer (vocal cord paralysis, lymphadenopathy)*
Thyroid function tests
Chest radiograph if suspect cancer
Chest radiograph showing airway deviation→axial CT or MRI

* Obtain computed tomography (CT) or magnetic resonance imaging (MRI).

The use of pre-operative CT imaging in thyroid goitre surgery is debatable.[17] In our practice, when clinical examination suggests thyroid enlargement it is frequently used as part of a pre-operative work-up. CT scan of the neck and chest is recommended for evaluating goitres with a retrosternal component. Useful information derived from this imaging modality includes the extent of the lesion, the likely effect on RLN position, location within the thorax, relationship to vital vascular structures and severity of tracheal/oesophageal deviation or compression. Iodinated contrast-enhanced CT should only be performed once a euthyroid state is confirmed by laboratory assay as the contrast load may precipitate acute thyrotoxicosis in patients with subclinical hyperthyroidism. Iodinated contrast CT also delays the use of post-operative RAI therapy should this adjuvant treatment be required.

Pre-operative evaluation of vocal cord movement is an underutilized test which is quick, inexpensive and provides the surgeon with critical clinical information which may affect surgical decision making. It also allows both surgeon and patient to be more informed regarding possible outcomes in the upcoming surgery and should be routinely performed in all patients undergoing thyroid surgery (Table 8.2)

SURGICAL CONSIDERATIONS

Most goitres are soft, compressible and therefore amenable to considerable manipulation during surgery. Goitres caused by the fibrotic variant of Hashimoto's thyroiditis are much more challenging to mobilize. Thus goitre consistency (as well as goitre size) is a significant factor in addition to size when contemplating surgery.

Retrosternal goitre

Retrosternal goitres present particular surgical challenges (see Table 8.1). The majority extend into the anterior mediastinum occupying a position anterior to the RLN, subclavian and innominate blood vessels. The relationship between the thyroid gland and RLN is therefore no different from that encountered in routine thyroid surgery.

We offer a new classification for retrosternal goitres (see Table 8.1). When a goitre extends into the posterior mediastinum (type IIA and IIB), the trachea and great vessels are pushed superficial to the mass.[6] The mass rests posterior or deep to the innominate vein, contents of the carotid sheath, innominate and subclavian arteries, RLN and inferior thyroid artery.[6] The resulting relationship between the RLN and thyroid mass, with the recurrent laryngeal nerve running on the anterior or ventral surface of the gland, is the opposite of the expected relationship between these structures. In this anterior position, the nerve is at greater risk of traction or transection injury even with an experienced thyroid surgeon. Type IIA posterior mediastinal goitres remain ipsilateral. Type IIB goitres cross the midline passing behind the oesophagus (type IIB1) or trachea (type IIB2). The latter usually occurs in a left-sided goitre which crosses into the right posterior mediastinum due to deflection off the aortic arch (see Fig. 8.1).

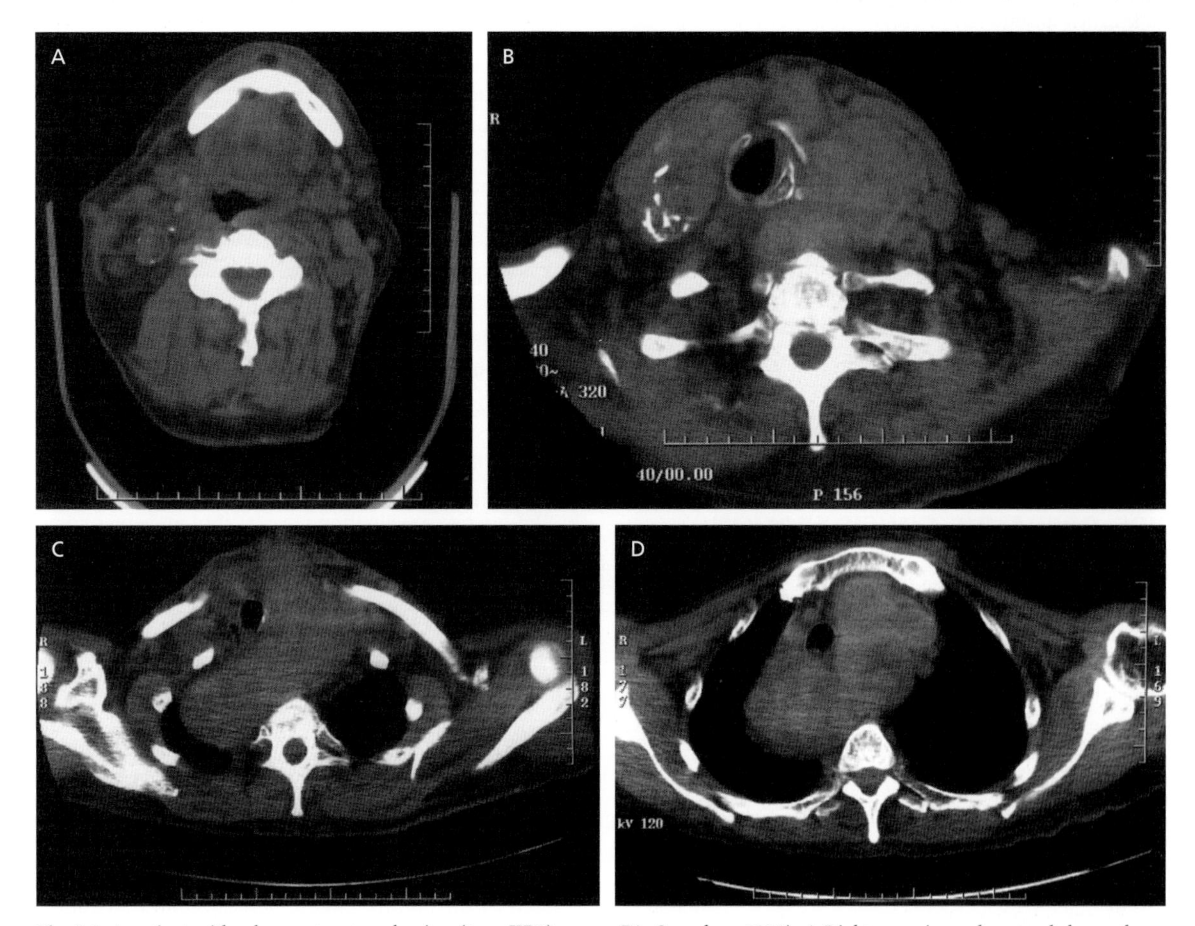

Fig. 8.1 A patient with a large retrosternal goitre (type IIB2). The thyroid mass extends into the left chest, crosses behind the trachea into the right chest and extends between the trachea and oesophagus. The specimen weighed 450 g and was 15 cm in greatest diameter. Transcervical resection was possible without the need for sternotomy. Intra-operative nerve monitoring was employed, and there was normal vocal cord motion post-operatively (adapted from Randolph GW. Surgery of the thyroid and parathyroid glands. Philadelphia, PA: Saunders, 2003). **A** Right superior pole extends beneath the sternocledomastoid muscle to the level of the mandible. **B** At the level of the cricoid cartilage, the goitre is present bilaterally in the neck. **C** At the level of the thoracic inlet, the left thyroid lobe extends into the left chest behind the trachea into the right thorax. **D** The mass extends retrosternally along the left lateral trachea abutting both left and right lung fields and splaying the great vessels.

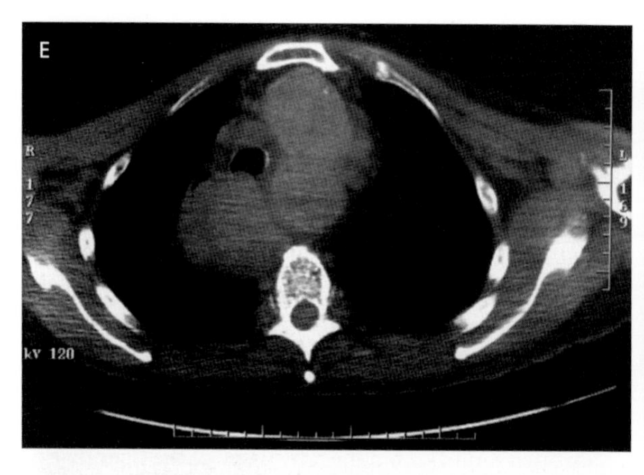

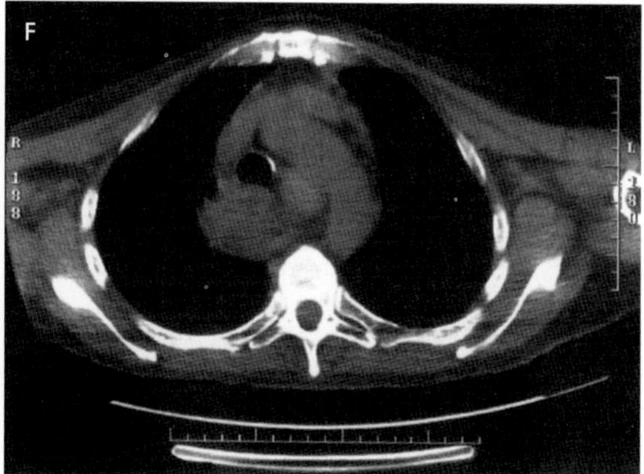

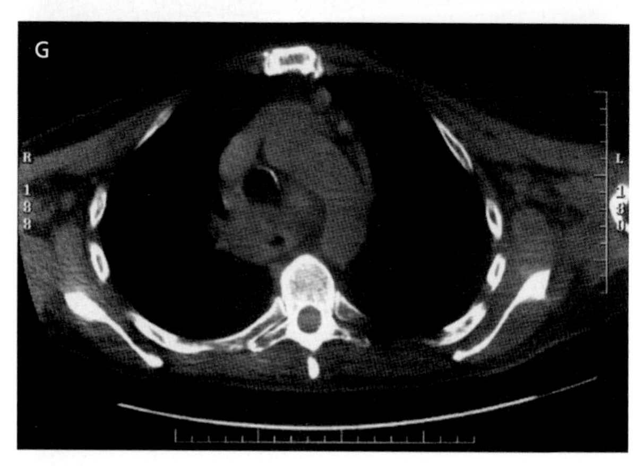

Fig. 8.1 *Continued* **E** The distal segment of the retrosternal mass has several lobulations. The innominate artery is seen anterior to the trachea. The goitre abuts the vertebral column posteriorly. **F** The inferior extent of the goitre is shown, deep to the level of the aortic arch. The mass infiltrates between trachea and oesophagus. **G** The mass extends between trachea and oesophagus, terminating just above the azygous vein and right main bronchus.

The vast majority of retrosternal goitres are removed through a neck incision without the need for a sternotomy. Manoeuvres to aid mobilization of a retrosternal goitre include division of the thyroid isthmus, adequate neck extension and bimanual retraction (Fig. 8.2). Cystic lesions can be aspirated to decrease goitre volume.

Rarely (<1% of retrosternal cases), an isolated thyroid goitre occurs within the mediastinum which is completely discontinuous from normal thyroid gland located in the neck.[18] Possible explanations for this unusual finding include embryological fragmentation and hyperdescent, exophytic nodule formation or 'parasitic' nodule formation in the context of previous surgery.[6] The blood supply often arises from the mediastinum rather than the neck. It may arise from the aorta, thyrocervical trunk, subclavian, internal mammary or innominate arteries. Venous drainage occurs via corresponding intrathoracic veins. Safe removal requires the expertise of an experienced thoracic surgeon.

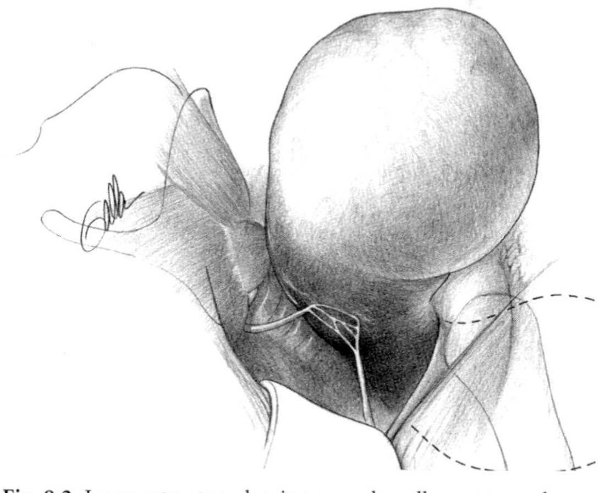

Fig. 8.2 Large retrosternal goitres may be adherent to and splay the RLN so that blind delivery without neural dissection may result in excessive nerve tension and vocal cord paralysis. A superior approach to the RLN is recommended in challenging cases (from Randolph GW. Surgery of the thyroid and parathyroid glands. Philadelphia, PA: Saunders, 2003).

Thyroid surgery

The following outline describes the standard thyroidectomy approach. The patient is positioned supine with the neck extended by means of a shoulder roll or inflatable pillow. A transverse incision is made in a relaxed skin tension line approximately 1 cm below the cricoid. Subplatysmal flaps are elevated up to the thyroid notch and down to the clavicles. A midline vertical incision is made in the superficial layer of the deep cervical fascia and the strap muscles are separated by blunt dissection. If it is necessary to divide them, do so superiorly to preserve innervation by the ansa cervicalis.

Dissection proceeds laterally along the thyroid capsule with the thyroid lobe retracted antero-medially. Division of the middle thyroid vein improves lateral exposure whilst identification of the cricoid cartilage and trachea aids anatomic orientation. The superior pole neurovascular pedicle is identified by sweeping the lobe inferomedially. Dissection continues along the capsule to avoid injury to the external branch of the superior laryngeal nerve (SLN) which should be routinely identified. Intraoperative nerve monitoring greatly facilitates the process (Fig. 8.3). The superior thyroid artery and vein are ligated as close as possible to the capsule to protect the nerve.

The superior parathyroid is often closely associated with the deep aspect of the superior pole and is sometimes located within the thyroid capsule. It must be dissected free with great care to prevent devascularization.

Attention is now focused on the inferior pole. The RLN is identified in the triangle formed by the trachea, common carotid artery and inferior border of the thyroid gland. Meticulous dissection should be performed in a direction parallel to the anticipated course of the nerve. The RLN can also be identified superiorly, to its entry into the larynx. In this approach, the location of the nerve tends to be more constant. When the mass distorts the usual anatomy, the nerve can be identified where it enters the larynx just posterior to the cricothyroid joint. The course of the nerve should be identified before dividing Berry's ligament because the main trunk or its branches may pass through the tough ligament fibres (Fig. 8.4).

The inferior thyroid artery and vein are divided as close as possible to the capsule. The inferior parathyroid glands often have a more variable location (see Chapter 16) and will be less frequently identified on the surface of the capsule compared with the superior glands. They are often found within the fatty tissue of the thyrothymic tract. The goitre specimen should be examined for capsular parathyroid glands. Fatty tissue and any clefts

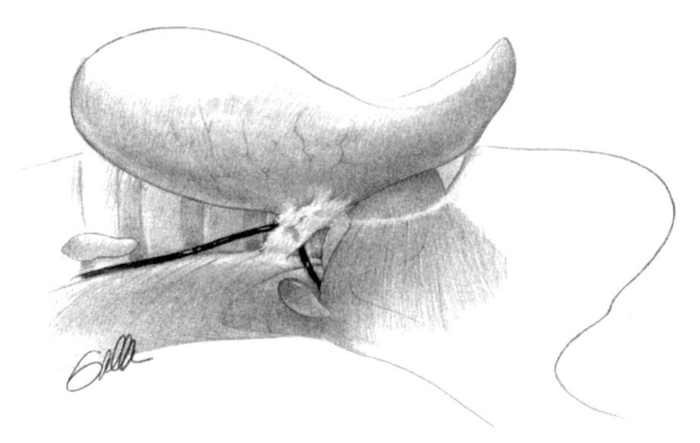

Fig. 8.4 Relationship of the recurrent laryngeal nerve and the ligament of Berry can result in traction injury to the recurrent laryngeal nerve at the level of the ligament of Berry if there is significant ventral retraction before the nerve is freed. (from Randolph GW. Surgery of the thyroid and parathyroid glands. Philadelphia, PA: Saunders, 2003).

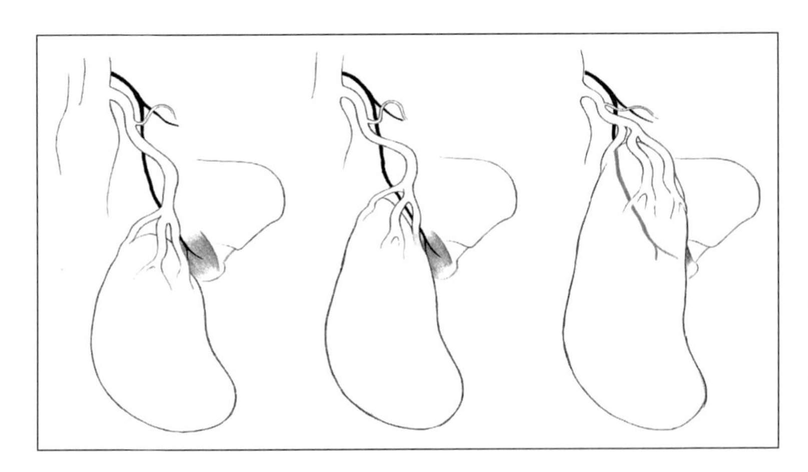

Fig. 8.3 Goiterous enlargement of the superior pole can result in the superior pole becoming closely associated with the external branch of the superior laryngeal nerve (from Randolph GW. Surgery of the thyroid and parathyroid glands. Philadelphia, PA: Saunders, 2003).

within the goitre are carefully assessed. If a parathyroid gland is identified it is diced into 1 mm pieces and re-implanted into the sternocleidomastoid muscle. The location is marked with a surgical clip.

The thyroid lobe is then divided at the isthmus. When performing a total thyroidectomy, the contralateral lobe is dissected in a similar fashion and the entire thyroid removed en bloc. Meticulous haemostasis is achieved in the surgical field, the strap muscles are re-approximated and the incision closed. Several well-designed prospective, randomized studies question the benefit of drain insertion following thyroidectomy.[19] In our practice a drain is used infrequently.

Minimally invasive, video-assisted thyroidectomy (MIT) is gaining popularity, and numerous publications report its efficacy in appropriate cases.[20,21] Selection criteria include:

- nodules <3 cm in size within a gland with a total volume <20 ml
- patients without previous neck surgery
- no thyroiditis.

The technique has mainly been used to remove small benign thyroid lesions, micropapillary cancers with no nodal disease and to perform thyroidectomy in *RET* oncogene carriers prior to the onset of clinical disease rather than goitre. The main advantage of MIT is improved cosmesis due to a shorter incision.

In contrast to the open approach, MIT requires the patient to be positioned supine without hyperextending the neck. This more neutral position facilitates identification of the RLN which appears more clearly when it is not stretched by neck extension. The procedure requires two assistants: one at the head of the operating table who retracts and a second assistant who holds the endoscope. A transverse skin incision 1.5 cm in length is made 2 cm above the sternal notch. Skin flaps are often not raised. As with the open approach, a longitudinal incision is made in the superficial layer of the deep cervical fascia and the strap muscles are bluntly dissected away from the thyroid. A 30° 5 mm or 7 mm videoscope is introduced into the incision and the thyrotracheal groove is dissected with 2 mm instruments using the endoscope to visualize the area of dissection. The thyroid lobe is retracted inferiorly and medially to identify the superior pole neurovascular bundle. The lobe is retracted medially to identify the RLN using the posterior border of the thyroid lobe as a landmark. At this stage, the lower and mid thyroid lobe is delivered ventrally through the wound. Next, the superior pole is rotated and retracted out of the wound and the ligament of Berry is divided, utilizing a standard direct loupe-assisted technique. Following meticulous haemostasis and RLN stimulation, the incision is closed with a single deep stitch and a skin sealant. A drain is not routinely used. Surgeons with considerable experience performing MIT report operative times comparable with traditional thyroidectomy.

SURGICAL COMPLICATIONS AND MANAGEMENT

Post-operative complications include haematoma, seroma, injury to the RLN or SLN, and hypoparathyroidism. Less common complications include wound infection, pneumothorax and chylous fistula.

An expanding haematoma can cause life-threatening airway compression post-operatively. The surgical incision must be opened at the bedside and the haematoma evacuated. The airway must be secured immediately and the patient returned to theatre for exploration and control of the bleeding site. In most cases an obvious bleeding vessel is not visualized at the time of exploration.[22]

Seromas occur in the early post-operative period and are more common with large goitres due to the greater associated dead space which is created following resection. Needle aspiration is usually sufficient treatment for this complication.

Injury to the external branch of the superior laryngeal nerve will impede function of the cricothyroid muscle and can lead to difficulty raising the volume and the pitch of the voice. Such voice changes are well tolerated in most patients but may seriously affect those who use their voice professionally, e.g. public speakers, performers and singers.[23] The diagnosis can be confirmed with electromyography. Treatment involves speech therapy.

Recurrent laryngeal nerve injury occurs along a spectrum. Stretch injury to the nerve with immediate paresis occurs in 7% of thyroid operations while permanent paralysis occurs less frequently.[24,25] Risk of injury is increased when there is thyroiditis, retrosternal extension or previous thyroid surgery. If neural transection injury is recognized intra-operatively, we advocate immediate re-anastomosis with a fine non-absorbable suture (10-0 Nylon). An alternative is to anastomose the distal end of the nerve to the ansa cervicalis innervating the strap musculature. Primary neural repair helps to prevent vocal fold atrophy, although the long-term functional results are questionable. Associated post-operative glottic dysfunction includes: (1) a strong adductor functional predominance and (2) synkinetic vocal cord motion with paradoxical inward adductor motion during inspiration.[27–29]

Unilateral injury may result in a breathy and quiet voice. If the SLN is also injured, the vocal cord may be bowed and the glottis rotated to the affected side. Following RLN injury dysphagia may also occur. This usually presents with aspiration due to decreased supraglottic sensation and reduced protective adductor function. Vocal cord dysfunction can take 6–12 months to resolve completely. In the interim, injection medialization laryngoplasty of the affected vocal fold with a temporary substance (gelfoam, micronized acellular dermal collagen or hyaluronic acid) can restore a functional voice. Some authorities advocate more long-lasting substances such as autologous fat or hydroxyapatite. The procedure is performed transorally by direct laryngoscopy or transcutaneously through the cricothyroid membrane. Both techniques require precise injection just lateral to the vocal process of the arytenoid cartilage to medialize the immobile vocal cord. Permanent vocal fold medialization procedures should not be attempted until at least 1 year post-operatively, after which time spontaneous nerve recovery is unlikely. Medialization laryngoplasty (also termed thyroplasty) is possible using a permanent implant to medialize the vocal fold through a window in the thyroid cartilage. Arytenoid medialization can also achieve good results.[30] Both procedures can be performed under local or general anaesthesia, and significantly improve vocal function for these patients.

Bilateral RLN injury is usually immediately obvious. There is stridor and upper airway compromise which requires immediate intubation or tracheostomy. It may also manifest in a delayed fashion. When cord paresis is permanent, arytenoidectomy and/or transverse cordotomy can be performed to improve the airway and facilitate tracheostomy decannulation. Improvement in the airway is achieved at the expense of a weak voice and increased aspiration risk.

Transient hypocalcaemia occurs in 7–25% of patients undergoing thyroid surgery.[31,32] The relatively high rate of post-operative hypocalcaemia reflects the sensitivity of the parathyroid glands and their blood supply to surgical manipulation. Symptomatic hypocalcaemia usually becomes evident 24–48 hours after surgery. If temporary, it tends to resolve within a few weeks. Permanent hypoparathyroidism has been reported in 0.4–13.8% of patients and arises following significant injury of the parathyroid glands. An increased risk of hypoparathyroidism is associated with excision of a large thyroid mass or locally advanced thyroid cancer as both conditions require extensive peri-thyroidal dissection.

Symptoms of hypocalcaemia initially include peri-oral and extremity parasthaesia. When left untreated, this progresses to tetany, bronchospasm, mental status changes, laryngospasm and arrhythmias. Routine post-operative serum calcium is monitored for 24–48 hours following total thyroidectomy. If serum calcium falls below 7 μg/dl or the patient becomes markedly symptomatic then intravenous replacement therapy is indicated (10 ml of 10% calcium gluconate and 5% dextrose). This should be titrated to serum calcium measurements and to symptoms. Less severe hypocalcaemia can be managed with oral supplementation of 2–6 g of calcium carbonate per day and calcitriol 0.25–0.5 μg twice daily. The UK/European regime is outlined in further detail in Chapters 13 and 17.

Early prediction of hypocalcaemia following thyroidectomy is possible by checking early post-operative serum calcium trends or parathyroid hormone (PTH) levels. The slope of the first two serum calcium values has an 85% positive predictive value.[33] Several studies have shown that the serum PTH level checked several hours after thyroidectomy has good sensitivity and specificity for predicting symptomatic hypocalcaemia.[34–36] In one study, a single PTH threshold (65% decrease compared with pre-operative levels) checked 6 hours following thyroidectomy had a sensitivity of 96.4% and specificity of 91.4% for detecting hypocalcaemia.[37] Further development and utilization of the PTH assay is likely to improve post-operative management of patients who have undergone total and completion thyroidectomy. Patients identified as low risk for hypocalcaemia may be discharged earlier, while high risk patients can be treated before developing the hypocalcaemic sequalae which contribute to significant patient morbidity and prolonged admission.

EVIDENCE APPRAISAL

The US Preventive Services Taskforce has provided general categories for levels of evidence in medicine, with the randomized controlled clinical trial being the highest quality evidence, i.e. Level I. Level II studies are well-designed controlled studies, but not randomized. Level III evidence comprises expert opinion and descriptive reports.

Several of the works cited in this chapter (references 15, 27, 29 and 26*) derive from expert anatomical study and do not neatly fit into this system. However, these are of great value to the physician and surgeon and should not be overlooked. Others (references 2, 6* and 9) represent considerable contributions that comprise years of research and experience as well as scholarly review of the evidence from numerous well-designed studies that have rightly impacted clinical decision making. A good number are, in our opinion, quality case–control and cohort (Level II) studies (references 16, 30, 32*, 34 and 36) that provide relevant and useful conclusions included in the text. One study (reference 19*) clearly demonstrates how Level I methodology may be applied in a targeted fashion to answer a discrete yet meaningful question with impact upon surgical patient management. (Those references marked with an asterisk are of particular relevance.)

REFERENCES

1. Rojeski MT, Gharib H. Nodular thyroid disease: evaluation and management. N Engl J Med 1985;313:428–36.
2. Burch HB. Evaluation and management of the solid thyroid nodule. Endocrinol Metab Clin North Am 1995;24:663–710.
3. Gharib H, Goellner JR. Evaluation of nodular thyroid disease. Endocrinol Metabl Clin North Am 1988;17:511.
4. Tuttle RM, Lemar H, Burch HB. Clinical features associated with an increased risk of thyroid malignancy in patients with follicular neoplasia by fine needle aspiration. Thyroid 1998;8:377.
5. Anders HJ. Compression syndromes caused by substernal goiters. Postgrad Med J 1998;74:327.
6. Randolph GW. Surgery of the thyroid and parathyroid glands. Philadelphia, PA: Saunders, 2003: 74.
7. Falk SA. Hyperthyroidism: a surgeon's perspective. In: English GM, ed. Otolaryngology. Philadelphia: Harper & Row, 1985:86–91.
8. Dobyns BM *et al.* Malignant and benign neoplasms of the thyroid in patients treated for hyperthyroidism: a report of the cooperative thyrotoxicosis therapy follow up study. J Clin Endocrinol Metab 1974;38:976.
9. Cusick EL, Krukowski ZH, Matheson NA. Outcome of surgery for Graves' disease re-examined. Br J Surg 1987;74:780.
10. Reid DJ. Hyperthyroidism and hypothyroidism complicating the treatment of thyrotoxicosis. Br J Surg 1987;74: 1060.
11. Wilson R, McKillop JH, Henderson N, *et al.* The ability of the serum thyrotrophin receptor antibody (TRAb) index and HLA status to predict long-term remission of thyrotoxicosis following medical therapy for Graves' disease. Clin Endocrinol (Oxf) 1986;25:151.
12. Kasuga Y, Sugenoya A, Kobayashi S, *et al.* Clinical evaluation of the response to surgical treatment of Graves' disease. Surg Gynecol Obstet 1990;170:327.
13. Falk SA, Birken EA, Ronquillo A. Graves' disease associated with histologic Hashimoto's thyroiditis. Otolaryngol Head Neck Surg 1985;93:86.
14. Gittoes NJL, Franklin JA. Hyperthyroidism: current treatment guidelines. Drugs 1998;55:543.
15. Reinhoff WF. The histologic changes brought about in cases of exophthalmic goiter by the administration of iodine. Bull Johns Hopkins Hosp 1925;37:385.
16. Lennquist S, Jörtsö E, Anderberg B, *et al.* Beta blockers compared with antithyroid drugs as preoperative treatment in hyperthyroidism: drug tolerance, complications, and postoperative thyroid function. Surgery 1985;98:1141.
17. Buckley JA, Stark P. Intrathoracic mediastinal thyroid goiter: imaging manifestations. AJR Am J Roentgenol 1999; 173:471.
18. Shahian DM, Rossi RL. Posterior mediastinal goiter. Chest 1988;94:599.
19. Lee SW, Choi EC, Lee YM, *et al.* Is lack of placement of drains after thyroidectomy with central neck dissection safe? A prospective, randomized study. Laryngoscope 2006;116: 1632–5.
20. Terris DJ, Gourin CG, Chin E. Minimally invasive thyroidectomy: basic and advanced techniques. Laryngoscope 2006;116:350–6.
21. Miccoli P, Materazzi G. Minimally invasive, video-assisted thyroidectomy (MIVAT). Surg Clin North Am 2004;84: 735–41.
22. Matory YL, Spiro RH. Wound bleeding after head and neck surgery. J Surg Oncol 1993;53:17.
23. Loré JM Jr, Kokocharov SI, Kaufman S, *et al.* Thirty-eight-year evaluation of a surgical technique to protect the external branch of the superior laryngeal nerve during thyroidectomy. Ann Otol Rhinol Laryngol 1998;107: 1015.
24. Max MH, Scherm M, Bland KI. Early and late complications after thyroid surgery. South Med J 1983;76:977.
25. Harness JK, Fung L, Thompson NW, *et al.* Total thyroidectomy: complications and technique. World J Surg 1986; 10:781.
26. Henry JF, Audiffret J, Denizot A. The non-recurrent inferior laryngeal nerve: review of 33 cases including two on the left. Surgery 1988;104:977.
27. Sato F, Ogura JH. Neurorrhaphy of the recurrent laryngeal nerve. Laryngoscope 1978;88:1034.
28. Crumley RL. Laryngeal synkinesis: its significance to the laryngologist. Ann Otol Rhinol Laryngol 1989;98:87.
29. Rubio A, Fernández MR, Figols J, *et al.* Experimental study on neurorrhaphy of recurrent laryngeal nerve in dogs. J Laryngol Otol 1996;110:748.
30. Billante CR, Spector B, Hudson M, *et al.* Voice outcome following thyroplasty in patients with cancer-related vocal fold paralysis. Auris Nasus Larynx 2001;28:315–21.
31. Glinoer D, Andry G, Chantrain G, *et al.* Clinical aspects of early and late hypocalcemia after thyroid surgery. Eur J Surg Oncol 2000;26:571–7.

32. Hundahl SA, Cady B, Cunningham MP, *et al.* Initial results from a prospective cohort study of 5583 cases of thyroid carcinoma treated in the United States during 1996. US and German Thyroid Cancer Study Group. An American College of Surgeons Commission on cancer patient care/evaluation study. Cancer 2000;89:202–17.
33. Husein M, Hier MP, Al-Abdulhadi K, *et al.* Predicting calcium status post thyroidectomy with early calcium levels. Otolaryngol Head Neck Surg 2002;127:289–93.
34. Lo CY, Luk JM, Tam SC. Applicability of intraoperative parathyroid hormone assay during thyroidectomy. Ann Surg 2002;236:564–9.
35. Lindblom P, Westerdahl J, Bergenfelz ••. Low parathyroid hormone levels after thyroid surgery: a feasible predictor of hypocalcemia. Surgery 2002;131:515–20.
36. McLeod IK, Arciero C, Noordzij JP, *et al.* The use of rapid parathyroid hormone assay in predicting postoperative hypocalcemia after total or completion thyroidectomy. Thyroid 2006;16:259–65.
37. Noordzij JP, Lee SL, Bernet VJ, *et al.* Early prediction of hypocalcemia after thyroidectomy using parathyroid hormone: an analysis of pooled individual patient data from 9 observational studies. J Am Coll Surg 2007;205:748–54.

MULTIPLE CHOICE QUESTIONS

Select more than one option where appropriate.

1. All of the following have been reported to lead to acute enlargement of thyroid goitre except:
A. Pregnancy
B. Iodine deficiency
C. Corticosteroid therapy
D. Haemorrhage

2. Surgery for non-toxic multinodular goitre has the following advantage(s):
A. Provides pathological examination
B Hyperthyroidism may be cured
C. It may lower the risk of treatment-related complications
D. All of the above

3. The following are all indications for surgery for benign goitre except:
A. Cosmesis
B. Aerodigestive compression
C. Palpable mass
D. Retrosternal extension

4. Regarding minimally invasive video-assisted thyroidectomy (MIT):
A. Typically a drain is inserted
B. The main advantage of this procedure is a shorter operating time
C. Patients who have had prior neck surgery are good candidates for MIT
D. A minimum of two assistants is required
E. Patients with a nodule <3 cm are good candidates for MIT

5. A retrosternal goitre:
A. Usually extends into the posterior mediastinum
B. Is usually superficial to important neurovascular structures
C. Is often fibrotic and difficult to mobilize
D. Derives a blood supply predominantly from thoracic vessels rather than neck vessels
E. Usually requires a sternotomy in order to access the goitre for excision

Answers

1. C
2. D
3. C
4. D, E
5. B

9 Oncogenesis and molecular targeted therapy in thyroid cancer

Kepal N. Patel[1] & Bhuvanesh Singh[2]

[1] Division of Endocrine Surgery, New York University School of Medicine, New York, NY, USA
[2] Head and Neck Service, Memorial Sloan-Kettering Cancer Center, New York, NY, USA

KEY POINTS

- Molecular studies have identified a number of abnormalities associated with progression and de-differentiation of thyroid carcinoma
- These distinct molecular events are associated with specific stages of tumour development
- A better understanding of the mechanisms involved in thyroid cancer pathogenesis will help translate these discoveries into improved patient care
- Novel treatments are being developed based on our improved understanding of this disease process
- Several clinical trials, currently in progress, have been initiated to assess the role of these novel therapies in aggressive thyroid carcinoma

INTRODUCTION

Cancers of thyroid gland origin are the most common endocrine malignancies and account for the majority of endocrine cancer-related deaths each year.[1,2] More than 90% of thyroid carcinomas are derived from follicular cells. A minority are of C-cell (parafollicular) origin; medullary thyroid carcinoma (MTC). Most thyroid carcinomas can be effectively managed by surgical resection with or without radioactive iodine ablation. However, a subset of tumours behave aggressively, leading to significant morbidity and mortality. The majority of patients with poorly differentiated and anaplastic thyroid cancers succumb to their disease despite aggressive treatment. During the past decade, our knowledge of the genetics and molecular pathways involved in oncogenesis has increased dramatically. Several molecular abnormalities have been identified which contribute to thyroid follicular/parafollicular cell transformation. They are the focus of current investigation as putative therapeutic targets.

A Practical Manual of Thyroid and Parathyroid Disease, 1st Edition. Edited by Asit Arora, Neil Tolley & R. Michael Tuttle.

THYROID CANCER OF FOLLICULAR CELL ORIGIN

Thyroid cancers derived from thyroid follicular epithelial cells (thyrocytes) are broadly classified as well-differentiated (WDTC), poorly differentiated (PDTC) and undifferentiated or anaplastic (ATC). WDTCs such as papillary and follicular thyroid cancer (FTC) behave in an indolent fashion and usually have an excellent prognosis. In contrast, ATC is highly aggressive and often rapidly fatal. PDTC is morphologically and behaviourally intermediate between WDTC and ATC. Accumulating evidence suggests that thyrocyte-derived thyroid carcinomas constitute a biological continuum progressing from the highly curable WDTC to the frequently incurable ATC.[3,4] PDTC and aggressive variants of WDTC such as tall and columnar cell serve as intermediates in the progression model.[5,6] Clinical, epidemiological and pathological evidence supports this concept of step-wise progression and de-differentiation.[7] The gradual loss of papillary and follicular growth patterns and simultaneous increase in a solid growth pattern, with increased mitoses, necrosis and nuclear pleomorphism, is frequently observed in aggressive thyroid carcinomas.[8,9] A majority of these tumours exhibit residual foci of differentiated thyroid carcinoma.

Since aggressive carcinomas such as PDTC and ATC result in significant morbidity and mortality, it is important to identify the molecular mechanisms driving the de-differentiation of WDTC. In the last decade there has been an explosion of genetic information available, particularly relating to the molecular alterations involved in the pathogenesis of thyroid carcinoma. Genetic alterations and mutations in factors regulating thyrocyte growth and differentiation play a prominent role.

Receptor tyrosine kinases

RET/PTC

The *RET* (*re*arranged during *t*ransfection) proto-oncogene is a 21-exon gene located on the long arm of chromosome 10 (10q11.2) which encodes a tyrosine kinase receptor. RET was the first activated receptor tyrosine kinase to be identified in thyroid cancer. It consists of an extracellular domain with a ligand-binding site, a transmembrane domain and an intracellular domain. RET is activated by interaction with a multicomponent complex which includes a soluble ligand family, glial-derived neurotrophic factors (GDNFs) and a family of cell surface-bound co-receptors; GDNF family receptors α (GFRα).[10] Ligand binding results in autophosphorylation of the protein on tyrosine residues. This activates several signalling pathways including extracellular-regulated kinase (ERK, also known as mitogen-activated protein kinase (MAPK) kinase 1 and 3), phosphatidylinositol 3-kinase (PI3K), MAPK p38 and C-JUN kinase (JNK, also known as MAPK kinase 8) (Fig. 9.1).[11,12]

RET is normally expressed in the developing central and peripheral nervous system and is necessary for renal organogenesis and enteric neurogenesis.[13] It is not usually expressed in the thyroid follicular cell.[14] Re-arrangements of the *RET* gene, '*RET/PTC* re-arrangements' occur in papillary thyroid carcinoma (PTC). The unique spatial proximity of translocation-prone gene loci favours this and explains why *RET* re-arrangements are specific for thyroid tumours.[15–18] Although more than 10 re-arrangements have been described, *RET/PTC1*, *RET/PTC2* and *RET/PTC3* account for the vast majority.[19,20] In each of these, the upstream (5′) component of a 'housekeeping' (or ubiquitously expressed) gene drives expression of the tyrosine kinase domain of RET. Expression of RET/PTC

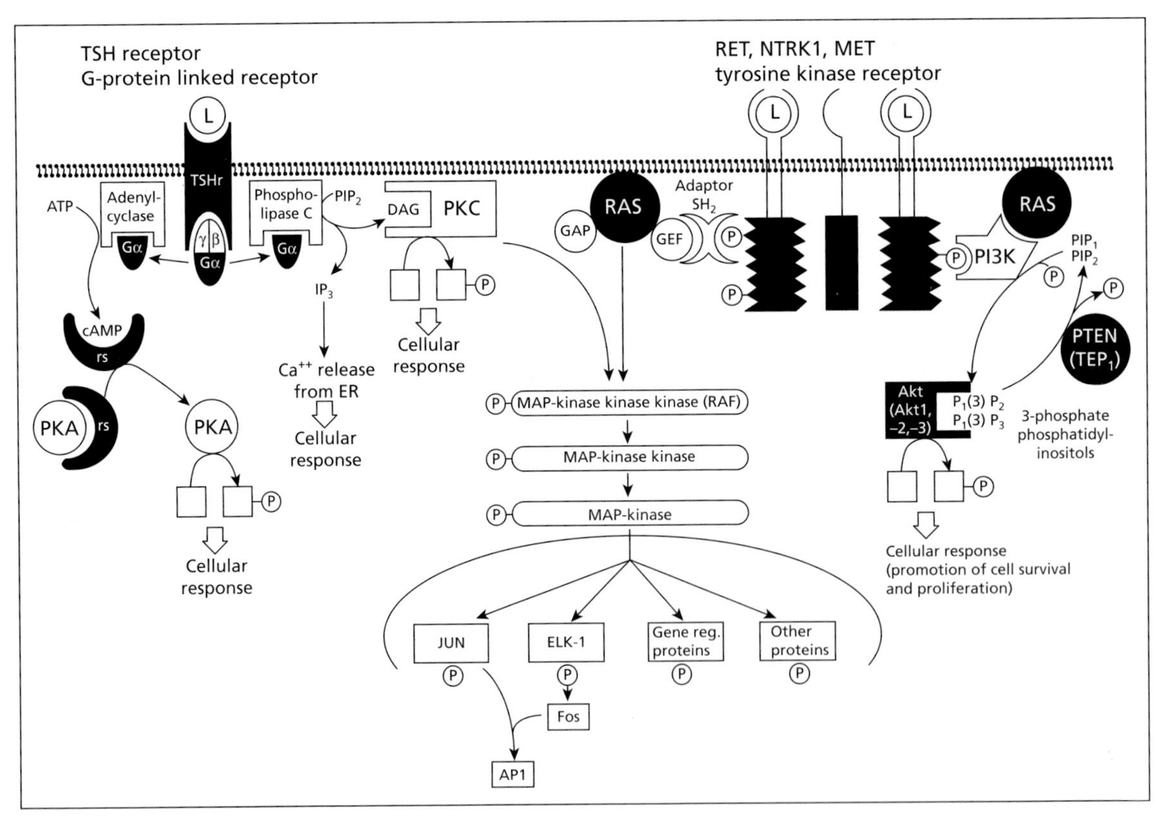

Fig. 9.1 Many of the molecular alterations associated with thyroid tumours involve common signalling pathways. With kind permission from Springer Science+Business Media: Molecular pathobiology of thyroid neoplasms. Endocr Pathol, 2002. 13(4): 271–88. Tallini, G.

Table 9.1 Average prevalence of specific genetic alterations in various types of thyroid carcinoma reported in the literature

	Papillary	Follicular	Poorly differentiated	Anaplastic
BRAF	42%	0%	10%	15%
RAS	10%	40%	35%	50%
RET/PTC	30%	0%	9%	0%
PAX8-PPARγ	<1%	35%	0%	0%
P53	2%	7%	20%	65%
β-Catenin	0%	0%	18%	66%

chimeric proteins is facilitated by heterologous promoters provided by the fused genes resulting in constitutive, ligand-independent RET receptor tyrosine kinase activation in papillary cancer cells.[21–23]

In the adult population, *RET* re-arrangements have been identified in 2.6–34% of PTC (Table 9.1).[24–33] In the paediatric population, *RET/PTC1* and *RET/PTC3* re-arrangements have been found in up to 80% of PTC.[34,35] Initial studies showed that this was particularly evident in children exposed to radiation following the Chernobyl nuclear accident or when there was prior external irradiation for treatment of benign diseases of the head and neck.[28,36–38] However, recent data suggest that re-arrangements frequently occur regardless of radiation history.[39]

The role of *RET* re-arrangements in PTC oncogenesis is convincingly demonstrated in transgenic mice with targeted overexpression of *RET/PTC1* and *RET/PTC3*. These mice develop thyroid tumours with microscopic features similar to human papillary carcinomas.[30,40,41] *RET/PTC* re-arrangements probably represent early genetic changes leading to the development of PTC.[32,42] However, several studies have shown that re-arrangements are associated with PTC which does not progress to PDTC or ATC.[17,43] Fewer than 10% of PDTCs are positive for *RET/PTC* re-arrangements, suggesting that fusion proteins play a minor role in tumour progression.[44]

The recent success in the treatment of chronic myelogenous leukaemia with imatinib mesylate, an inhibitor of constitutively activated ABL kinase, has generated considerable interest in therapeutic protein kinase inhibitors. Several compounds have recently been developed that exhibit significant inhibitory activity on RET kinase, which may prove clinically beneficial for RET-induced thyroid carcinomas.[45]

NTRK1

The neurotrophic receptor tyrosine kinase gene *NTRK1* (also known as *TRK* and *TRKA*) is located on chromosome 1q22 and encodes the receptor for nerve growth factor. It was the second identified subject of chromosomal re-arrangement in thyroid tumorigenesis. NTRK1 expression is typically restricted to neurons of sensory spinal and cranial ganglia of neural-crest origin and regulates neuronal growth and survival.[11] The activated receptor initiates several signal transduction cascades, including the ERK, PI3K and the phospholipase Cγ (PLCγ) pathways.[46]

As with *RET*, *NTRK1* undergoes similar oncogenic activation by chromosomal re-arrangements that fuse the *NTRK1* tyrosine kinase domain to the 5′-terminal region of heterologous genes. The resulting chimeric protein exhibits constitutively active tyrosine kinase activity. Several NTRK1 chimeric proteins have been described in thyroid cancer (TRK, TRK-T1, TRK-T2 and TRK-T3).[47–49] *NTRK1* oncogenes appear to be restricted to PTC but are found with a lower prevalence (~10%) than that reported for *RET/PTC*. The prevalence of *NTRK1* re-arrangements is approximately 3% in post-Chernobyl PTCs.[50,51]

MET proto-oncogene

The *MET* gene encodes a transmembrane protein acting as the receptor for hepatocyte growth factor/scatter factor (HGF/SF). HGF/SF is a powerful mitogen for epithelial cells, including thyroid follicular cells.[52] They induce a variety of tissue-specific changes including epithelial cell dissociation, migration, invasion, growth and polarity. Increased expression of MET is thought to be due to transcriptional or post-transcriptional regulation. PTC typically expresses very high levels of the MET protein.[53–56] Furthermore, *RET* and *RAS* have both been shown to induce *MET* overexpression in primary thyroid cell cultures, suggesting that *MET* may modulate their tumorigenic effects.[57] Although some studies have shown that increased *MET* expression in PTC is associated with advanced stage and poor prognosis,[55,58] others have found decreased *MET* expression in aggressive PTC, PDTC and ATC.[56,59]

Signal transduction proteins

RAS

Three *RAS* genes, H-*RAS*, K-*RAS* and N-*RAS*, synthesize a family of 21 kDa proteins that play an important role in tumorigenesis.[60] The RAS proteins exist in two different forms: an inactive form bound to guanosine diphosphate (GDP) and an active form that exhibits guanosine triphosphatase (GTPase) activity. Their function is to convey signals originating from tyrosine kinase membrane receptors to a cascade of MAPKs. This activates the transcription of target genes involved in cell proliferation, survival and apoptosis (Fig. 9.1).[60] Oncogenic RAS activation occurs due to point mutations which fix the protein in an activated state, resulting in chronic stimulation of downstream targets, genomic instability, additional mutations and malignant transformation.[61]

Mutations in all three *RAS* genes occur in both benign and malignant thyroid tumours. They are common in follicular carcinoma, PDTC and ATC, but occur less frequently in PTC (Table 9.1).[62–68] The frequency of mutations in the follicular variant of PTC (FVPTC) is high, similar to that of follicular carcinoma.[69,70] This suggests that the FVPTC may occupy an intermediate position between follicular tumours and classic PTC. The role of oncogenic RAS in thyroid tumour progression awaits clarification. Some studies show a similar prevalence of *RAS* mutations in benign and malignant thyroid neoplasms, suggesting that RAS activation may represent an early event.[62,71] Other studies have shown that *RAS* mutations, specifically at codon 61 of N-*RAS*, are involved with tumour progression and aggressive clinical behaviour.[68,72–77] Transgenic mice with thyroid-specific mutant *RAS* expression develop thyroid hyperplasia and carcinoma.[78] The presence of *RAS* mutations appears to predict poor outcome for WDTC independent of tumour stage, while PDTC and ATC often harbour multiple *RAS* mutations.[77] These mutations probably represent an intermediate event in the progression of thyroid carcinoma.

BRAF

A significant recent development in thyroid cancer genetics is the identification of the BRAF-activating point mutation which is the most common molecular defect in PTC.[39] There are three isoforms of serine-threonine kinase RAF in mammalian cells: ARAF, BRAF and CRAF or RAF-1. BRAF is expressed in haematopoietic cells, neurons and testes, and is also the predominant isoform in thyroid follicular cells.[39,79] Most of the genetic alterations in thyroid cancer exert their oncogenic effect via activation of the MAPK pathway. The RAF isoforms activate the MAPK/ERK kinase (MEK) cascade (Fig. 9.1).[80] This is a key component in the MAPK pathway responsible for activating transcription of genes involved in cell proliferation, survival and apoptosis.[80] When constitutively activated, the MAPK pathway leads to tumorigenesis.[81] Among the three isoforms, BRAF is the most potent activator of the MAPK pathway.[82,83]

The BRAF-activating point mutation in thyroid cancer is almost exclusively a thymine–adenine transversion at position 1799 (T1799A) in exon 15. This leads to a valine–glutamate substitution at residue 600 (V600E) and subsequent constitutive activation of the BRAF kinase.[84,85] The *BRAF* mutation is reported in 29–83% of PTC, making it the most common oncogene identified in sporadic PTC (Table 9.1).[39,86–94] It appears to be limited to PTC, PDTC and ATC.[39] and has not been found in follicular carcinoma or benign thyroid neoplasms. Some studies have shown a 'non-V600E' *BRAF* mutation in follicular adenomas and FVPTC.[87,95,96]

The high frequency and specificity of the *BRAF* mutation suggests a fundamental role in the initiation of PTC tumorigenesis. This is supported by further studies which show that a subset of papillary microcarcinomas harbour the *BRAF* mutation and that this oncogene may be activated during tumour initiation.[89] Transgenic mice with thyroid-specific expression of mutated BRAF develop PTC which progresses to PDTC.[101] This confirms that *BRAF* mutation may be a tumour-initiating early event in PTC and suggests a step-wise progression of PTC to PDTC and ATC. The *BRAF* mutation has been found in approximately 15% of PDTC and ATC.[89,91] *BRAF* mutation-positive ATC is probably derived from *BRAF* mutation-positive PTC. The co-existence of PTC and ATC in the same tumour, both of which harbour the *BRAF* mutation, supports this theory.[39,89,93,99,100]

PTCs with *BRAF* mutation have distinct phenotypic and biological properties. They behave more aggressively and carry a poorer prognosis.[93] The tall cell variant usually harbours the *BRAF* mutation.[39,69,89] PTCs with *BRAF* mutation tend to present at an advanced stage with extrathyroidal extension, exhibit locoregional recurrence and are less responsive to radioactive iodine.[89,91,97,98]

A new mechanism of BRAF activation has recently been identified which involves inversion of chromosome 7q leading to an in-frame fusion between *BRAF* and the *AKAP9* gene.[102] This activating re-arrangement generates a constitutively active oncoprotein which is more common in PTC associated with radiation exposure.[103]

Although *RAS* and *BRAF* mutations both activate the MAPK pathway, the latter appears to be a marker for papillary thyroid carcinomas whereas *RAS* mutations are more often found in FTC or FVPTC. This suggests that the RAS and BRAF oncoproteins activate distinct sets of downstream effectors. *BRAF* mutations, *RAS* mutations and *RET/PTC* re-arrangements all appear to be mutually exclusive in PTC.[69,86,87]

PI3K/AKT/*PTEN*

PI3K/AKT signalling results in cell growth and inhibition of apoptosis mediated by phosphorylation of downstream targets by the serine threonine kinase AKT. The PI3K/AKT pathway is negatively regulated by *PTEN* but activated by *RAS* and *RET/PTC* (Fig. 9.1). Mutations of the tumour suppressor gene *PTEN* have been identified in up to 25% of sporadic follicular adenomas and carcinomas but rarely in PTC.[104–106] Germline *PTEN* gene mutations have been identified in patients with Cowden's syndrome, an autosomal dominant condition characterized by multiple hamartomas of skin, intestine, breast and thyroid (described in further detail in a later section).[107,108]

Nuclear receptors and cell cycle regulation

PAX8-PPARγ

The *PAX8* gene encodes a transcription factor essential for the genesis of thyroid follicular cell lineages and regulation of thyroid-specific gene expression. The peroxisome proliferator-activated receptor γ (PPARγ) is a member of the nuclear hormone receptor superfamily that includes thyroid hormone, retinoic acid, and androgen and oestrogen receptors.[52] The *PAX8-PPARγ* re-arrangement leads to in-frame fusion of exon 7, 8 or 9 of *PAX8* on 2q13 with exon 1 of *PPARγ* on 3p25.[109] The exact mechanism by which this re-arrangement imparts a carcinogenic phenotype is not fully understood. It appears that PAX8-PPARγ chimeric protein inactivates the wild-type PPARγ, a putative tumour suppressor.[109,110]

PAX8-PPARγ re-arrangement is involved in the development of FTC occurring in 33% of these tumours (Table 9.1).[7,111–115] However, it also occurs in follicular adenomas and is not specific for carcinoma.[111] It has not been detected in PDTC or ATC and its role in tumour progression is not well defined.

Cyclin D1

Cell cycle regulators govern growth activity. 'Progression' factors (cyclin D1, cyclin E1, cyclin-dependent kinases (CDKs) and E2Fs) and competitor factors (retinoblastoma protein RB, $p16^{INK4A}$, $p21^{CIP1}$, $p27^{KIP1}$ and p53) regulate transition from G1 to S phase. Overexpression of cyclin D1 has been documented in PTC and FTC. Expression of cyclin D1 and cyclin E1 is observed in 30–76% of papillary thyroid carcinomas.[116–120] Furthermore, cyclin D1 overexpression correlates with metastatic spread in PTC, and significant overexpression of cyclin D1 is also observed in ATC.[121–123] Upregulation of transcription or a post-transcriptional event is the likely mechanism.[121]

p53

The *p53* gene encodes a nuclear transcription factor that plays a central role in the regulation of the cell cycle, DNA repair and apoptosis.[124] As the 'policeman' of the genome, *p53* is overexpressed following cellular exposure to DNA-damaging agents and causes transient cell cycle arrest, presumably to allow for DNA repair.[125] If the damage is severe, it initiates apoptosis to prevent replication of the flawed cell.[7] Cells with impaired *p53* function are likely to accumulate genetic damage and exhibit a selective advantage for clonal expansion. Alterations in the *p53* tumour suppressor gene occur by deletion or inactivating point mutations, usually involving exons 5–8. The end result is progressive genome destabilization, additional mutations and propagation of malignant clones. This represents the most frequent genetic damage in human cancer and it usually occurs as a late tumorigenic event.[52]

Among thyroid tumours, *p53* mutations are generally restricted to PDTC and ATC.[126,127] Point mutations of *p53* occur in approximately 60% of ATC and in 25% of PDTC (Table 9.1).[126–132] Tumours containing both well-differentiated and anaplastic components exhibit *p53* mutations in the anaplastic component only.[126,130,133] These findings support the hypothesis that *p53* inactivation serves as a second hit, triggering tumour de-differentiation and progression to PDTC and ATC. Transgenic mice with thyroid-specific *RET/PTC* re-arrangements develop PTC, but when crossed with $p53^{-/-}$ mice, the progeny succumb to rapidly growing PDTC and ATC.[134,135] Conversely, the recovery of wild-type *p53* in cultured ATC cells leads to re-expression of thyroid-specific genes and the re-ability to respond to thyroid-stimulating hormone (TSH).[136,137] It is therefore unlikely that *p53* mutation is an initiating event in PDTC or ATC; rather it is a late event that contributes to the evolution of the transformed phenotype.

Cell surface adhesion molecules

Cadherins

Cadherins belong to a family of single transmembrane calcium-dependent cell–cell adhesion proteins.[11] There are three classical cadherins: neuronal (N)-, placental (P)- and epithelial (E)-cadherin. E-cadherin is highly expressed in normal thyroid and benign adenomas. Its expression is thought to be regulated by gene promoter methylation.[141] E-cadherin is required for normal epithelial differentiation and suppresses tumour spread and invasion. Expression is maintained in some well-differentiated minimally invasive thyroid carcinomas. In widely invasive, anaplastic, recurrent or metastatic thyroid carcinomas, expression is low or absent.[138–140]

β-Catenin

β-Catenin, a cytoplasmic protein encoded by the *CTNNB1* gene, plays an important role in E-cadherin-mediated cell–cell adhesion. It is also an integral intermediate in the wingless (Wnt) signalling pathway.[142] Point mutations in exon 3 of the gene stabilize the protein and make it insensitive to degradation by the adenomatous polyposis coli (APC) multiprotein complex. This results in accumulation of β-catenin and activation of target gene expression. β-Catenin upregulates the transcriptional activity of cyclin D1, C-*MYC*, C-*JUN* and other genes. Point mutations in exon 3 have been reported in up to 25% of PDTC and 66% of ATC, but not in WDTC (Table 9.1).[143,144] This suggests that these mutations represent a late event in the tumour progression model and directly trigger de-differentiation.

Fibronectin

Fibronectin is an extracellular matrix protein that regulates cell adhesion, migration, invasion and metastasis. Fibronectin expression is upregulated in WDTC compared with normal thyroid tissue.[145,146] In contrast, reduced fibronectin expression is documented in transformed cell lines and at the periphery of invasive WDTC.[147] The tumour suppressor *PTEN* has been shown to increase fibronectin-mediated cell adhesion.[148]

CD44

CD44 is a polymorphic family of integral membrane proteoglycans and glycoproteins involved in cell–cell adhesion, cell–matrix adhesion, cell migration and tumour metastasis. Multiple different CD44 isoforms exist as a result of alternative mRNA splicing. Variant CD44 molecules are expressed widely throughout the body on epithelial cells in a tissue-specific pattern.[149,150] Significant levels of CD44 protein are expressed on the plasma membranes of papillary thyroid cancer cells.[151] PTC exhibits specific patterns of aberrant CD44 mRNA splicing. These aberrations are postulated to affect the function of CD44 protein molecules and might regulate PTC growth patterns and metastatic potential.[152,153]

DNA methylation

Epigenetic alterations, i.e. changes around a gene which alter gene expression without affecting the nucleotide sequence, play a fundamental role in the regulation of human gene expression.[154] Mechanisms include DNA methylation and histone modifications. Gene promoter methylation, particularly near a transcription start site, usually results in silencing of the gene.[155,156]

Aberrant methylation and hence inappropriate silencing of tumour suppressor genes is common in thyroid tumours. Examples of these genes include *PTEN*, *RASSF1A*, tissue inhibitor of metalloproteinase-3 (*TIMP3*), *SLC5A8*, death-associated protein kinase (*DAPK*) and retinoic acid receptor β2 (*RAR 2*). These tumour suppressor genes have well-established functions and it is likely that silencing them plays an important role in thyroid tumorigenesis.[157–161]

Other molecular factors

Angiogenic factors

Vascular endothelial growth factor (VEGF) plays a critical role in angiogenesis. Increased expression of VEGF has been reported in thyroid carcinomas.[162–164] VEGF overexpression correlates with the density of lymphatics and lymph node metastasis, and may contribute to the papillary morphogenesis of PTC.[165,166] Abrogation of VEGF activity with an anti-VEGF monoclonal antibody inhibits the growth of ATC and PTC xenografts in nude mice.[167,168]

Growth factors

Several growth factors have been described in thyroid neoplasms. These include transforming growth factor-α (TGF-α), epidermal growth factor (EGF), insulin-like growth factor (IGF-1) and fibroblast growth factors 1 and 2 (FGF-1 and FGF-2). They have been shown to stimulate thyroid cell proliferation and are overexpressed in benign and malignant thyroid neoplasms.[169] Growth factor overexpression is likely to be a secondary rather than a primary event in thyroid cancer pathogenesis.

TSH receptor and G-proteins

Activating mutations of the TSH receptor have been described in toxic hyperfunctioning adenomas.[170] Adenomas rarely exhibit malignant behaviour, supporting the idea that activation of the adenylate cyclase pathway maintains the differentiated thyrocyte phenotype. Activating mutations in the TSH receptor are quite rare in WDTC and PDTC.[171]

When TSH binds to its membrane receptor, a conformational change occurs in the TSH receptor allowing it to bind trimeric G-proteins. This results in dissociation of the Gsα subunit from the G-protein complex, allowing Gsα to stimulate adenylate cyclase and produce cAMP. The cAMP exerts its downstream effects by activating cAMP-dependent protein kinase A (PKA) which catalyses the transfer of phosphate groups from adenosine triphosphate (ATP) to specific serine or threonine residues of selected proteins (Fig. 9.1). The oncogene *gsp* encodes the Gsα subunit, and is commonly mutated in hyperfunctioning adenomas.[170] Activating *gsp* mutations have occasionally been described in thyroid cancers. However, this is rare, and it is likely that *gsp* must be activated in concert with another oncogene to promote cancer formation.

Genomic instability

Thyroid cancers accumulate a number of alterations at the genomic level and it is likely that this plays a crucial role in tumour progression.[174] Chromosome instability has been identified in follicular adenomas and carcinomas. These tumours are frequently aneuploid with a high prevalence of loss of heterozygosity (LOH) involving multiple chromosomal regions. PTC cells exhibit less frequent LOH.[172,173] This contrasting pattern of chromosome instability suggests that these two distinct types of thyroid cancer occur through discrete molecular pathways.

Certain genetic aberrations (MAPK activation and *p53* inactivation) appear to render rapidly dividing cells more susceptible to further genetic damage. As additional mutations are acquired, cells may attain a growth advantage, evade apoptosis and continue to proliferate, accumulating further genetic damage. This 'multiple hit' theory predicts a multistep process of clonal evolution in thyroid neoplasms (Fig. 9.2).

Genetic syndromes associated with non-medullary thyroid carcinoma

The prevalence of thyroid cancer is increased in certain genetic syndromes. This group includes Cowden's syndrome, Gardner's syndrome, familial adenomatous polyposis (FAP) and familial papillary thyroid cancer syndromes.[175–178]

Cowden's syndrome is an autosomal dominant disorder resulting from a germline mutation of the *PTEN* gene. Mucocutaneous manifestations include trichilemmomas, oral papillomas, and acral and palmo-plantar keratoses. Thyroid nodules or thyroiditis are present in 60–70% of patients. Affected patients have an increased incidence of endometrial and thyroid carcinomas. The lifetime risk of thyroid cancer, which is mostly FTC, approaches 10%.

Thyroid tumours associated with FAP are often a cribiform variant of PTC and are clinically detectable in 2% of patients.[179]

MEDULLARY THYROID CARCINOMA

Medullary thyroid carcinomas (MTCs) arise from the parafollicular or C cells of the thyroid. These tumours are uncommon and account for 15% of all thyroid malignancies. Approximately 80% of MTCs are sporadic, whereas the remainder appear to be familial.[10]

The tumours in patients with sporadic MTC vary considerably in size but are usually unilateral and sometimes arise from a somatic *RET* mutation in a single cell. In contrast, familial MTC tumours are frequently bilateral, multicentric and almost always result from a germline *RET* mutation that affects all cells.[180]

Familial MTC is an autosomal dominant disorder that occurs in three recognized forms: familial non-MEN medullary thyroid carcinoma (FMTC), MTC associated with multiple endocrine neoplasia type 2A syndrome (MEN2A) and MTC associated with MEN2B syndrome. The genetic predisposition to develop a familial MTC is conferred by a point mutation in the germline DNA that encodes the *RET* oncogene.[181] These mutations serve constitutively to activate the tyrosine kinase function of the *RET* gene product and predispose to the development of C-cell hyperplasia and multifocal MTC.

Several inherited *RET* mutations have been described in the three inherited medullary thyroid carcinoma syndromes, each demonstrating different mechanisms of oncogenic activation. In MEN2A, 98% of mutations are in the extracellular domain and involve changing a cysteine to a non-cysteine residue. Cysteine residues normally form intramolecular disulphide bonds. When one is mutated, the other forms an intermolecular bond with another mutant RET receptor, causing constitutive dimerization and activation of the receptor.[182–184] In MEN2B, 95–98% of patients demonstrate a point mutation in the kinase domain of *RET* that changes a

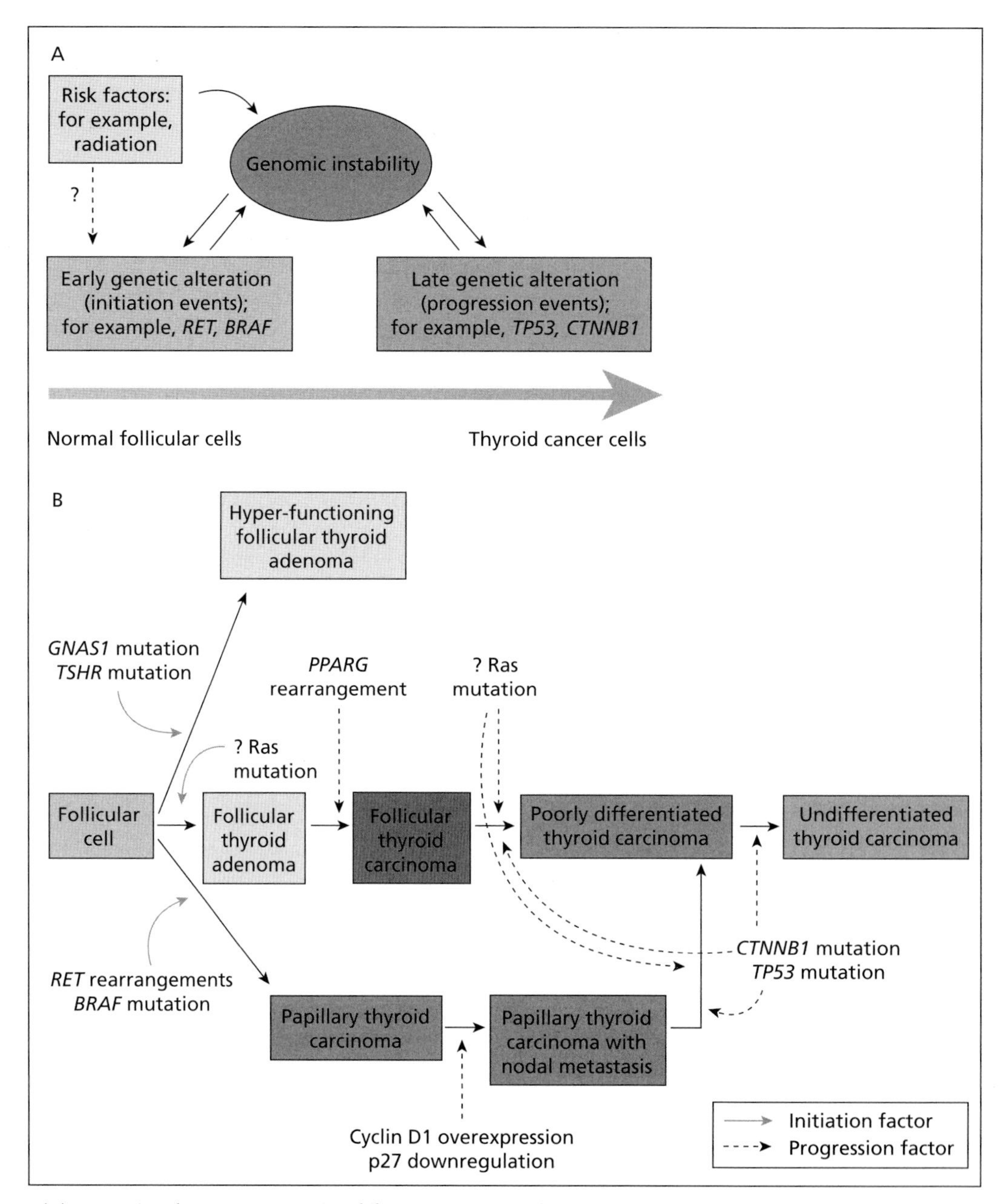

Fig. 9.2 (A) Interactions between genomic instability and genetic alterations promotes progression from well-differentiated to undifferentiated thyroid carcinoma. (B) Distinct pathways proposed for neoplastic proliferation of thyroid follicular cells. Hyperfunctioning follicular thyroid adenoma is almost always benign without propensity for progression. Reprinted by permission from Macmillan Publishers Ltd: Nature Reviews Cancer (6:292–306), copyright (2006).

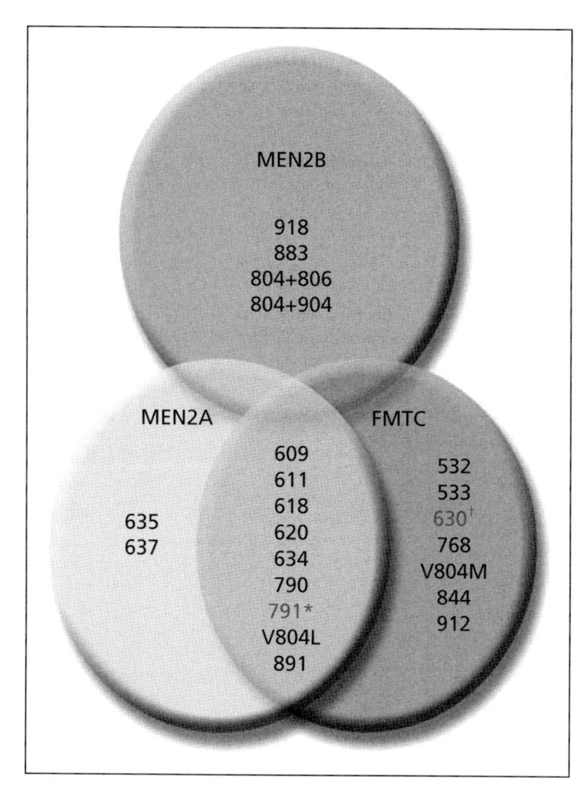

Fig. 9.3 Correlation of specific *RET* codon mutations with the phenotypic expression of hereditary MTC. *Development of pheochromocytoma has not been reported. †Distinction between MEN2A and FMTC cannot be made. Adapted from: Kouvaraki, MA, *et al.* RET proto-oncogene: a review and update of genotype-phenotype correlations in hereditary medullary thyroid cancer and associated endocrine tumors. Thyroid 2005;15:531–44.

methionine to a threonine. This initiates tyrosine kinase activity, although a ligand is still required for full activation of the receptor.[185] These different mechanisms of *RET* oncogene activation may account for the phenotypic variation between MEN2A and MEN2B. Known *RET* mutations in familial MTC and their biological aggressiveness are summarized in Fig. 9.3 and Plate 9.1.[186]

NEW MOLECULAR TARGETED THERAPIES IN THYROID CANCER

Thyroid cancer serves as a good model for targeted therapies. The retained expression and function of the TSH receptor and sodium–iodide symporter (NIS) in most thyroid cells enables levothyroxine and radioiodine to suppress TSH levels successfully following surgery. This has led to remarkable long-term survival rates for patients with early stage thyroid cancers, approaching 98% at 20 years.[187] However, this excellent prognosis is not shared by individuals with aggressive thyroid cancers (such as PDTC or ATC) because they de-differentiate, losing expression and function of both the TSH receptor and NIS. These tumours have increased rates of recurrence and metastasis and do not respond well to traditional non-targeted cytotoxic chemotherapeutic agents. This has led to the development of novel targeted therapies which utilize recent advances in our understanding of the critical pathways involved in thyroid cancer initiation and progression.

Hopes for identification of molecular treatment targets have been fuelled by the tyrosine kinase gene alterations BCR/Abl and the cKIT mutation for the tyrosine kinase inhibitor Gleevec.[188] The frequent presence of constitutively active tyrosine kinase genes in thyroid cancer makes them logical candidates for targeted treatment. RET and RAS/RAF/MAPK novel targeted therapies are all being developed. Recent examples include ZD6474 (Vandetanib, Astra Zeneca), a tyrosine kinase inhibitor, which blocks the activity of RET-derived oncoproteins. It successfully inhibited tumour growth of RET/PTC-transformed NIH-3T3 cells in nude mice.[189,190] In addition, ZD6474 is an orally bioavailable inhibitor of EGF receptor and VEGF signalling pathways, both of which may be involved in thyroid cancer pathogenesis.[191] Phase I clinical trials demonstrated that it was generally well tolerated, with adverse events including rash, diarrhoea and asymptomatic QTc prolongation.[192,193] An international, randomized, placebo-controlled phase II trial in MTC is now accruing patients. Given the high rates of activation of RET in PTC, phase II trials using ZD6474 are also planned.[194]

AMG706 is a potent oral, multikinase inhibitor that targets VEGF, platelet-derived growth factor (PDGF), KIT and RET receptors, and has anti-angiogenic and anti-tumour activity. In a pre-clinical study, it produced a statistically significant reduction in vascular blood flow in human tumour xenografts.[195] A phase II study of AMG706 in advanced thyroid cancer is ongoing.

PP1 and PP2 are pyrazolopyrimidines with a strong activity toward RET kinase. They are small molecule tyrosine kinase inhibitors which block RET/PTC signalling and abolish tumorigenic effects in experimental animals.[196,197]

Downstream of RET, the association of MAPK signalling members such as RAS and BRAF with aggressive thyroid cancer subtypes, along with their independent prognostic value, make them ideal subjects for targeted treatment. Both *in vitro* and *in vivo* studies showed that inhibition of oncogenic RAS and BRAF led to tumour shrinkage in several human tumour types.[198] The multikinase inhibitor BAY 43-9006 (Sorafenib, Bayer) was one of the first molecules to undergo clinical development. It is a potent competitive inhibitor of ATP binding and inhibits BRAF-stimulated DNA synthesis and cell proliferation whilst inducing apoptosis in thyroid cancer cells.[199] Sorafenib has also been shown to exert an anti-angiogenic effect by targeting the receptor tyrosine kinases VEGFR-2 and PDGFR and their associated signalling cascades.[200] Sorafenib inhibits BRAF signalling and growth of all thyroid cell lines carrying the *BRAF* mutation.[201] It also retarded the growth of ATC cell line xenografts in nude mice.[201,202] A huge phase I programme with Sorafenib has been carried out, and a phase II trial in thyroid carcinoma is planned.

Cytostatic suppression of MEK signalling further downstream along the MAPK cascade has been achieved with the MEK inhibitor CI-1040. It was found to abrogate tumour growth in BRAF mutant xenografts derived from various tumour types.[203] RAS and BRAF inhibition has been shown to result in re-differentiation with resultant re-expression of thyroid-specific genes, including the NIS gene.[204,205] MAPK inhibition may not only inhibit tumour growth, but also restore radioactive iodine avidity in a significant proportion of de-differentiated/advanced thyroid cancers.

In addition to MAPK signalling, several studies have assessed the feasibility of PI3K/AKT inhibition and p53 targeting in thyroid cancer. Furuya *et al.* demonstrated that LY294002, a potent PI3K inhibitor, reduced tumour cell proliferation and blocked metastatic spread of thyroid tumours in a mouse model of follicular thyroid cancer.[206] Treatment of thyroid cancer cells with the AKT inhibitor KP372-1 also suppressed cell proliferation and induced apoptosis in thyroid cancer cells.[207] Other promising agents include histone deacetylase inhibitors and PPARγ expression ligands.[208–214]

It is hoped that these efforts will substantially improve the outcome of patients with aggressive, refractory, metastatic disease. Numerous clinical trials are currently underway to assess the viability of targeting some of the pathways described in this chapter (Table 9.2).

Table 9.2 Ongoing clinical trials on molecular targeting of thyroid cancer at the NCI (http://www.cancer.gov/clinicaltrials/search)

Phase II/III Study of Combretastatin and Paclitaxel/Carboplatin in the Treatment of Anaplastic Thyroid Cancer (OXC4T4-302)
Phase I/II study of Vandetanib in Treating Young Patients With Medullary Thyroid Cancer NCI-07-C-0189
Phase II study of FR901228 in Treating Patients With Recurrent and/or Metastatic Thyroid Cancer That Has Not Responded to Radioactive Iodine MSKCC-04059
Phase II study of Rosiglitazone in Treating Patients With Locoregionally Extensive or Metastatic Thyroid Cancer UCSF-03201
Phase II Study of Irinotecan in Patients With Metastatic or Inoperable Locoregional Medullary Thyroid Cancer JHOC-J0459
Phase II study of Bortezomib in Treating Patients With Metastatic Thyroid Cancer That Did Not Respond to Radioactive Iodine Therapy MDA-2004-0059
Phase II study of Sorafenib in Treating Patients With Advanced Anaplastic Thyroid Cancer CASE-5304
Phase II Trial Evaluating Gleevec in Patients With Anaplastic Thyroid Carcinoma UMCC 2003-044
Phase II study of Lenalidomide in Treating Patients With Metastatic Thyroid Cancer That Has Not Responded to Radioactive Iodine and Cannot Be Removed By Surgery UKMC-05-0701-F3R
Phase II Study of Sunitinib Malate in Patients With Iodine I 131-Refractory, Unresectable Well-Differentiated Thyroid Cancer or Medullary Thyroid Cancer UCCRC-NCI-7735
Phase II study of Sorafenib in Treating Patients With Metastatic, Locally Advanced, or Recurrent Medullary Thyroid Cancer OSU-06054
Phase II Study Of AG-013736 In Patients With Doxorubicin-Refractory Or Intolerant Thyroid Cancer A4061027. An efficacy phase II Study Comparing ZD6474 to Placebo in Medullary Thyroid Cancer D4200C00058
Phase II study of Sunitinib and Imaging Procedures in Treating Patients With Thyroid Cancer FHCRC-6494
Phase I study of NGR-TNF in Treating Patients With Advanced Solid Tumors EORTC-16041

EVIDENCE APPRAISAL

This chapter is unique in that most of the evidence is based on laboratory data. There is no level of evidence to assign these data. Most of the experiments were well designed with adequate controls and validation studies. There are very few data based on clinical trials because the trials are still in phase I or II.

REFERENCES

1. Sarlis NJ, Benvenga S. Molecular signaling in thyroid cancer. Cancer Treat Res 2004;122:237–64.
2. Sarlis NJ. Expression patterns of cellular growth-controlling genes in non-medullary thyroid cancer: basic aspects. Rev Endocr Metab Disord 2000;1:183–96.
3. Venkatesh YS, *et al.* Anaplastic carcinoma of the thyroid. A clinicopathologic study of 121 cases. Cancer 1990;66:321–30.
4. Carcangiu ML, *et al.* Anaplastic thyroid carcinoma. A study of 70 cases. Am J Clin Pathol 1985;83:135–58.
5. Carcangiu ML, Zampi G, Rosai J. Poorly differentiated ('insular') thyroid carcinoma. A reinterpretation of Langhans' 'wuchernde Struma'. Am J Surg Pathol 1984;8:655–68.
6. Sakamoto A, Kasai N, Sugano H. Poorly differentiated carcinoma of the thyroid. A clinicopathologic entity for a high-risk group of papillary and follicular carcinomas. Cancer 1983;52:1849–55.
7. Nikiforov YE. Genetic alterations involved in the transition from well-differentiated to poorly differentiated and anaplastic thyroid carcinomas. Endocr Pathol 2004;15:319–27.
8. Rosai J, Saxen EA, Woolner L. Undifferentiated and poorly differentiated carcinoma. Semin Diagn Pathol 1985;2:123–36.
9. Hunt JL, *et al.* Molecular evidence of anaplastic transformation in coexisting well-differentiated and anaplastic carcinomas of the thyroid. Am J Surg Pathol 2003;27:1559–64.
10. DeLellis RA. Pathology and genetics of thyroid carcinoma. J Surg Oncol 2006;94:662–9.
11. Kondo T, Ezzat S, Asa SL. Pathogenetic mechanisms in thyroid follicular-cell neoplasia. Nat Rev Cancer 2006;6:292–306.
12. Airaksinen MS, Saarma M. The GDNF family: signalling, biological functions and therapeutic value. Nat Rev Neurosci 2002;3:383–94.
13. Neumann S, *et al.* Lack of correlation for sodium iodide symporter mRNA and protein expression and analysis of sodium iodide symporter promoter methylation in benign cold thyroid nodules. Thyroid 2004;14:99–111.
14. Viglietto G, *et al.* RET/PTC oncogene activation is an early event in thyroid carcinogenesis. Oncogene 1995;11:1207–10.
15. Nikiforova MN, *et al.* Proximity of chromosomal loci that participate in radiation-induced rearrangements in human cells. Science 2000;290:138–41.
16. Roccato E, *et al.* Proximity of TPR and NTRK1 rearranging loci in human thyrocytes. Cancer Res 2005;65:2572–6.
17. Santoro M, *et al.* Ret oncogene activation in human thyroid neoplasms is restricted to the papillary cancer subtype. J Clin Invest 1992;89:1517–22.
18. Santoro M, *et al.* Involvement of RET oncogene in human tumours: specificity of RET activation to thyroid tumours. Br J Cancer 1993;68:460–4.
19. Santoro M, *et al.* Gene rearrangement and Chernobyl related thyroid cancers. Br J Cancer 2000;82:315–22.
20. Vecchio G, Santoro M. Oncogenes and thyroid cancer. Clin Chem Lab Med 2000;38:113–6.
21. Moretti F, Nanni S, Pontecorvi A. Molecular pathogenesis of thyroid nodules and cancer. Baillieres Best Pract Res Clin Endocrinol Metab 2000;14:517–39.
22. Learoyd DL, *et al.* RET/PTC and RET tyrosine kinase expression in adult papillary thyroid carcinomas. J Clin Endocrinol Metab 1998;83:3631–5.
23. De Vita G, *et al.* Expression of the RET/PTC1 oncogene impairs the activity of TTF-1 and Pax-8 thyroid transcription factors. Cell Growth Differ 1998;9:97–103.
24. Ishizaka Y, *et al.* Detection of retTPC/PTC transcripts in thyroid adenomas and adenomatous goiter by an RT-PCR method. Oncogene 1991;6:1667–72.
25. Jhiang SM, *et al.* Detection of the PTC/retTPC oncogene in human thyroid cancers. Oncogene 1992;7:1331–7.
26. Sugg SL, *et al.* ret/PTC-1, -2, and -3 oncogene rearrangements in human thyroid carcinomas: implications for metastatic potential? J Clin Endocrinol Metab 1996;81:3360–5.
27. Delvincourt C, *et al.* Ret and trk proto-oncogene activation in thyroid papillary carcinomas in French patients from the Champagne–Ardenne region. Clin Biochem 1996;29:267–71.
28. Bounacer A, *et al.* High prevalence of activating ret proto-oncogene rearrangements, in thyroid tumors from patients who had received external radiation. Oncogene 1997;15:1263–73.
29. Bongarzone I, *et al.* Frequent activation of ret protooncogene by fusion with a new activating gene in papillary thyroid carcinomas. Cancer Res 1994;54:2979–85.
30. Santoro M, *et al.* Development of thyroid papillary carcinomas secondary to tissue-specific expression of the RET/PTC1 oncogene in transgenic mice. Oncogene 1996;12:1821–6.
31. Cheung CC, *et al.* Analysis of ret/PTC gene rearrangements refines the fine needle aspiration diagnosis of thyroid cancer. J Clin Endocrinol Metab 2001;86:2187–90.
32. Nikiforov YE. RET/PTC rearrangement in thyroid tumors. Endocr Pathol 2002;13:3–16.
33. Fagin JA. Perspective: lessons learned from molecular genetic studies of thyroid cancer—insights into pathogenesis and tumor-specific therapeutic targets. Endocrinology 2002;143:2025–8.
34. Bongarzone I, *et al.* Age-related activation of the tyrosine kinase receptor protooncogenes RET and NTRK1 in papillary thyroid carcinoma. J Clin Endocrinol Metab 1996;81:2006–9.
35. Nikiforov YE, *et al.* Distinct pattern of ret oncogene rearrangements in morphological variants of radiation-

induced and sporadic thyroid papillary carcinomas in children. Cancer Res 1997;57:1690–4.
36. Klugbauer S, *et al.* A new form of RET rearrangement in thyroid carcinomas of children after the Chernobyl reactor accident. Oncogene 1996;13:1099–102.
37. Klugbauer S, *et al.* High prevalence of RET rearrangement in thyroid tumors of children from Belarus after the Chernobyl reactor accident. Oncogene 1995;11:2459–67.
38. Fugazzola L, *et al.* Oncogenic rearrangements of the RET proto-oncogene in papillary thyroid carcinomas from children exposed to the Chernobyl nuclear accident. Cancer Res 1995;55:5617–20.
39. Xing M. BRAF mutation in thyroid cancer. Endocr Relat Cancer 2005;12:245–62.
40. Jhiang SM, *et al.* Targeted expression of the ret/PTC1 oncogene induces papillary thyroid carcinomas. Endocrinology 1996;137:375–8.
41. Powell DJ Jr, *et al.* The RET/PTC3 oncogene: metastatic solid-type papillary carcinomas in murine thyroids. Cancer Res 1998;58:5523–8.
42. Tallini G, Asa SL. RET oncogene activation in papillary thyroid carcinoma. Adv Anat Pathol 2001;8:345–54.
43. Tallini G, *et al.* RET/PTC oncogene activation defines a subset of papillary thyroid carcinomas lacking evidence of progression to poorly differentiated or undifferentiated tumor phenotypes. Clin Cancer Res 1998;4:287–94.
44. Santoro M, *et al.* RET activation and clinicopathologic features in poorly differentiated thyroid tumors. J Clin Endocrinol Metab 2002;87:370–9.
45. Lanzi C, *et al.* Inhibition of transforming activity of the ret/ptc1 oncoprotein by a 2-indolinone derivative. Int J Cancer 2000;85:384–90.
46. Miller FD, Kaplan DR. On Trk for retrograde signaling. Neuron 2001;32:767–70.
47. Greco A, Roccato E, Pierotti MA. TRK oncogenes in papillary thyroid carcinoma. Cancer Treat Res 2004;122:207–19.
48. Bongarzone I, *et al.* RET/NTRK1 rearrangements in thyroid gland tumors of the papillary carcinoma family: correlation with clinicopathological features. Clin Cancer Res 1998;4:223–8.
49. Pierotti MA. Chromosomal rearrangements in thyroid carcinomas: a recombination or death dilemma. Cancer Lett 2001;166:1–7.
50. Beimfohr C, *et al.* NTRK1 re-arrangement in papillary thyroid carcinomas of children after the Chernobyl reactor accident. Int J Cancer 1999;80:842–7.
51. Rabes HM, *et al.* Pattern of radiation-induced RET and NTRK1 rearrangements in 191 post-Chernobyl papillary thyroid carcinomas: biological, phenotypic, and clinical implications. Clin Cancer Res 2000;6:1093–103.
52. Tallini G. Molecular pathobiology of thyroid neoplasms. Endocr Pathol 2002;13:271–88.
53. Di Renzo MF, *et al.* Expression of the Met/HGF receptor in normal and neoplastic human tissues. Oncogene 1991;6:1997–2003.
54. Di Renzo MF, *et al.* Overexpression of the c-MET/HGF receptor gene in human thyroid carcinomas. Oncogene 1992;7:2549–53.
55. Di Renzo MF, *et al.* Overexpression of the c-MET/HGF receptor in human thyroid carcinomas derived from the follicular epithelium. J Endocrinol Invest 1995;18:134–9.
56. Ruco LP, *et al.* Expression of Met protein in thyroid tumours. J Pathol 1996;180:266–70.
57. Ivan M, *et al.* Activated ras and ret oncogenes induce overexpression of c-met (hepatocyte growth factor receptor) in human thyroid epithelial cells. Oncogene 1997;14:2417–23.
58. Chen BK, *et al.* Overexpression of c-Met protein in human thyroid tumors correlated with lymph node metastasis and clinicopathologic stage. Pathol Res Pract 1999;195:427–33.
59. Belfiore A, *et al.* Negative/low expression of the Met/hepatocyte growth factor receptor identifies papillary thyroid carcinomas with high risk of distant metastases. J Clin Endocrinol Metab 1997;82:2322–8.
60. Barbacid M. ras genes. Annu Rev Biochem 1987;56:779–827.
61. Finney RE, Bishop JM. Predisposition to neoplastic transformation caused by gene replacement of H-ras1. Science 1993;260:1524–7.
62. Lemoine NR, *et al.* High frequency of ras oncogene activation in all stages of human thyroid tumorigenesis. Oncogene 1989;4:159–64.
63. Namba H, *et al.* H-ras protooncogene mutations in human thyroid neoplasms. J Clin Endocrinol Metab 1990;71:223–9.
64. Suarez HG, *et al.* Presence of mutations in all three ras genes in human thyroid tumors. Oncogene 1990;5:565–70.
65. Karga H, *et al.* Ras oncogene mutations in benign and malignant thyroid neoplasms. J Clin Endocrinol Metab 1991;73:832–6.
66. Manenti G, *et al.* Selective activation of ras oncogenes in follicular and undifferentiated thyroid carcinomas. Eur J Cancer 1994;30A:987–93.
67. Meinkoth JL. Biology of Ras in thyroid cells. Cancer Treat Res 2004;122:131–48.
68. Vasko V, *et al.* Specific pattern of RAS oncogene mutations in follicular thyroid tumors. J Clin Endocrinol Metab 2003;88:2745–52.
69. Adeniran AJ, *et al.* Correlation between genetic alterations and microscopic features, clinical manifestations, and prognostic characteristics of thyroid papillary carcinomas. Am J Surg Pathol 2006;30:216–22.
70. Di Cristofaro J, *et al.* Molecular genetic study comparing follicular variant versus classic papillary thyroid carcino-

mas: association of N-ras mutation in codon 61 with follicular variant. Hum Pathol 2006;37:824–30.
71. Namba H, Rubin SA, Fagin JA. Point mutations of ras oncogenes are an early event in thyroid tumorigenesis. Mol Endocrinol 1990;4:1474–9.
72. Basolo F, *et al.* N-ras mutation in poorly differentiated thyroid carcinomas: correlation with bone metastases and inverse correlation to thyroglobulin expression. Thyroid 2000;10:19–23.
73. Motoi N, *et al.* Role of ras mutation in the progression of thyroid carcinoma of follicular epithelial origin. Pathol Res Pract 2000;196:1–7.
74. Hara H, *et al.* N-ras mutation: an independent prognostic factor for aggressiveness of papillary thyroid carcinoma. Surgery 1994;116:1010–6.
75. Ezzat S, *et al.* Prevalence of activating ras mutations in morphologically characterized thyroid nodules. Thyroid 1996;6:409–16.
76. Esapa CT, *et al.* Prevalence of Ras mutations in thyroid neoplasia. Clin Endocrinol (Oxf) 1999;50:529–35.
77. Garcia-Rostan G, *et al.* ras mutations are associated with aggressive tumor phenotypes and poor prognosis in thyroid cancer. J Clin Oncol 2003;21:3226–35.
78. Rochefort P, *et al.* Thyroid pathologies in transgenic mice expressing a human activated Ras gene driven by a thyroglobulin promoter. Oncogene 1996;12:111–8.
79. Daum G, *et al.* The ins and outs of Raf kinases. Trends Biochem Sci 1994;19:474–80.
80. Chang F, *et al.* Signal transduction mediated by the Ras/Raf/MEK/ERK pathway from cytokine receptors to transcription factors: potential targeting for therapeutic intervention. Leukemia 2003;17:1263–93.
81. Peyssonnaux C, Eychene A. The Raf/MEK/ERK pathway: new concepts of activation. Biol Cell 2001;93:53–62.
82. Mercer KE, Pritchard CA. Raf proteins and cancer: B-Raf is identified as a mutational target. Biochim Biophys Acta 2003;1653:25–40.
83. Sithanandam G, *et al.* B-raf and a B-raf pseudogene are located on 7q in man. Oncogene 1992;7:795–9.
84. Kumar R, *et al.* BRAF mutations in metastatic melanoma: a possible association with clinical outcome. Clin Cancer Res 2003;9:3362–8.
85. Davies H, *et al.* Mutations of the BRAF gene in human cancer. Nature 2002;417:949–54.
86. Kimura ET, *et al.* High prevalence of BRAF mutations in thyroid cancer: genetic evidence for constitutive activation of the RET/PTC–RAS–BRAF signaling pathway in papillary thyroid carcinoma. Cancer Res 2003;63:1454–7.
87. Soares P, *et al.* BRAF mutations and RET/PTC rearrangements are alternative events in the etiopathogenesis of PTC. Oncogene 2003;22:4578–80.
88. Trovisco V, *et al.* BRAF mutations are associated with some histological types of papillary thyroid carcinoma. J Pathol 2004;202:247–51.
89. Nikiforova MN, *et al.* BRAF mutations in thyroid tumors are restricted to papillary carcinomas and anaplastic or poorly differentiated carcinomas arising from papillary carcinomas. J Clin Endocrinol Metab 2003;88:5399–404.
90. Fukushima T, *et al.* BRAF mutations in papillary carcinomas of the thyroid. Oncogene 2003;22:6455–7.
91. Namba H, *et al.* Clinical implication of hot spot BRAF mutation, V599E, in papillary thyroid cancers. J Clin Endocrinol Metab 2003;88:4393–7.
92. Xu X, *et al.* High prevalence of BRAF gene mutation in papillary thyroid carcinomas and thyroid tumor cell lines. Cancer Res 2003;63:4561–7.
93. Cohen Y, *et al.* BRAF mutation in papillary thyroid carcinoma. J Natl Cancer Inst 2003;95:625–7.
94. Kim KH, *et al.* Mutations of the BRAF gene in papillary thyroid carcinoma in a Korean population. Yonsei Med J 2004;45:818–21.
95. Lima J, *et al.* BRAF mutations are not a major event in post-Chernobyl childhood thyroid carcinomas. J Clin Endocrinol Metab 2004;89:4267–71.
96. Trovisco V, *et al.* Type and prevalence of BRAF mutations are closely associated with papillary thyroid carcinoma histotype and patients' age but not with tumour aggressiveness. Virchows Arch 2005;446:589–95.
97. Xing M, *et al.* BRAF mutation predicts a poorer clinical prognosis for papillary thyroid cancer. J Clin Endocrinol Metab 2005;90:6373–9.
98. Vasko V, *et al.* High prevalence and possible de novo formation of BRAF mutation in metastasized papillary thyroid cancer in lymph nodes. J Clin Endocrinol Metab 2005. 90:5265–9.
99. Begum S, *et al.* BRAF mutations in anaplastic thyroid carcinoma: implications for tumor origin, diagnosis and treatment. Mod Pathol 2004;17:1359–63.
100. Cohen Y, *et al.* Mutational analysis of BRAF in fine needle aspiration biopsies of the thyroid: a potential application for the preoperative assessment of thyroid nodules. Clin Cancer Res 2004;10:2761–5.
101. Knauf JA, *et al.* Targeted expression of BRAFV600E in thyroid cells of transgenic mice results in papillary thyroid cancers that undergo dedifferentiation. Cancer Res 2005;65:4238–45.
102. Ciampi R, *et al.* Oncogenic AKAP9–BRAF fusion is a novel mechanism of MAPK pathway activation in thyroid cancer. J Clin Invest 2005;115:94–101.
103. Ciampi R, Nikiforov YE. RET/PTC rearrangements and BRAF mutations in thyroid tumorigenesis. Endocrinology 2007;148:936–41.
104. Halachmi N, *et al.* Somatic mutations of the PTEN tumor suppressor gene in sporadic follicular thyroid tumors. Genes Chromosomes Cancer 1998;23:239–43.
105. Dahia PL, *et al.* Somatic deletions and mutations in the Cowden disease gene, PTEN, in sporadic thyroid tumors. Cancer Res 1997;57:4710–3.

106. Bruni P, *et al.* PTEN expression is reduced in a subset of sporadic thyroid carcinomas: evidence that PTEN growth-suppressing activity in thyroid cancer cells mediated by p27kip1. Oncogene 2000;19:3146–55.
107. Longy M, Lacombe D. Cowden disease. Report of a family and review. Ann Genet 1996;39:35–42.
108. Di Cristofano A, *et al.* Pten is essential for embryonic development and tumour suppression. Nat Genet 1998;19:348–55.
109. Kroll TG, *et al.* PAX8–PPARgamma1 fusion oncogene in human thyroid carcinoma [corrected]. Science 2000;289:1357–60.
110. Ying H, *et al.* Mutant thyroid hormone receptor beta represses the expression and transcriptional activity of peroxisome proliferator-activated receptor gamma during thyroid carcinogenesis. Cancer Res 2003;63:5274–80.
111. Marques AR, *et al.* Expression of PAX8–PPAR gamma 1 rearrangements in both follicular thyroid carcinomas and adenomas. J Clin Endocrinol Metab 2002;87:3947–52.
112. Nikiforova MN, *et al.* PAX8–PPARgamma rearrangement in thyroid tumors: RT-PCR and immunohistochemical analyses. Am J Surg Pathol 2002;26:1016–23.
113. Cheung L, *et al.* Detection of the PAX8–PPAR gamma fusion oncogene in both follicular thyroid carcinomas and adenomas. J Clin Endocrinol Metab 2003;88:354–7.
114. Dwight T, *et al.* Involvement of the PAX8/peroxisome proliferator-activated receptor gamma rearrangement in follicular thyroid tumors. J Clin Endocrinol Metab 2003;88:4440–5.
115. Castro P, *et al.* PAX8–PPARgamma rearrangement is frequently detected in the follicular variant of papillary thyroid carcinoma. J Clin Endocrinol Metab 2006;91:213–20.
116. Basolo F, *et al.* Cyclin D1 overexpression in thyroid carcinomas: relation with clinico-pathological parameters, retinoblastoma gene product, and Ki67 labeling index. Thyroid 2000;10:741–6.
117. Lazzereschi D, *et al.* Cyclin D1 and cyclin E expression in malignant thyroid cells and in human thyroid carcinomas. Int J Cancer 1998;76:806–11.
118. Zou M, *et al.* Inverse association between cyclin D1 overexpression and retinoblastoma gene mutation in thyroid carcinomas. Endocrine 1998;8:61–4.
119. Saiz AD, *et al.* Immunohistochemical expression of cyclin D1, E2F-1, and Ki-67 in benign and malignant thyroid lesions. J Pathol 2002;198:157–62.
120. Brzezinski J, *et al.* Cyclin E expression in papillary thyroid carcinoma: relation to staging. Int J Cancer 2004;109:102–5.
121. Khoo ML, *et al.* Cyclin D1 protein expression predicts metastatic behavior in thyroid papillary microcarcinomas but is not associated with gene amplification. J Clin Endocrinol Metab 2002;87:1810–3.
122. Khoo ML, *et al.* Overexpression of cyclin D1 and underexpression of p27 predict lymph node metastases in papillary thyroid carcinoma. J Clin Endocrinol Metab 2002;87:1814–8.
123. Wang S, *et al.* The role of cell cycle regulatory protein, cyclin D1, in the progression of thyroid cancer. Mod Pathol 2000;13:882–7.
124. Farid NR, Shi Y, Zou M. Molecular basis of thyroid cancer. Endocr Rev 1994;15:202–32.
125. Segev DL, Umbricht C, Zeiger MA. Molecular pathogenesis of thyroid cancer. Surg Oncol 2003;12:69–90.
126. Donghi R, *et al.* Gene p53 mutations are restricted to poorly differentiated and undifferentiated carcinomas of the thyroid gland. J Clin Invest 1993;91:1753–60.
127. Dobashi Y, *et al.* Stepwise participation of p53 gene mutation during dedifferentiation of human thyroid carcinomas. Diagn Mol Pathol 1994;3:9–14.
128. Fagin JA, *et al.* High prevalence of mutations of the p53 gene in poorly differentiated human thyroid carcinomas. J Clin Invest 1993;91:179–84.
129. Nakamura T, *et al.* p53 gene mutations associated with anaplastic transformation of human thyroid carcinomas. Jpn J Cancer Res 1992;83:1293–8.
130. Ito T, *et al.* Genetic alterations in thyroid tumor progression: association with p53 gene mutations. Jpn J Cancer Res 1993;84:526–31.
131. Ho YS, *et al.* p53 gene mutation in thyroid carcinoma. Cancer Lett 1996;103:57–63.
132. Takeuchi Y, *et al.* Mutations of p53 in thyroid carcinoma with an insular component. Thyroid 1999;9:377–81.
133. Matias-Guiu X, *et al.* p53 in a thyroid follicular carcinoma with foci of poorly differentiated and anaplastic carcinoma. Pathol Res Pract 1996;192:1242–9; discussion 1250–1.
134. La Perle KM, Jhiang SM, Capen CC. Loss of p53 promotes anaplasia and local invasion in ret/PTC1-induced thyroid carcinomas. Am J Pathol 2000;157:671–7.
135. Powell DJ Jr, *et al.* Altered gene expression in immunogenic poorly differentiated thyroid carcinomas from RET/PTC3p53–/– mice. Oncogene 2001;20:3235–46.
136. Moretti F, *et al.* p53 re-expression inhibits proliferation and restores differentiation of human thyroid anaplastic carcinoma cells. Oncogene 1997;14:729–40.
137. Fagin JA, *et al.* Reexpression of thyroid peroxidase in a derivative of an undifferentiated thyroid carcinoma cell line by introduction of wild-type p53. Cancer Res 1996;56:765–71.
138. Brabant G, *et al.* E-cadherin: a differentiation marker in thyroid malignancies. Cancer Res 1993;53:4987–93.
139. Scheumman GF, *et al.* Clinical significance of E-cadherin as a prognostic marker in thyroid carcinomas. J Clin Endocrinol Metab 1995;80:2168–72.
140. Kato N, *et al.* E-cadherin expression in follicular carcinoma of the thyroid. Pathol Int 2002;52:13–8.
141. Soares P, *et al.* E-cadherin gene alterations are rare events in thyroid tumors. Int J Cancer 1997;70:32–8.

142. Abbosh PH, Nephew KP. Multiple signaling pathways converge on beta-catenin in thyroid cancer. Thyroid 2005; 15:551–61.
143. Garcia-Rostan G, *et al.* Beta-catenin dysregulation in thyroid neoplasms: down-regulation, aberrant nuclear expression, and CTNNB1 exon 3 mutations are markers for aggressive tumor phenotypes and poor prognosis. Am J Pathol 2001;158:987–96.
144. Miyake N, *et al.* Absence of mutations in the beta-catenin and adenomatous polyposis coli genes in papillary and follicular thyroid carcinomas. Pathol Int 2001;51:680–5.
145. Huang Y, *et al.* Gene expression in papillary thyroid carcinoma reveals highly consistent profiles. Proc Natl Acad Sci USA 2001;98:15044–9.
146. Wasenius VM, *et al.* Hepatocyte growth factor receptor, matrix metalloproteinase-11, tissue inhibitor of metalloproteinase-1, and fibronectin are up-regulated in papillary thyroid carcinoma: a cDNA and tissue microarray study. Clin Cancer Res 2003;9:68–75.
147. Ryu S, *et al.* Strong intracellular and negative peripheral expression of fibronectin in tumor cells contribute to invasion and metastasis in papillary thyroid carcinoma. Cancer Lett 1999;146:103–9.
148. Liu W, Asa SL, Ezzat S. 1alpha,25-Dihydroxyvitamin D3 targets PTEN-dependent fibronectin expression to restore thyroid cancer cell adhesiveness. Mol Endocrinol 2005;19: 2349–57.
149. Shefelbine SE, *et al.* Mutational analysis of the GDNF/RET–GDNFR alpha signaling complex in a kindred with vesicoureteral reflux. Hum Genet 1998;102:474–8.
150. Mackay CR, *et al.* Expression and modulation of CD44 variant isoforms in humans. J Cell Biol 1994;124:71–82.
151. Figge J, *et al.* Preferential expression of the cell adhesion molecule CD44 in papillary thyroid carcinoma. Exp Mol Pathol 1994;61:203–11.
152. Ermak G, *et al.* Restricted patterns of CD44 variant exon expression in human papillary thyroid carcinoma. Cancer Res 1996;56:1037–42.
153. Ermak G, *et al.* Deregulated alternative splicing of CD44 messenger RNA transcripts in neoplastic and nonneoplastic lesions of the human thyroid. Cancer Res 1995;55: 4594–8.
154. Xing M. Gene methylation in thyroid tumorigenesis. Endocrinology 2007;148:948–53.
155. Bird A. DNA methylation patterns and epigenetic memory. Genes Dev 2002;16:6–21.
156. Yoo CB, Jones PA. Epigenetic therapy of cancer: past, present and future. Nat Rev Drug Discov 2006;5:37–50.
157. Alvarez-Nunez F, *et al.* PTEN promoter methylation in sporadic thyroid carcinomas. Thyroid 2006;16:17–23.
158. Schagdarsurengin U, *et al.* Frequent epigenetic silencing of the CpG island promoter of RASSF1A in thyroid carcinoma. Cancer Res 2002;62:3698–701.
159. Xing M, *et al.* Early occurrence of RASSF1A hypermethylation and its mutual exclusion with BRAF mutation in thyroid tumorigenesis. Cancer Res 2004;64:1664–8.
160. Hoque MO, *et al.* Quantitative assessment of promoter methylation profiles in thyroid neoplasms. J Clin Endocrinol Metab 2005;90:4011–8.
161. Hu S, *et al.* Association of aberrant methylation of tumor suppressor genes with tumor aggressiveness and BRAF mutation in papillary thyroid cancer. Int J Cancer 2006;119: 2322–9.
162. Soh EY, *et al.* Vascular endothelial growth factor expression is higher in differentiated thyroid cancer than in normal or benign thyroid. J Clin Endocrinol Metab 1997;82: 3741–7.
163. Klein M, *et al.* Vascular endothelial growth factor gene and protein: strong expression in thyroiditis and thyroid carcinoma. J Endocrinol 1999;161:41–9.
164. Bunone G, *et al.* Expression of angiogenesis stimulators and inhibitors in human thyroid tumors and correlation with clinical pathological features. Am J Pathol 1999;155: 1967–76.
165. Yasuoka H, *et al.* VEGF-D expression and lymph vessels play an important role for lymph node metastasis in papillary thyroid carcinoma. Mod Pathol 2005;18: 1127–33.
166. Katoh R, *et al.* Expression of vascular endothelial growth factor (VEGF) in human thyroid neoplasms. Hum Pathol 1999;30:891–7.
167. Bauer AJ, *et al.* Systemic administration of vascular endothelial growth factor monoclonal antibody reduces the growth of papillary thyroid carcinoma in a nude mouse model. Ann Clin Lab Sci 2003;33:192–9.
168. Bauer AJ, *et al.* Vascular endothelial growth factor monoclonal antibody inhibits growth of anaplastic thyroid cancer xenografts in nude mice. Thyroid 2002;12:953–61.
169. Vella V, *et al.* The IGF system in thyroid cancer: new concepts. Mol Pathol 2001;54:121–4.
170. Russo D, *et al.* Genetic alterations in thyroid hyperfunctioning adenomas. J Clin Endocrinol Metab 1995;80: 1347–51.
171. Russo D, *et al.* Detection of an activating mutation of the thyrotropin receptor in a case of an autonomously hyperfunctioning thyroid insular carcinoma. J Clin Endocrinol Metab 1997;82:735–8.
172. Belge G, *et al.* Cytogenetic investigations of 340 thyroid hyperplasias and adenomas revealing correlations between cytogenetic findings and histology. Cancer Genet Cytogenet 1998;101:42–8.
173. Castro P, *et al.* Adenomas and follicular carcinomas of the thyroid display two major patterns of chromosomal changes. J Pathol 2005;206:305–11.
174. Sobrinho-Simoes M, *et al.* Molecular pathology of well-differentiated thyroid carcinomas. Virchows Arch 2005; 447:787–93.

175. Plail RO, *et al.* Adenomatous polyposis: an association with carcinoma of the thyroid. Br J Surg 1987;74:377–80.
176. Lote K, *et al.* Familial occurrence of papillary thyroid carcinoma. Cancer 1980;46:1291–7.
177. Liaw D, *et al.* Germline mutations of the PTEN gene in Cowden disease, an inherited breast and thyroid cancer syndrome. Nat Genet 1997;16:64–7.
178. Malchoff CD, Malchoff DM. The genetics of hereditary nonmedullary thyroid carcinoma. J Clin Endocrinol Metab 2002;87:2455–9.
179. Cameselle-Teijeiro J, Chan JK. Cribriform-morular variant of papillary carcinoma: a distinctive variant representing the sporadic counterpart of familial adenomatous polyposis-associated thyroid carcinoma? Mod Pathol 1999;12:400–11.
180. Wohllk N, *et al.* Relevance of RET proto-oncogene mutations in sporadic medullary thyroid carcinoma. J Clin Endocrinol Metab 1996;81:3740–5.
181. Fialkowski EA, Moley JF. Current approaches to medullary thyroid carcinoma, sporadic and familial. J Surg Oncol 2006;94:737–47.
182. Asai N, *et al.* Mechanism of activation of the ret proto-oncogene by multiple endocrine neoplasia 2A mutations. Mol Cell Biol 1995;15:1613–9.
183. Borrello MG, *et al.* RET activation by germline MEN2A and MEN2B mutations. Oncogene 1995;11:2419–27.
184. Santoro M, *et al.* Activation of RET as a dominant transforming gene by germline mutations of MEN2A and MEN2B. Science 1995;267:381–3.
185. Ichihara M, Murakumo Y, Takahashi M. RET and neuroendocrine tumors. Cancer Lett 2004;204:197–211.
186. Kouvaraki MA, *et al.* RET proto-oncogene: a review and update of genotype–phenotype correlations in hereditary medullary thyroid cancer and associated endocrine tumors. Thyroid 2005;15:531–44.
187. Hundahl SA, *et al.* A National Cancer Data Base report on 53,856 cases of thyroid carcinoma treated in the U.S., 1985–1995. Cancer 1998;83:2638–48.
188. Jones RL, Judson IR. The development and application of imatinib. Expert Opin Drug Saf 2005;4:183–91.
189. Carlomagno F, *et al.* ZD6474, an orally available inhibitor of KDR tyrosine kinase activity, efficiently blocks oncogenic RET kinases. Cancer Res 2002;62:7284–90.
190. Vidal M, *et al.* ZD6474 suppresses oncogenic RET isoforms in a Drosophila model for type 2 multiple endocrine neoplasia syndromes and papillary thyroid carcinoma. Cancer Res 2005;65:3538–41.
191. Hoffmann S, *et al.* Targeting the EGF/VEGF-R system by tyrosine-kinase inhibitors—a novel antiproliferative/antiangiogenic strategy in thyroid cancer. Langenbecks Arch Surg 2006;391:589–96.
192. Tamura T, *et al.* A phase I dose-escalation study of ZD6474 in Japanese patients with solid, malignant tumors. J Thorac Oncol 2006;1:1002–9.
193. Heymach JV. ZD6474—clinical experience to date. Br J Cancer 2005;92 Suppl 1:S14–20.
194. Holden SN, *et al.* Clinical evaluation of ZD6474, an orally active inhibitor of VEGF and EGF receptor signaling, in patients with solid, malignant tumors. Ann Oncol 2005;16:1391–7.
195. Milano A, *et al.* New molecular targeted therapies in thyroid cancer. Anticancer Drugs 2006;17:869–79.
196. Carlomagno F, *et al.* The kinase inhibitor PP1 blocks tumorigenesis induced by RET oncogenes. Cancer Res 2002;62:1077–82.
197. Carlomagno F, *et al.* Efficient inhibition of RET/papillary thyroid carcinoma oncogenic kinases by 4-amino-5-(4-chloro-phenyl)-7-(t-butyl)pyrazolo[3,4-d]pyrimidine (PP2). J Clin Endocrinol Metab 2003;88:1897–902.
198. Gollob JA, *et al.* Role of Raf kinase in cancer: therapeutic potential of targeting the Raf/MEK/ERK signal transduction pathway. Semin Oncol 2006;33:392–406.
199. Karasarides M, *et al.* B-RAF is a therapeutic target in melanoma. Oncogene 2004;23:6292–8.
200. Wilhelm SM, *et al.* BAY 43-9006 exhibits broad spectrum oral antitumor activity and targets the RAF/MEK/ERK pathway and receptor tyrosine kinases involved in tumor progression and angiogenesis. Cancer Res 2004;64:7099–109.
201. Salvatore G, *et al.* BRAF is a therapeutic target in aggressive thyroid carcinoma. Clin Cancer Res 2006;12:1623–9.
202. Kim S, *et al.* Sorafenib inhibits the angiogenesis and growth of orthotopic anaplastic thyroid carcinoma xenografts in nude mice. Mol Cancer Ther 2007;6:1785–92.
203. Solit DB, *et al.* BRAF mutation predicts sensitivity to MEK inhibition. Nature 2006;439:358–62.
204. Durante C, *et al.* BRAF mutations in papillary thyroid carcinomas inhibit genes involved in iodine metabolism. J Clin Endocrinol Metab 2007;92:2840–3.
205. Riesco-Eizaguirre G, *et al.* The oncogene BRAF V600E is associated with a high risk of recurrence and less differentiated papillary thyroid carcinoma due to the impairment of Na+/I– targeting to the membrane. Endocr Relat Cancer 2006;13:257–69.
206. Furuya F, *et al.* Inhibition of phosphatidylinositol 3′ kinase delays tumor progression and blocks metastatic spread in a mouse model of thyroid cancer. Carcinogenesis 2007;28:2451–8.
207. Mandal M, *et al.* The Akt inhibitor KP372-1 suppresses Akt activity and cell proliferation and induces apoptosis in thyroid cancer cells. Br J Cancer 2005;92:1899–905.
208. Shao Y, *et al.* Apoptotic and autophagic cell death induced by histone deacetylase inhibitors. Proc Natl Acad Sci USA 2004;101:18030–5.
209. Della Ragione F, *et al.* Genes modulated by histone acetylation as new effectors of butyrate activity. FEBS Lett 2001;499:199–204.
210. Ueda H, *et al.* Action of FR901228, a novel antitumor bicyclic depsipeptide produced by Chromobacterium

violaceum no. 968, on Ha-ras transformed NIH3T3 cells. Biosci Biotechnol Biochem 1994;58:1579–83.

211. Glick RD, *et al.* Hybrid polar histone deacetylase inhibitor induces apoptosis and CD95/CD95 ligand expression in human neuroblastoma. Cancer Res 1999;59:4392–9.
212. Kelly WK, *et al.* Phase I study of an oral histone deacetylase inhibitor, suberoylanilide hydroxamic acid, in patients with advanced cancer. J Clin Oncol 2005;23:3923–31.
213. Kelly WK, *et al.* Phase I clinical trial of histone deacetylase inhibitor: suberoylanilide hydroxamic acid administered intravenously. Clin Cancer Res 2003;9:3578–88.
214. Kersten S, Desvergne B, Wahli W. Roles of PPARs in health and disease. Nature 2000;405:421–4.

MULTIPLE CHOICE QUESTIONS

Select the single most appropriate option.

1. The *RET* proto-oncogene is a 21-exon gene located on the proximal arm of chromosome:
A. 14
B. 11
C. 10
D. 2

2. Mutation of what gene is most prevalent in sporadic forms of papillary thyroid cancer?
A. *RET*
B. *RAS*
C. *BRAF*
D. *p53*

3. p53 seems to be associated with which stage of thyroid tumour development?
A. Early
B. Intermediate
C. Late
D. Not involved

4. What percentage of medullary thyroid carcinomas are familial?
A. 1%
B. 20%
C. 50%
D. 80%

5. MEN2A consists of all of the below EXCEPT:
A. Medullary thyroid carcinoma
B. Pheochromocytoma
C. Pancreatic neoplasia
D. Parathyroid neoplasia

Answers

1. C
2. C
3. C
4. B
5. C

10 An overview of the management of thyroid cancer

R. Michael Tuttle

Joan and Sanford I. Weill Medical College of Cornell University, Memorial Sloan Kettering Cancer Center, New York, USA

KEY POINTS

- While clinically evident recurrence may develop in 15–20% of thyroid cancer patients, 30-year disease-specific survival rates exceed 90%
- Risk stratification in thyroid cancer is an active, evolving, ongoing process which uses clinical follow-up data to modify (either increase or decrease) the initial risk estimates derived from the established staging systems
- While we usually emphasize estimates of the risk of recurrence and disease-specific death, it is the risk of failing our initial treatments that is the primary determinant of adverse clinical outcome
- Total thyroidectomy is the preferred operation for all but the smallest papillary thyroid cancer confined to the thyroid
- Based on clinical data in the first several years following initial therapy, response to therapy is classified as excellent (no evidence of disease), acceptable (minimal residual disease versus persistent normal thyroid cells) or incomplete (persistent, clinically significant disease)

INTRODUCTION

Thyroid cancer accounts for more than 90% of all endocrine malignancies even though it represents less than 1% of all human cancers. Thyroid cancer is often considered a rare disease, yet the estimated number of new cases diagnosed in the USA in 2008 exceeds the number of cases of stomach, liver, ovary, brain myeloma, pharynx, larynx, testis and bone cancer (Table 10.1).[1] Outcome in thyroid cancer patients ranges from clinically insignificant disease, detected as an incidental finding at autopsy, to very aggressive disease with 5-year disease-specific mortality rates as high as a 50%. The latter occurs in older patients presenting with distant metastases,[2] although the vast majority of patients experience an excellent overall disease-specific survival. This is evidenced by the relatively low number of deaths from thyroid cancer in 2008 compared with other solid malignancies.

Thyroid cancer arises either from thyroid follicular cells (papillary, follicular, anaplastic thyroid cancers) or from other cells within the thyroid gland such as lymphocytes (primary thyroid lymphoma) or neuroendocrine C cells (medullary thyroid cancer). In most large series, thyroid cancer arising from thyroid follicular cells accounts for 90–95% of all primary thyroid cancers. Papillary thyroid cancer accounts for the vast majority of these (>90%), while follicular thyroid cancer constitutes 5–8% and anaplastic cancer 1–2% of cases. Rarely, malignancies such as renal cell carcinoma, lung cancer, breast cancer or melanoma metastasize to the thyroid gland, usually as part of widespread disseminated metastatic disease.

An overall 10-year survival rate of 98% was demonstrated in a cohort of 15 698 thyroid cancer patients followed in the US Surveillance Epidemiology and End Results (SEER) tumour registry at the National Cancer Institute.[3] This included 92% 10-year survival for papillary thyroid cancer, 89% for follicular thyroid cancer, 80% for medullary thyroid cancer and 13% for anaplastic thyroid cancer. Other retrospective studies have shown 40-year survival rates of 94% for papillary thyroid cancer and 84% for follicular thyroid cancer.[4]

While the disease-specific mortality for thyroid cancer has remained stable over the last 25 years, the SEER data indicate a dramatic rise in the incidence of thyroid cancer between 1975 and 2001.[5] Further analysis by Davies and Welch demonstrates that this increase is due to the 2.9-fold increase in papillary thyroid cancer between 1988 and 2002. There was no significant change detected in follicular, medullary or anaplastic thyroid cancer over the same time frame.[6] Taking into account this increased incidence, as many as 1 in 127 men and women will be diagnosed with thyroid cancer during their lifetime.[3] While the aetiology of this dramatic increase in incidence remains unclear, it is interesting to note that approximately

A Practical Manual of Thyroid and Parathyroid Disease, 1st Edition. Edited by Asit Arora, Neil Tolley & R. Michael Tuttle.

Table 10.1 Estimated number of new cases and disease-specific deaths in 2008 in the USA

	New cases	Deaths
Lung	215 020	161 840
Breast	184 450	40 930
Prostate	186 320	28 660
Lymphoma	74 340	20 510
Bladder	68 810	14 100
Melanoma	62 480	8420
Uterine	51 170	11 340
Kidney	54 390	13 010
Leukaemia	44 270	21 710
Pancreas	37 680	34 290
Thyroid	37 340	1590
Stomach	21 500	10 880
Liver	21 370	18 410
Ovary	21 650	15 520
Brain	21 810	13 070
Myeloma	19 920	10 690
Pharynx	12 410	2200
Larynx	12 250	3670
Testis	8090	380
Bone	2380	1470

Data from the American Cancer Society, Cancer Facts and Figures, 2008.

half the thyroid cancer cases were less than 1 cm at diagnosis, and 87% were less than 2 cm at diagnosis.[6] It is likely that the increasingly widespread use of cross-sectional imaging in the head and neck may have led to an apparent increase in incidence of previously subclinical disease. More intensive clinical evaluation with high resolution thyroid ultrasound (US) and the widespread availability of US-guided fine needle aspiration (FNA) would also be expected to increase the incidence of previously non-apparent microscopic thyroid cancer.

Further epidemiological studies are required to exclude other causative factors. Although radiation is the best known risk factor for development of thyroid cancer, it seems unlikely that the low level fall-out from the atomic weapons testing programme is responsible for the increased incidence.[7] Most patients diagnosed in the current decade were born after atmospheric testing ended. Likewise, the worldwide exposure to fall-out from the Chernobyl accident is below the level which is considered a significant risk (except in countries immediately downwind of the accident). Other risk factors such as occupational exposure, dietary habits, lifestyle, parity and genetic predisposition have been described, but are much less well studied.[8]

INITIAL PRESENTATION

Thyroid cancer usually presents as an asymptomatic, painless mass in the neck detected by either the patient or their healthcare professional. Women are affected more commonly that men, with a ratio of approximately 2:1 for papillary thyroid cancer. It is important to note that thyroid function tests (thyroid-stimulating hormone (TSH), T4 levels) are almost universally normal. Normal thyroid function provides little, if any, information regarding structural thyroid disease (thyroid nodules) and does not exclude the presence of malignancy.

Since thyroid nodules may be present in nearly 50% of the adult population and less than 5–10% of these nodules are malignant,[9] the challenge is to identify and treat the few cases of thyroid cancer in the sea of benign thyroid nodules. Clinical factors which increase the likelihood of a nodule being malignant include rapid growth, local compressive symptoms, male gender, ipsilateral vocal cord paralysis, family history of thyroid cancer, history of radiation exposure during childhood, a hard/fixed nodule and palpable cervical lymphadenopathy. Differentiated thyroid cancer can be part of one of several relatively rare clinical syndromes such as Gardner's syndrome, familial adenomatous polyposis, Carney complex and Cowden's syndrome.[10]

Because only a minority of thyroid cancer patients present with signs or symptoms diagnostic of thyroid cancer, the diagnosis is usually made on FNA of the thyroid nodule.[9] FNA has a high specificity and sensitivity for detecting malignant thyroid nodules and remains the mainstay for the diagnosis of thyroid cancer (see Chapter 3).

At the time of diagnosis, thyroid cancer is localized to the thyroid in approximately 60% of cases. In 34% of cases there is regional lymph node involvement, and distant metastases occur in 5% of cases.[3] These registry data are consistent with retrospective cohort studies which report clinically apparent regional lymph node involvement in 20–50% of patients.[4,11–14] When meticulous neck dissection is performed, as many as 70–80% of patients harbour microscopic lymph node metastases at diagnosis.[15,16] Distant metastasis at diagnosis is found in only 2–5% of cases in these retrospective series.[4,14,17,18]

CLINICAL OUTCOMES

As discussed above, 10-year survival rates in excess of 98% and 30-year survival rates in excess of 90–95% are reported in most large series of thyroid cancer patients. Despite this relatively low disease-specific mortality rate, the risk of recurrent disease can be as high as 20–30% over a 30- to 40-year follow-up period.[4,18] In the Ohio State follow-up cohort, 24% of the patients had a clinically evident recurrence at a median of 17 years of follow-up. This included 18% with local recurrence in the neck (74% lymph node metastasis, 20% thyroid bed recurrence and 6% recurrence in neck muscle or trachea) and 8% with recurrence in sites outside the neck (distant metastases). Data from the Mayo Clinic demonstrate a 14% recurrence rate over a 40-year follow-up period with similar excellent overall disease-specific survival.[19]

While most clinically evident recurrences can be adequately treated with further surgery, radioactive iodine (RAI) or external beam irradiation (EBRT), as many as 8% of patients with local recurrence and up to 50% of patients with distant metastatic recurrence die of thyroid cancer.[4] It is likely that the more sensitive follow-up tests currently used will result in early detection of small volume recurrent disease which can therefore be more adequately treated, reducing the relatively high disease-specific mortality rates.

In many cancers, the risk of recurrence is tightly linked to the risk of disease-specific survival. This is true in older thyroid cancer patients (>45 years at diagnosis), where the risk of recurrence does indeed parallel the risk of disease-specific mortality.[4] However, many patients at high risk of disease recurrence have a low risk of disease-specific mortality (e.g. young patients with well-differentiated papillary thyroid cancer presenting with several positive cervical lymph nodes). As a result, staging systems designed to predict the risk of disease-specific death are unlikely to provide useful information regarding risk of recurrence in young thyroid cancer patients. Thus it is imperative to be very specific about which outcomes are being predicted by the various staging systems currently used to guide thyroid cancer management.

RISK STRATIFICATION

In keeping with the general trend in oncology, in the last several years there has been an increased emphasis on using individual estimates of risk to tailor recommendations for both initial therapy and follow-up in thyroid cancer patients.[9,20–29] However, it is important to emphasize that risk assessment is an ongoing process that uses new data obtained during follow-up to modify initial risk assessment.[26,28] These ongoing risk estimates provide the basis for new recommendations regarding the need for additional therapy or continued observation. Ongoing risk estimates should guide the intensity and modalities of the long-term follow-up paradigm.

What risks are we trying to predict?

Staging systems have traditionally been employed to predict the risk of disease-specific mortality as the primary clinical endpoint. However, the risk of recurrence (local or distant) is usually substantially higher than the risk of death in most thyroid cancer patients. Thus it is desirable to predict the risk of recurrence in addition to the risk of death. What we are really trying to predict is the failure of our initial therapy which then results in either recurrence or disease-specific death. In our view, it is both the underlying biology of the specific tumour and the effectiveness of initial therapy that determines long-term clinical outcome.

Initial risk stratification

For many years, a small set of clinical and histopathological features have been used in several staging systems to predict accurately the risk of death from thyroid cancer.[24,30–37] Some of these are 'patient-related' factors (age, gender) while others are considered 'tumour-related' factors (size of the primary tumour, histology, gross extrathyroidal extension, completeness of resection, cervical lymph node involvement or distant metastasis). A comparison of the 14 most commonly used staging systems revealed that each one demonstrated good ability to predict cause-specific survival in differentiated thyroid cancer.[38] Two additional scoring systems specifically designed to predict risk of recurrence have recently been published.[39,40]

Limitations of our current staging systems

Current staging systems are designed to predict risk of disease-specific death but may not accurately reflect the risk of either persistent disease after initial therapy or clinically evident disease recurrence. In addition, most of the current staging systems do not include variables reflecting the effectiveness (or ineffectiveness) of initial therapies that are given in an effort to make a significant impact on recurrence and mortality rates.

Furthermore, most of the current staging systems do not incorporate specific histological subtypes of thyroid cancer (e.g. tall cell variant, columnar variant, Hurthle cell variant) or molecular characteristics (specific tumour mutations) of the primary tumour that may convey an increased risk beyond that seen in classic papillary thyroid cancer. While the size of the primary tumour is the major determinant of clinical outcome, the presence of vascular invasion, extrathyroidal (or extranodal) extension, lymphatic involvement and adverse histological subtypes of thyroid cancer (such as the tall cell variant, columnar variant, insular variant and poorly differentiated subtypes) may also be associated with an increased risk of recurrence and/or death. Therefore, regardless of size of the primary, these additional features increase the estimate for risk of recurrence and death which often leads to more aggressive additional therapies.

Over the last several years, our understanding of the molecular biology of thyroid cancer has increased dramatically.[41] This is outlined in further detail in Chapter 9. Several authors have suggested that the presence of specific molecular abnormalities can provide important information as to the risk of recurrence.[42–44] For example, it has recently been demonstrated that tumours harbouring *BRAF* mutations appear to display a more aggressive clinical course.[45,46] Since many pathology departments now offer molecular analysis of malignancy it is likely that molecular profiling will be added to our risk stratification schemes in years to come.

One of the major problems inherent in the current staging systems is that they do not evolve over time. The patient is assigned a stage within the first few weeks after initial therapy and there are no provisions for modifying this initial risk as new data are accumulated over time during follow-up. From a clinical perspective, most of our follow-up testing can be viewed as data that evaluate the effectiveness of our initial therapy that can be used either to increase or to decrease our initial risk estimates. For most patients, the most important response to therapy variables are the serum thyroglobulin (Tg) and neck US performed in the first few years after initial therapy.

Recently Welsch *et al.* proposed a multiparameter scoring system designed to predict recurrence-free survival. This is based on 25 clinical factors that incorporate the standard initial clinical factors (e.g. age, gender, histology, size of the primary, extrathyroidal extension, lymph node status) with several responses to therapy predictors (e.g. RAI avidity, [^{18}F]fluorodeoxyglucose positron emission tomography (FDG-PET) positivity, site of distant metastases and post-operative serum Tg measurements).[40]

Finally, the current staging systems do not incorporate a variable that reflects disease-free survival. Using our current highly sensitive detection techniques, the vast majority of patients with persistent or recurrent thyroid cancer are identified in the first few years after initial therapy. It seems likely that the risk of death from thyroid cancer and the risk of clinically evident recurrence should decrease as a function of disease-free survival.

The net effect is that in our current staging systems the initial risk estimate remains unchanged for the entire life of the patient regardless of how well they respond to initial therapy or how long they have been free of disease. This approach to staging does not reflect clinical practice or the biology of thyroid cancer. Continuing to follow this traditional approach will result in a higher than necessary risk estimate for high risk patients that have an excellent response to initial therapy and a lower than appropriate risk estimate for low risk patients failing to respond to our initial therapy.

Practical aspects of initial risk stratification

Our approach to initial risk stratification begins with gathering all pertinent clinical data obtained pre-operatively, intra-operatively or in the first few weeks post-operatively that can be used to provide the best clinical estimates of the risk. These primarily include the data outlined in Table 10.2.

Since the completeness of surgical resection is a major response to therapy variable, it is critical that all the members of the disease management team have a good understanding of the intra-operative findings. Often, completeness of surgical resection cannot be determined by the pathology report alone. For example, a pathology report that notes 'positive margins' or 'extrathyroidal

Table 10.2 Initial risk stratification

Age at diagnosis
Histology
Size of the primary tumour
Lymph node status
Multifocality
Vascular invasion
Extrathyroidal extension
Completeness of surgical resection
Presence of distant metastases
Post-operative serum thyroglobulin

Table 10.3 Risk of death from thyroid cancer

	Very low risk	Low risk	Intermediate risk	High risk
Age at diagnosis	<45 years	<45 years	Young patients (<45 years) Classic PTC > 4 cm Or vascular invasion Or extrathyroidal extension Or worrisome histology of any size†	>45 years
Primary tumour size	<1 cm	1–4 cm	Older patients (>45 years) Classic PTC < 4 cm Or extrathyroidal extension Or worrisome histology <1–2 cm confined to the thyroid†	>4 cm classic PTC
Histology	Classic PTC, confined to the thyroid gland*	Classic PTC, confined to the thyroid gland*	Histology in conjunction with age as above	Worrisome histology >1–2 cm†
Completeness of resection	Complete resection	Complete resection	Complete resection	Incomplete tumour resection
Lymph node involvement	None apparent	Present or absent‡	Present or absent‡	Present or absent‡
Distant metastasis	None apparent	None apparent	None apparent	Present
Risk of failing initial therapy	Very low	Low	Intermediate	High

* Confined to the thyroid gland with no evidence of vascular invasion or extrathyroidal extension.
† Worrisome histologies includes histological subtypes of papillary thyroid cancer such as tall cell variant, columnar variant, insular variant and poorly differentiated thyroid cancers.
‡ Cervical lymph node metastases in older patients, but probably not in younger patients, may confer an increased risk of death from disease.

extension' could reflect either (1) minor extension into perithyroidal adipose tissue or minor invasion into strap muscles that was completely resected, or (2) the surgical margin of gross disease that was not completely resectable. Obviously, the risk stratification and subsequent therapeutic recommendations in these two situations differ dramatically depending on other details of the pathology report and clinical situation.

The clinical parameters described in Table 10.2 are then used to quantify both the risk of death from thyroid cancer and the risk of developing a clinically evident recurrence for each individual patient. The risk of death is stratified into very low, low, intermediate or high risk (Table 10.3) while the risk of recurrence is classified as low, intermediate or high (Table 10.4).[26,28] The combination of the risk of death from thyroid cancer with the risk of clinical recurrence provides our best initial assessment of the likely clinical outcome in specific patients.

While most patients have a neck US and chest radiograph (CXR) prior to surgery, additional use of cross-sectional imaging studies is not routinely recommended unless the patient is at an increased risk for distant metastasis.[9,22] Since patients classified as high risk for recurrence and death are also at significant risk for distant metastasis, cross-sectional imaging of the lungs and brain is recommended to identify other sites of disease that may need therapy or close observation. Likewise, aggressive histologies such as Hurthle cell carcinoma, tall cell or poorly differentiated variants of papillary thyroid may concentrate RAI poorly and therefore are often better detected with FDG-PET scanning rather than RAI scanning.[9,47,48] It is important to avoid intravenous contrast

Table 10.4 Risk stratification for the likelihood of clinically evident recurrence from thyroid cancer following complete resection of primary tumour in patients with no evidence of distant metastases at initial evaluation*

	Low risk	Intermediate risk	High risk
Age at diagnosis	Any age	20–60 years	<20 or >60 years
Primary tumour size	<1 cm†	1–4 cm	>4 cm‡
Histology	Classic PTC confined to the thyroid gland	Classic PTC, minor extrathyroidal extension or vascular invasion	Other than classic PTC, gross extrathyroidal extension or vascular invasion
Lymph node involvement	None apparent	Present or absent	Present
Risk of failing initial therapy	Low	Intermediate	High

* Patients with incomplete tumour resection or distant metastasis at diagnosis are very likely to have persistent disease even after aggressive initial therapy. They are not included in this risk stratification scheme and are dealt with differently from the more usual patient without evidence of distant metastasis in which all gross evidence of disease has been resected.

† PTC < 1 cm with known local lymph node metastases would be classified as intermediate risk.

‡ Patients less than 20 years of age with lymph node metastases are considered to have high risk of recurrence regardless of the size of the primary tumour.

containing iodine in patients who are likely to require RAI since the large amount of stable iodine present in CT contrast will render RAI ineffective for at least 2–3 months.

In addition to estimating the risk of death and the risk of recurrence, it is also important to determine the risk of failing a proposed initial therapy. The goal is to provide the minimal effective therapy and the least intensive follow-up that is likely to result in good clinical outcomes. As such, patients at low risk of recurrence and low risk of death who are likely to respond to minimal therapy do not require aggressive treatment and follow-up. However, if a minimal therapeutic approach is considered unlikely to be effective, more aggressive initial therapy is recommended. For example, patients unlikely to have an acceptable response to lobectomy are offered total thyroidectomy. Patients unlikely to respond to total thyroidectomy alone may also receive RAI, EBRT or both depending upon the clinical setting. Finally, patients unlikely to respond to these initial treatment interventions are considered for systemic therapy. Recommendation for more aggressive therapy is based on a combination of the estimates of risk for recurrence and death as well as the risk of failing a proposed therapy.

Before proceeding with a more aggressive surgical or radiotherapy approach, it is important to be confident that the proposed therapy will have a meaningful clinical impact (response to therapy estimate) with an acceptable short-term and long-term complication rate. Unfortunately, some high risk patients with persistent disease do not respond to additional surgery or further doses of RAI. In these cases, well meaning attempts at 'aggressive therapy' are more likely to cause complications and side effects rather than produce a meaningful clinical benefit. By balancing the risk of adverse outcome with the efficacy of therapy and the likelihood of complications from our treatments, we can arrive at a shared decision with the patient.

Initial treatment recommendations

Risk stratification begins before the patient has thyroid surgery. It is an ongoing, evolving process that begins with the diagnosis of thyroid cancer and continues through all phases of treatment and follow-up. In our view, the decision regarding the extent of surgery, use of RAI for remnant ablation and/or use of EBRT cannot be based on a mathematical equation or series of complicated tables. It is a joint decision between the patient and the disease management team which strikes the best balance between necessary effective therapy and the likely side effects of that therapy. Our general approach to initial treatment decision making based on risk of recurrence and risk of death is outlined in Table 10.5.

Most of the published guidelines recommend total thyroidectomy as the initial procedure of choice in patients with biopsy-proven papillary thyroid cancer.[27] In most large series, a total thyroidectomy is associated with statistically significantly lower recurrence rates than thyroid lobectomy.[4,19,34] However, a unilateral lobectomy achieves the same excellent disease-specific survival in patients who are at very low or low risk of dying from

Table 10.5 Initial therapeutic recommendations

Risk of death	Risk of decurrence	Initial surgery	RAI remnant ablation
Very low	Low	Lobectomy or total thyroidectomy	Not required
Low	Low	Lobectomy or total thyroidectomy	Not required
Low	Intermediate	Total thyroidectomy	For selected patients*
Low	High	Total thyroidectomy	Yes
Intermediate	Intermediate	Total thyroidectomy	For most patients
Intermediate	High	Total thyroidectomy	Yes
High	Intermediate	Total thyroidectomy	Yes
High	High	Total thyroidectomy	Yes

* Selected patients would probably include patients with primary size of the tumour >2–3 cm, documented lymph node metastases, extrathyroidal extension or vascular invasion. Radioactive iodine (RAI) is used in an effort to decrease recurrence with little impact on disease-specific mortality.

thyroid cancer (see Table 10.1).[23] With careful follow-up (primarily neck US), the few recurrences that may develop years later in low risk patients initially treated with less than total thyroidectomy are usually readily detectable and easily treated with additional surgery with or without post-operative RAI. Therefore, less than total thyroidectomy is still considered an acceptable surgical option for patients at low risk of dying from thyroid cancer.

In rare cases, the final pathology report may result in upstaging a patient who was initially deemed low risk based on pre-operative and intra-operative findings. If this is the case then a completion thyroidectomy is recommended. For example, a patient with a 1.5 cm tumour who was tentatively staged as low risk prior to and during surgery may require a subsequent completion thyroidectomy if the histopathology report reveals worrisome features (e.g. microscopic vascular invasion, adverse histological subtype, microscopic extrathyroidal extension). Because the final pathology report is required for an accurate final risk assessment, several authorities advocate a total thyroidectomy in all patients with a pre-operative diagnosis of well-differentiated thyroid cancer.

From a practical perspective, the extent of initial surgery is often influenced by the follow-up methods and paradigms that will be used by the referring endocrinologists. If RAI ablation is planned, then total thyroidectomy is required to minimize the volume of normal thyroid tissue that would preferentially concentrate the RAI and prevent detection/therapy of metastatic lesions. In addition, total thyroidectomy and RAI ablation has the added benefit of resulting in serum Tg levels that are either very low or undetectable. The maximum sensitivity and specificity of serum Tg is achieved when all normal thyroid tissue has been destroyed (total thyroidectomy and RAI ablation). While this is not required in patients at low to intermediate risk for recurrence, many endocrinologists are more comfortable following thyroid cancer patients previously treated with total thyroidectomy and RAI ablation. As such, they often prefer total thyroidectomy and RAI ablation in nearly all but the very low risk patients.

Case study 1

A patient at low risk of death and low risk of recurrence:

- 33-year-old female
- 8 mm unifocal well-differentiated PTC, entirely confined to the thyroid, completely resected with no vascular invasion, extrathyroidal extension or apparent lymph node involvement
- adequate therapy with either lobectomy or total thyroidectomy. RAI ablation is unlikely to have any significant impact on either recurrence or disease-specific survival in these low risk patients.

Case study 2

A patient at low risk of death but high risk of recurrence:

- 33-year-old female
- 3 cm multifocal, well-differentiated PTC with gross extrathyroidal extension
- all visible disease completely resected
- vascular invasion and lymph node involvement
- serum Tg 35 ng/ml with a TSH of 10 mIU/ml 2 weeks post-operatively
- likely to benefit from RAI in terms of decreased rates of recurrence and persistent disease although little expected impact on their already excellent survival outcome.

Case study 3

A patient at low risk of death but intermediate risk of recurrence:

- 33-year-old female
- 2 cm multifocal well-differentiated PTC completely resected with minor extrathyroidal extension noted following careful pathology review. No vascular invasion or apparent lymph node involvement
- this group continues to be the focus of controversy regarding the initial management of thyroid cancer. We usually offer RAI ablation to patients with a primary size of the tumour >2–3 cm, documented lymph node metastases, extrathyroidal extension or vascular invasion
- presence of tumour multifocality, even in microcarcinomas <1 cm, is a risk factor for lymph node recurrence but is probably not a risk factor for death from thyroid cancer.[11,49] If RAI is used in these intermediate risks patients, it is given in an attempt to decrease the risk of recurrence and persistent disease with little expectation of a survival benefit.

Given the detailed pathology reviews that we now receive, it is important to determine if minimal focal extrathyroidal extension or minor vascular invasion has significant prognostic significance. We may be upstaging these patients (and therefore overtreating them with RAI) based on the assumption that these minor histological features are independent factors which predict an adverse outcome. However, until more definitive data become available, RAI continues to be offered to patients at low risk of death but intermediate risk of recurrence.

Case study 4

A patient at intermediate risk of death from disease and high risk of recurrence:

- 35-year-old male with 6 cm classic PTC with microscopic vascular invasion, extrathyroidal extension and extensive lymph node involvement
- 61-year-old male with 1.5 cm poorly differentiated thyroid cancer, entirely confined to the thyroid with minor extrathyroidal extension and lymph node involvement but without vascular invasion.

Case study 5

A patient at high risk of death from disease:

- 65-year-old male
- 5 cm poorly differentiated thyroid cancer with gross extrathyroidal extension, microscopic vascular invasion, extensive lymph node involvement and pulmonary metastases on initial pre-operative CXR.

In general, there is less controversy regarding the use of RAI in patients at intermediate risk of death from disease and high risk of recurrence or patients at a high risk of death.

Case study 6

A patient at intermediate risk of death and intermediate risk of recurrence:

- 55-year old female with 3 cm well-differentiated PTC entirely confined to the thyroid with 1/23 lymph nodes involved
- 23-year-old female with 2 cm well-differentiated thyroid cancer confined to the thyroid with a single focus of microscopic vascular invasion but without extrathyroidal extension or apparent lymph node involvement
- this group is usually offered RAI ablation although this is done on a case by case basis.

Evaluating response to initial therapy

In keeping with the theme of ongoing risk assessment, recommendations regarding follow-up investigations are also based on initial risk assessments and then modified as new data become available (Table 10.6).[50] The goal is to identify those patients with persistent disease that may require additional therapy, but equally importantly to identify those patients that are probably cured of thyroid cancer so that excessive additional treatments and follow-up studies can be avoided. Usually by 1–2 years after initial therapy it is possible to differentiate accurately between patients who have had an excellent response to therapy and those that still have persistent disease.

Patients at low risk of death and low risk of recurrence can be followed with suppressed Tg without the need for a stimulated Tg value. Since most of these patients will not have received RAI ablation, the stimulated Tg value is of little clinical value. Even though neck US is very unlikely to be positive in these very low risk patients, we continue to recommend at least one follow-up US over the first 2 years primarily for patient reassurance. Further studies are needed in this very low risk population because it is possible that the US will reveal more false-positive findings than true disease and could result in additional unnecessary testing or treatment.

Patients at low risk of death but intermediate to high risk of recurrence are followed slightly more closely with suppressed Tg measurement every 6 months, a stimulated Tg at 12–18 months after initial therapy and an US

Table 10.6 Routine follow-up recommendations during the first two post-operative years for patients without evidence of distant metastases or gross residual disease at initial evaluation

Risk of death	Risk of recurrence	Suppressed Tg	Stimulated Tg	Neck US	Other imaging
Very low	Low	6, 12, 24 months	Not required	12–24 months	Not required
Low	Low	6, 12, 24 months	Not required	12–24 months	Not required
Low	Intermediate	Q 6 months	12–18 months	12, 24 months	Consider diagnostic WBS at 12–18 months if suppressed Tg > 1 ng/ml or stimulated Tg > 10 ng/ml
Low	High	Q 6 months	12–18 months	12, 24 months	Consider diagnostic WBS at 12–18 months if suppressed Tg > 1 ng/ml or stimulated Tg > 10 ng/ml
Intermediate	Intermediate	Q 6 months	12–18 months	12, 24 months	Consider diagnostic WBS at 12–18 months. Other imaging not required unless response to therapy is less than excellent
Intermediate	High	Q 6 months	12–18 months	12, 24 months	Consider diagnostic WBS at 12–18 months. Other imaging not required unless response to therapy is less than excellent
High	Intermediate	Q 6 months	12–18 months	12, 24 months	Consider diagnostic WBS at 12–18 months. FDG-PET, RAI scans, other cross-sectional imaging
High	High	Q 6 months	12–18 months	12, 24 months	Consider diagnostic WBS at 12–18 months. FDG-PET, RAI scans, other cross-sectional imaging

Q-every 6 months

done at 12 and 24 months. This group usually consists of young patients with well-differentiated thyroid cancer which produces Tg and is usually RAI avid. Recurrence usually occurs in cervical lymph nodes. Therefore, a follow-up paradigm that emphasizes serum Tg and neck US is effective at detecting persistent or recurrent disease. A diagnostic RAI scan may also be useful to identify the source of persistent significantly elevated Tg levels (suppressed Tg > 1 ng/ml or stimulated Tg > 10 ng/ml).

Patients at intermediate risk of death (young patients with PTC > 4 cm, or older patients with 1–4 cm PTC) and either intermediate (1–4 cm PTC) or high risk (>4 cm PTC) of recurrence often require follow-up studies beyond serum Tg and neck US. While additional cross-sectional or functional imaging is not recommended for all of these patients, we maintain a low threshold for considering these additional tests if there is less than an excellent response to initial therapy over the first 2 years. Even though the yield of diagnostic whole-body scanning (WBS) is low in these patients, the finding of RAI-avid disease allows for additional RAI therapy which is a potentially important additional treatment in this group.

Patients at high risk of death (older patients, well-differentiated PTC > 4 cm, or poorly differentiated PTC > 2 cm with gross extrathyroidal extension, incomplete tumour resection or distant metastases) and either intermediate or high risk of recurrence routinely require follow-up testing beyond serum Tg and neck US. These are usually older patients with poorly differentiated thyroid cancer which is less likely to be RAI avid. Therefore, additional functional imaging (FDG-PET) and cross-sectional imaging of the brain, neck and chest is often recommended as part of our initial staging in these high risk patients. Furthermore, the FDG-PET scan provides important prognostic information and can serve as a valuable response to therapy predictor. Metastatic lesions that are strongly positive on FDG-PET seldom respond to RAI alone[51] and often require additional surgery, EBRT or systemic therapy.

Response to therapy variables generally involves data accumulated over months to years after initial therapy although we have increasingly used a post-operative serum Tg prior to RAI ablation as a very early 'response to therapy' marker. The post-operative serum Tg can be used as a reflection of the likelihood of persistent thyroid tissue or alert the clinician to the presence of distant metastases before RAI scanning. The precise cut-off value used depends on the post-operative TSH and the time

Table 10.7 Therapeutic outcomes

	Excellent response*	Acceptable response	Incomplete response
Oncology correlates	Complete remission	Minimal residual disease versus residual normal thyroid cells	Persistent disease
Suppressed Tg†	Undetectable	Detectable but <1 ng/ml	>1 ng/ml
Stimulated Tg†	Undetectable	<10 ng/mL	>10 ng/ml
Trend in suppressed Tg‡	Remains undetectable	Declining	Stable or rising
Anti-Tg antibodies	Absent	Absent or declining	Persistent or rising
Neck examination	Normal	Normal	Palpable disease
Neck ultrasonography	No evidence of disease	Non-specific changes in thyroid bed Probable inflammatory lymph nodes Stable millimetre sized cervical lymph nodes even if abnormal by US criteria	Evidence of structurally significant recurrent/persistent disease in the thyroid bed (>1 cm) Cervical lymph nodes (>1 cm), or distant metastases, particularly if structurally progressive or FDG1avid
Diagnostic RAI WBS§	No evidence for RAI-avid disease	No evidence for RAI-avid disease Very faint uptake in thyroid bed only	Persistent/recurrent RAI-avid disease present
Cross-sectional imaging (MRI, CT)§	No evidence of disease	Non-specific changes	Structural disease present
FDG-PET scanning§	No evidence of disease	Non-specific changes consistent with normal variants or inflammatory changes	FDG-avid disease present

* Patients deemed to have an excellent or acceptable response to therapy generally warrant observation without additional specific therapy while patients with an incomplete response are likely to require additional evaluation and treatment.
† Stimulated and suppressed Tg value cut-offs optimized for patients treated with total thryoidectomy and RAI remnant ablation.
‡ While most sensitive and specific in patients treated with total thyroidectomy and RAI remnant ablation, a rising Tg over time should also prompt further evaluation in patients treated with less than total thyroidectomy or with total thyroidectomy without RAI remnant ablation. This highlights the crucial importance of measuring serum Tg in the same laboratory in order to ensure samples are comparable over time.
§ While these studies are not routinely recommended for patients without additional high risk features or clinical suspicion of persistent/recurrent disease, results from these studies can be used as additional response to therapy measures.

since surgery; like Welsh *et al.*,[40] we use a serum Tg cut-off value of 10 ng/ml obtained about 2 weeks post-operatively. A Tg level higher than 10 ng/ml raises the suspicion of either a larger than expected thyroid remnant after total thyroidectomy or the presence of distant metastases. Tg < 10 ng/ml is reassuring and reflects adequate surgical resection of the tumour with either small volume residual disease or normal thyroid bed remnant.

Possible therapeutic outcomes

From a clinical standpoint we define three possible therapeutic outcomes: excellent, acceptable and incomplete (Table 10.7).[26,28] In oncology terms, these outcomes could be considered complete remission (excellent response), minimal residual disease versus residual normal thyroid (acceptable) and persistent disease (incomplete response). The intention of this table is not to imply that all patients with thyroid cancer need all of these follow-up modalities. Rather, it is a way to risk-stratify the results obtained when the test is done in the appropriate patient population as described in the section above.

The optimal outcome would be an excellent response to therapy in which the patient has no biochemical or structural evidence of disease. The risk of death and even the risk of recurrence should be very low in these patients. Therefore, follow-up testing after the initial 2-year evaluation period can be less intense and probably will just require a suppressed Tg yearly and perhaps a neck US every few years. Patients with an excellent response to therapy are expected to have a better outcome than may have been predicted by their initial staging.

With the more widespread use of highly sensitive detection tools, we have identified a large cohort of patients with persistent low level Tg values or millimetre sized abnormal cervical lymph nodes with no evidence of disease progression. Some of these patients have persistent low level disease (minimal residual disease) while others have persistent normal thyroid cells after RAI ablation. Some authorities advocate additional therapy to these patients with an acceptable, but not excellent, response to therapy. We feel that most of the patients in the 'acceptable response to therapy' outcome can be followed with observation alone. Additional therapy is reserved for patients with evidence of structural disease progression or rising serum Tg.

In our experience, a large proportion of these patients followed with observation alone in this group eventually transition to excellent outcomes as their Tg values gradually become lower and eventually undetectable over time. Sometimes the lymph nodes enlarge or the Tg begins to rise, in which case their response is no longer 'acceptable' and additional imaging studies and therapies are considered. However, additional studies documenting a meaningful impact of additional therapy in this acceptable response group are required before we submit all of these relatively low risk patients to the potential side effects of additional surgery, RAI, EBRT or systemic therapy.

Patients with an incomplete response probably had a failure of initial therapy and are usually offered additional treatment. These patients are likely to have clinically significant persistent or progressive disease, so strong consideration for additional effective therapy is warranted.

CONCLUSIONS

In summary, we view risk stratification as an active, ongoing process that informs our decisions, beginning with the correct initial therapy through appropriate selection of tests for detection of recurrent or persistent disease. While we place importance on estimating the risk of recurrence and the risk of death from thyroid cancer, we view the risk of failing therapy as the primary determinant of clinical outcome. Therefore, our follow-up paradigm is designed to identify patients that have failed initial therapy in whom additional therapies are likely to offer a substantial clinical benefit. It is only through proper risk stratification that we can maximize the benefit of aggressive therapy in patients that are likely to benefit from it while minimizing potential complications and side effects in low risk patients destined to live a full, healthy, productive life following minimal therapeutic intervention.

EVIDENCE APPRAISAL

Over the last several years, several international thyroid organizations have published evidenced-based guidelines regarding the management of thyroid cancer. Unfortunately, for most of the controversial management topics (extent of initial surgery, extent of lymph node dissection, need for RAI ablation and follow-up detection strategies), there are no randomized prospective clinical trials. Therefore, most of the evidence presented in this chapter is Level III or Level IV, with most of the treatment recommendations based on retrospective cohorts and expert opinion.

REFERENCES

1. American Cancer Society. Cancer Facts and Figures 2008. 2008. (Accessed 1 July 2008, at www.cancer.org.)
2. Hundahl SA, Cady B, Cunningham MP, *et al.* Initial results from a prospective cohort study of 5583 cases of thyroid carcinoma treated in the united states during 1996. U.S. and German Thyroid Cancer Study Group. An American College of Surgeons Commission on Cancer Patient Care Evaluation study. Cancer 2000;89:202–17.
3. SEER Cancer Statistics Review, 1975–2005. 2008. (Accessed 1 July 2008, at http://seer.cancer.gov/csr/1975_2005.)
4. Mazzaferri EL, Kloos RT. Clinical review 128: current approaches to primary therapy for papillary and follicular thyroid cancer. J Clin Endocrinol Metab 2001;86:1447–63.
5. Davies L, Welch HG. Epidemiology of head and neck cancer in the United States. Otolaryngol Head Neck Surg 2006; 135:451–7.
6. Davies L, Welch HG. Increasing incidence of thyroid cancer in the United States, 1973–2002. JAMA 2006;295:2164–7.
7. Schneider AB, Sarne DH. Long-term risks for thyroid cancer and other neoplasms after exposure to radiation. Nat Clin Pract Endocrinol Metab 2005;1:82–91.
8. Nagataki S, Nystrom E. Epidemiology and primary prevention of thyroid cancer. Thyroid 2002;12:889–96.
9. Cooper DS, Doherty GM, Haugen BR, *et al.* Management guidelines for patients with thyroid nodules and differentiated thyroid cancer. Thyroid 2006;16:109–42.
10. Malchoff CD, Malchoff DM. Familial nonmedullary thyroid carcinoma. Cancer Control 2006;13:106–10.
11. Chow SM, Law SC, Chan JK, *et al.* Papillary microcarcinoma of the thyroid—prognostic significance of lymph node metastasis and multifocality. Cancer 2003;98:31–40.
12. Grebe SK, Hay ID. Thyroid cancer nodal metastases: biologic significance and therapeutic considerations. Surg Oncol Clin North Am 1996;5:43–63.
13. Ito Y, Uruno T, Nakano K, *et al.* An observation trial without surgical treatment in patients with papillary microcarcinoma of the thyroid. Thyroid 2003;13:381–7.

14. McConahey WM, Hay ID, Woolner LB, *et al.* Papillary thyroid cancer treated at the Mayo Clinic, 1946 through 1970: initial manifestations, pathologic findings, therapy, and outcome. Mayo Clin Proc 1986;61:978–96.
15. Arturi F, Russo D, Giuffrida D, *et al.* Early diagnosis by genetic analysis of differentiated thyroid cancer metastases in small lymph nodes. J Clin Endocrinol Metab 1997;82: 1638–41.
16. Qubain SW, Nakano S, Baba M, *et al.* Distribution of lymph node micrometastasis in pN0 well-differentiated thyroid carcinoma. Surgery 2002;131:249–56.
17. Hay ID. Papillary thyroid carcinoma. Endocrinol Metab Clin North Am 1990;19:545–76.
18. Mazzaferri EL, Jhiang SM. Long-term impact of initial surgical and medical therapy on papillary and follicular thyroid cancer. Am J Med 1994;97:418–28.
19. Hay ID, Thompson GB, Grant CS, *et al.* Papillary thyroid carcinoma managed at the Mayo Clinic during six decades (1940–1999): temporal trends in initial therapy and long-term outcome in 2444 consecutively treated patients. World J Surg 2002;26:879–85.
20. British Thyroid Association and Royal College of Physicians. Guidelines for the management of thyroid cancer in adults 2007. (Accessed 12 October 2009, at british-thyroid-association.org.)
21. Mazzaferri EL. Management of low-risk differentiated thyroid cancer. Endocr Pract 2007;13:498–512.
22. Pacini F, Schlumberger M, Dralle H, *et al.* European consensus for the management of patients with differentiated thyroid carcinoma of the follicular epithelium. Eur J Endocrinol 2006;154:787–803.
23. Shaha AR, Shah JP, Loree TR. Low-risk differentiated thyroid cancer: the need for selective treatment. Ann Surg Oncol 1997;4:328–33.
24. National Comprehensive Cancer Network. Clinical Practice Guidelines in Oncology, Thyroid Cancer V.1. 2009. (Accessed 12 October 2009, at http://www.nccn.org/professionals/physician_gls/PDF/thyroid.pdf.)
25. Thyroid Carcinoma Task Force. AACE/AAES medical/surgical guidelines for clinical practice: management of thyroid carcinoma. American Association of Clinical Endocrinologists. American College of Endocrinology. Endocr Pract 2001;7:202–20.
26. Tuttle RM, Leboeuf R. Follow up approaches in thyroid cancer: a risk adapted paradigm. Endocrinol Metab Clin North Am 2008;37:419–35.
27. Tuttle RM, Leboeuf R, Martorella AJ. Papillary thyroid cancer: monitoring and therapy. Endocrinol Metab Clin North Am 2007;36:753–78, vii.
28. Tuttle RM, Leboeuf R, Shaha A. Medical management of thyroid cancer: a risk adapted approach. J Surg Oncol 2008;97:712–6.
29. Watkinson JC. The British Thyroid Association guidelines for the management of thyroid cancer in adults. Nucl Med Commun 2004;25:897–900.
30. Byar DP, Green SB, Dor P, *et al.* A prognostic index for thyroid carcinoma. A study of the E.O.R.T.C. Thyroid Cancer Cooperative Group. Eur J Cancer 1979;15: 1033–41.
31. Cady B, Rossi R. An expanded view of risk-group definition in differentiated thyroid carcinoma. Surgery 1988;104: 947–53.
32. Dean DS, Hay ID. Prognostic indicators in differentiated thyroid carcinoma. Cancer Control 2000;7:229–39.
33. Hay ID, Bergstralh EJ, Goellner JR, *et al.* Predicting outcome in papillary thyroid carcinoma: development of a reliable prognostic scoring system in a cohort of 1779 patients surgically treated at one institution during 1940 through 1989. Surgery 1993;114:1050–7; discussion 7–8.
34. Hay ID, Grant CS, Taylor WF, *et al.* Ipsilateral lobectomy versus bilateral lobar resection in papillary thyroid carcinoma: a retrospective analysis of surgical outcome using a novel prognostic scoring system. Surgery 1987;102:1088–95.
35. Mazzaferri EL, Jhiang SM. Differentiated thyroid cancer long-term impact of initial therapy. Trans Am Clin Climatol Assoc 1994;106:151–68; discussion 68–70.
36. Shaha AR, Loree TR, Shah JP. Prognostic factors and risk group analysis in follicular carcinoma of the thyroid. Surgery 1995;118:1131–6; discussion 6–8.
37. Sherman SI, Brierley JD, Sperling M, *et al.* Prospective multicenter study of thyroid carcinoma treatment: initial analysis of staging and outcome. National Thyroid Cancer Treatment Cooperative Study Registry Group. Cancer 1998;83:1012–21.
38. Lang BH, Lo CY, Chan WF, *et al.* Staging systems for papillary thyroid carcinoma: a review and comparison. Ann Surg 2007;245:366–78.
39. Ito Y, Higashiyama T, Takamura Y, *et al.* Risk factors for recurrence to the lymph node in papillary thyroid carcinoma patients without preoperatively detectable lateral node metastasis: validity of prophylactic modified radical neck dissection. World J Surg 2007;31:2085–91.
40. Welsch M, Abeln M, Zaplatnikov K, *et al.* Multiparameter scoring system for the prognosis of differentiated thyroid cancer. Nuklearmedizin 2007;46:257–62; quiz N53–4.
41. Kondo T, Ezzat S, Asa SL. Pathogenetic mechanisms in thyroid follicular-cell neoplasia. Nat Rev Cancer 2006;6: 292–306.
42. Baloch ZW, LiVolsi VA. Prognostic factors in well-differentiated follicular-derived carcinoma and medullary thyroid carcinoma. Thyroid 2001;11:637–45.
43. Nikiforova MN, Nikiforov YE. Molecular genetics of thyroid cancer: implications for diagnosis, treatment and prognosis. Expert Rev Mol Diagn 2008;8:83–95.
44. Ward LS, Morari EC, Leite JL, *et al.* Identifying a risk profile for thyroid cancer. Arq Bras Endocrinol Metabol 2007;51: 713–22.
45. Kebebew E, Weng J, Bauer J, *et al.* The prevalence and prognostic value of BRAF mutation in thyroid cancer. Ann Surg 2007;246:466–70; discussion 70–1.

46. Lupi C, Giannini R, Ugolini C, *et al.* Association of BRAF V600E mutation with poor clinicopathological outcomes in 500 consecutive cases of papillary thyroid carcinoma. J Clin Endocrinol Metab 2007;92:4085–90.
47. Robbins RJ, Wan Q, Grewal RK, *et al.* Real-time prognosis for metastatic thyroid carcinoma based on 2-[18F]fluoro-2-deoxy-D-glucose-positron emission tomography scanning. J Clin Endocrinol Metab 2006;91:498–505.
48. Tuttle RM, Leboeuf R. Investigational therapies for metastatic thyroid carcinoma. J Natl Compr Canc Netw 2007;5: 641–6.
49. Baudin E, Travagli JP, Ropers J, *et al.* Microcarcinoma of the thyroid gland: the Gustave-Roussy Institute experience. Cancer 1998;83:553–9.
50. Tuttle RM. Risk adapted management of thyroid cancer. Endocr Pract 2008;14:764–74.
51. Wang W, Larson SM, Tuttle RM, *et al.* Resistance of [18f]-fluorodeoxyglucose-avid metastatic thyroid cancer lesions to treatment with high-dose radioactive iodine. Thyroid 2001;11:1169–75.

MULTIPLE CHOICE QUESTIONS

Select the single most appropriate option.

1. Which of the following is the most common endocrine malignancy?
A. Adrenocortical carcinoma
B. Thyroid cancer
C. Islet cell tumours of the pancreas
D. Pituitary carcinoma

2. Which of the following statements is NOT true?
A. Thyroid cancer is more common in women
B. Most thyroid cancers present as painless nodules
C. Thyroid function tests are almost always normal in patients presenting with thyroid cancer
D. Most thyroid cancer patients present with local compression symptoms or ipsilateral vocal cord paralysis

3. Which of the following are NOT used to estimate risk of death or risk of recurrence in our current staging systems?
A. Age
B. Size of the primary
C. Completeness of resection
D. Time from discovery of nodule to definite therapy

4. Joint decision making with a patient requires a thorough understanding of
A. Risk of recurrence
B. Risk of death from thyroid cancer
C. Risk of complications of proposed therapy
D. Likelihood of clinical benefit from proposed therapy
E. All of the above

5. Which of the following statements is true regarding recommendations for extent of initial surgery?
A. Total thyroidectomy is associated with a decreased risk of disease-specific death in all patients with papillary thyroid cancer
B. Total thyroidectomy is associated with the lowest recurrence rates in most retrospective series of thyroid cancer patients
C. Total thyroidectomy is required for all thyroid cancer patients since they all must be given RAI remnant ablation.

Answers

1. B
2. D
3. D
4. E
5. B

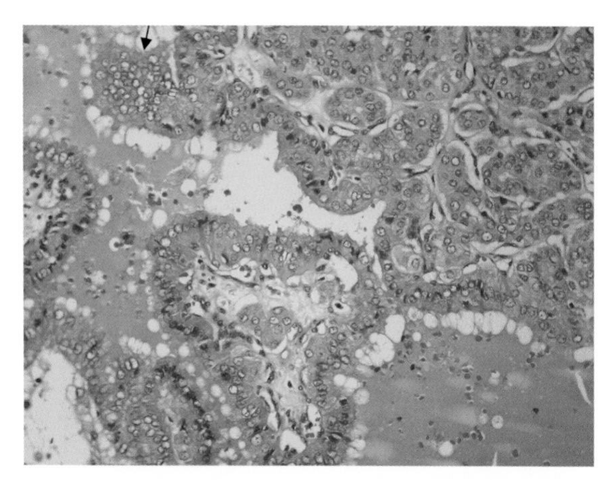

Plate 2.1 Papillae in papillary carcinoma; the epithelial cells show optically clear nuclei.

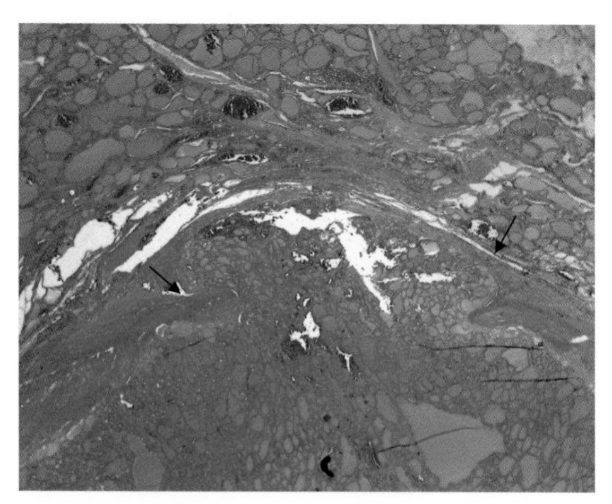

Plate 2.2 Capsular invasion (centre), diagnostic of follicular carcinoma.

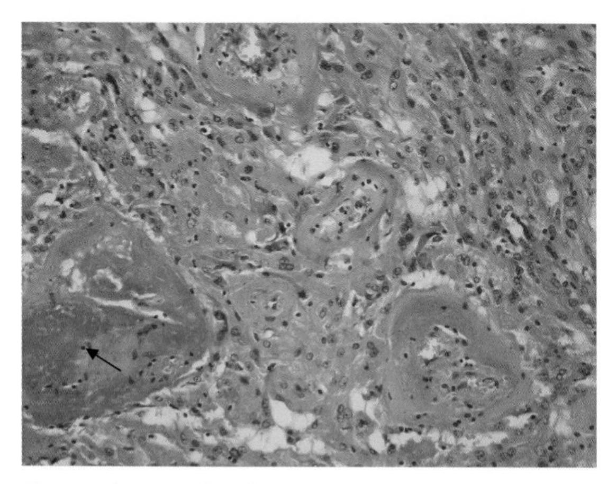

Plate 2.3 Sort spindle cells with accumulation of amyloid in medullary carcinoma.

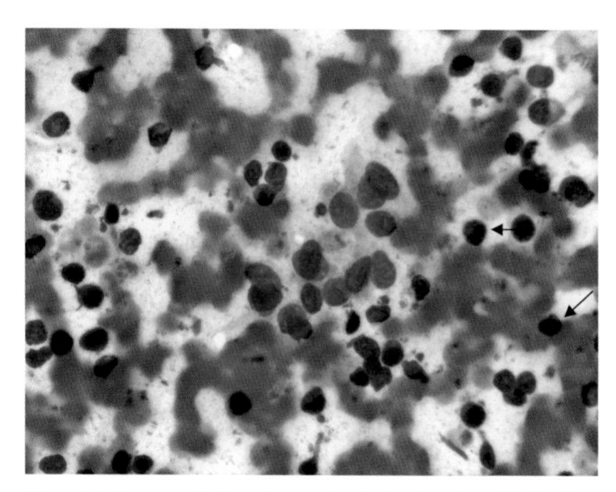

Plate 3.1 Low-grade lymphoma involving the thyroid gland. Numerous small lymphoid cells are present in addition to bland follicular epithelial cells.

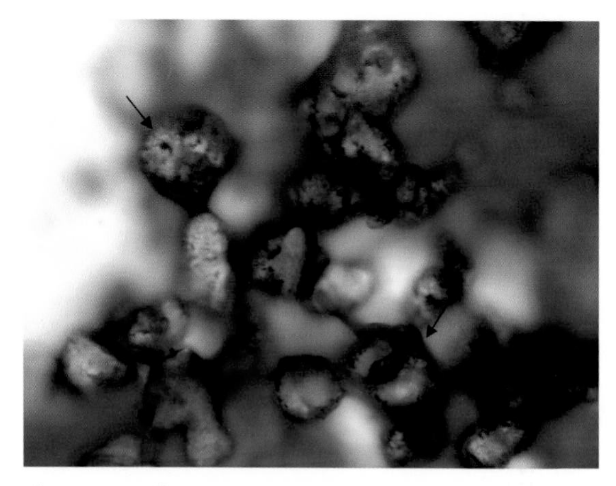

Plate 3.2 Papillary carcinoma. Psammomatous calcifications appear as semi-translucent spherical structures on May–Grünwald–Giemsa stain.

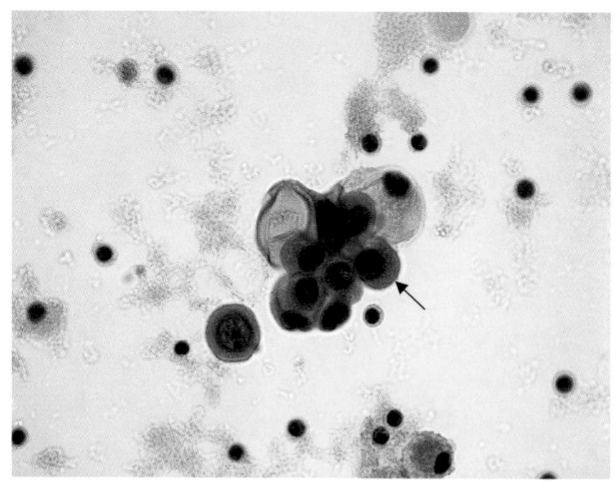

Plate 3.3 Papillary carcinoma. A rounded cluster of malignant epithelial cells with a scalloped outline, characteristic of metastatic papillary carcinoma within a lymph node (Papanicolaou stain).

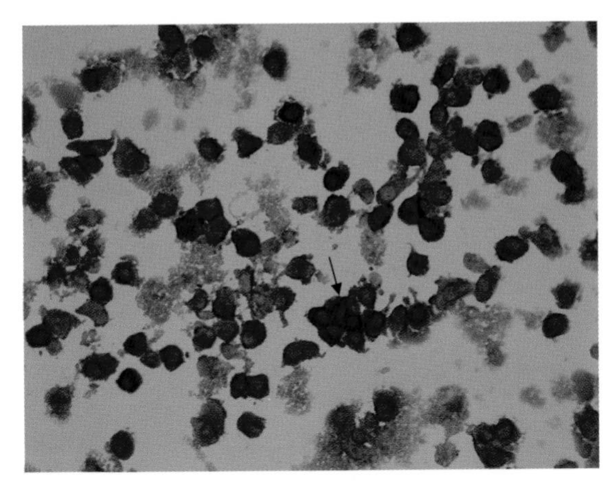

Plate 3.4 Medullary carcinoma of the thyroid, calcitonin stain. Immunocytochemistry for calcitonin is strongly positive in medullary carcinoma.

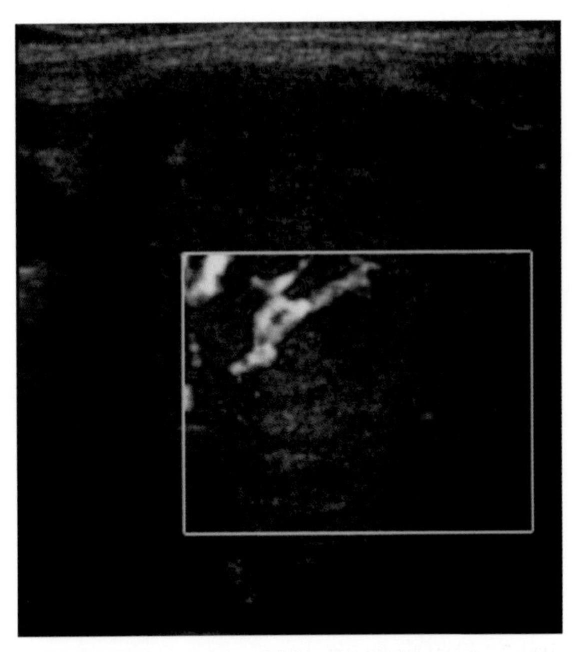

Plate 4.1 Thyroid nodule exhibiting internal (type 3) vascularity.

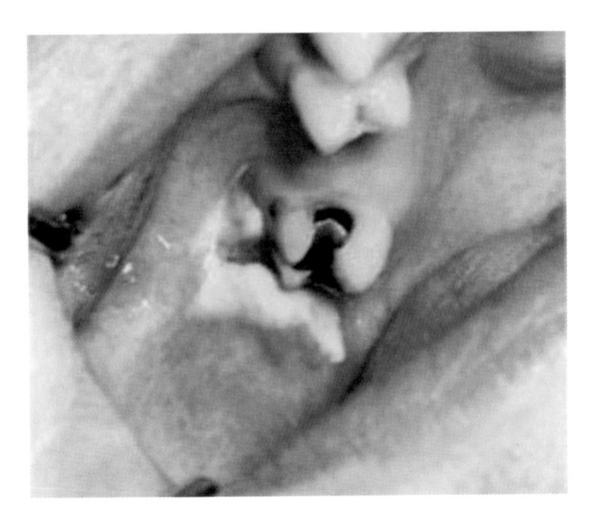

Plate 6.1 Side effects of thionamide therapy: an oral cavity ulcer resulting from agranulocytosis.

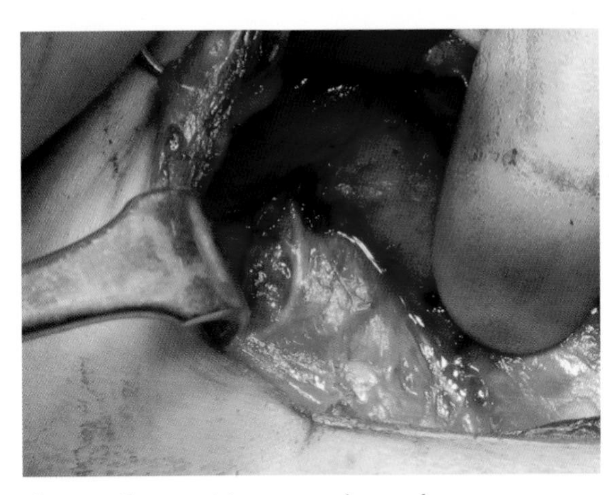

Plate 7.1 Aberrant right recurrent laryngeal nerve.

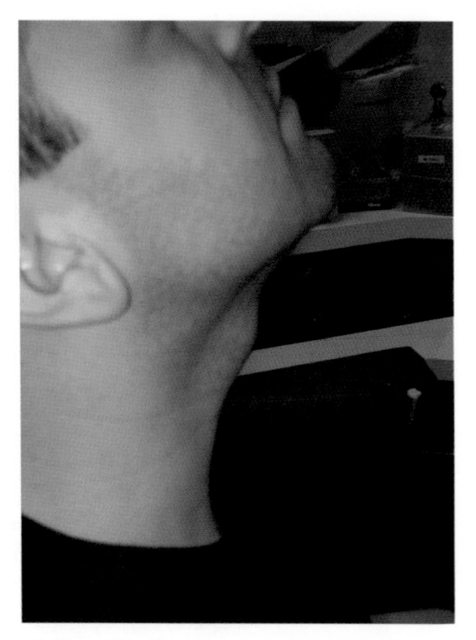

Plate 7.2 Thyroglossal cyst.

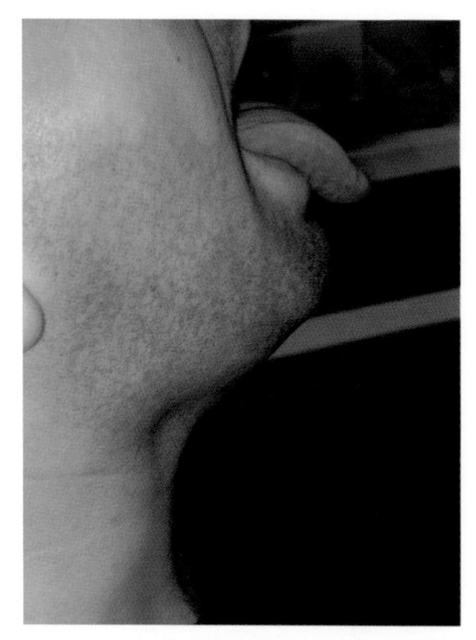

Plate 7.3 Ascent of a thyroglossal cyst on protrusion of the tongue.

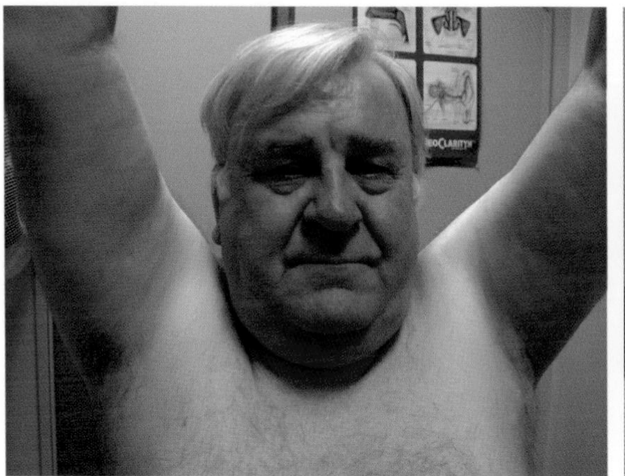

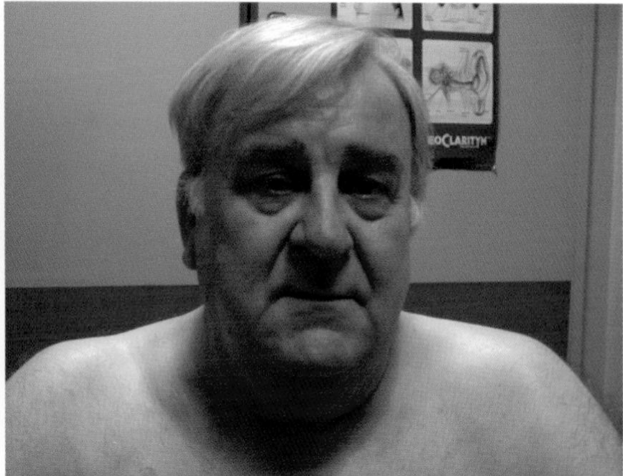

Plate 8.1 Physical examination demonstrating Pemberton's sign. When the patient has both arms elevated, the resultant facial congestion is indicative of increased pressure in the thoracic inlet caused by a large retrosternal goitre.

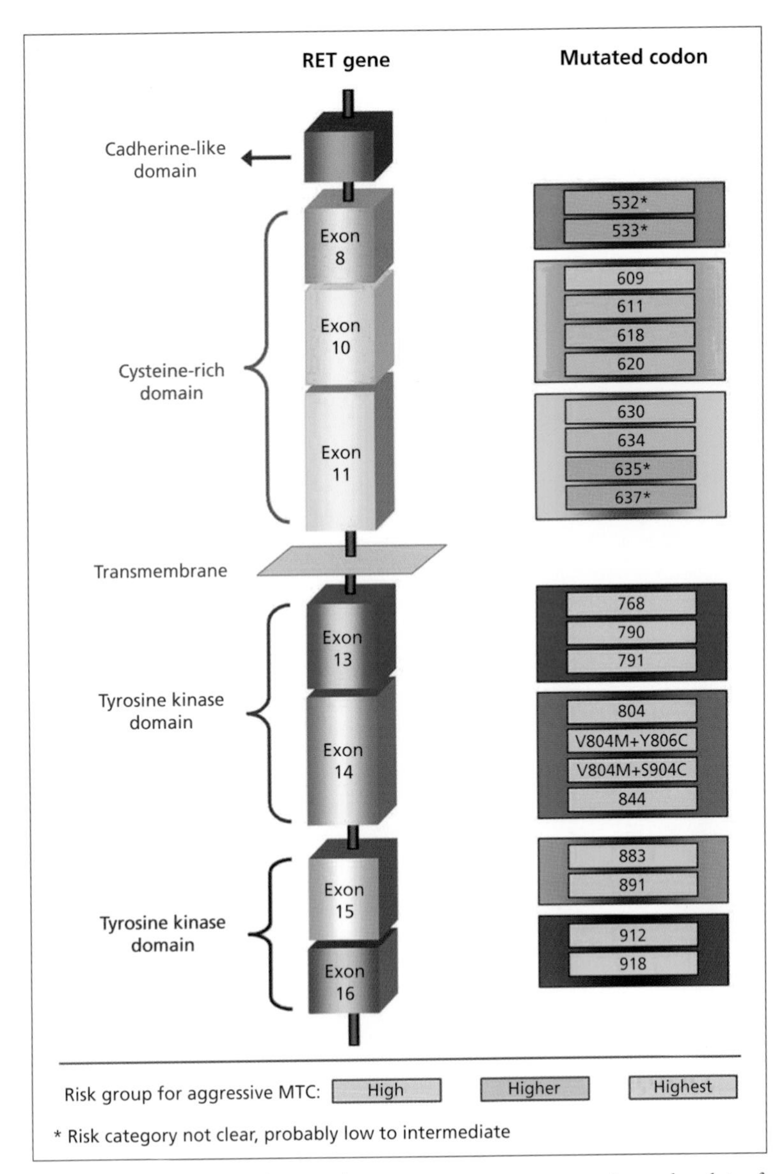

Plate 9.1 Schematic diagram of the *RET* gene and reported codons responsible for three levels of biologic aggressiveness of MTC. (Adapted from: Kouvaraki MA *et al.* RET proto-oncogene: a review and update of genotype-phenotype correlations in hereditary medullary thyroid cancer and associated endocrine tumors. Thyroid 2005;15:531–44.).

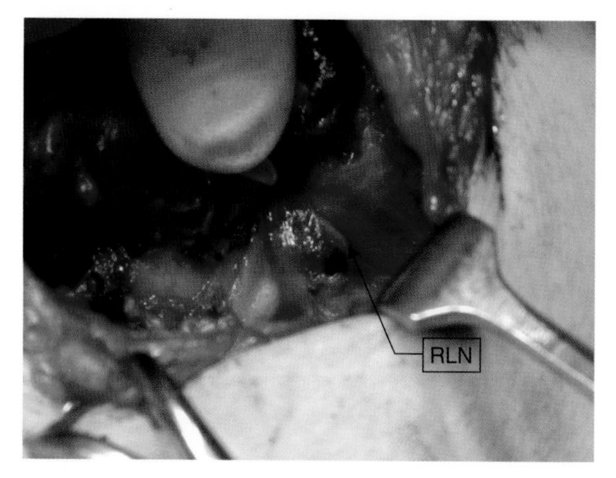

Plate 11.1 PTC central compartment lymph node metastases adjacent to the recurrent laryngeal nerve (annotated).

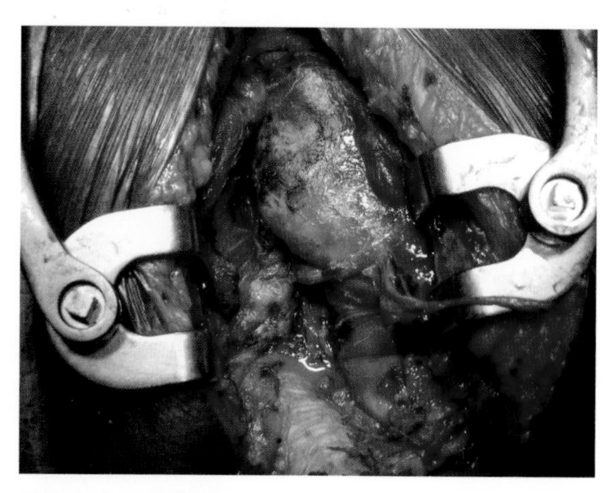

Plate 11.2 Medullary thyroid cancer requires aggressive surgical management with complete mediastinal (Level 7) clearance.

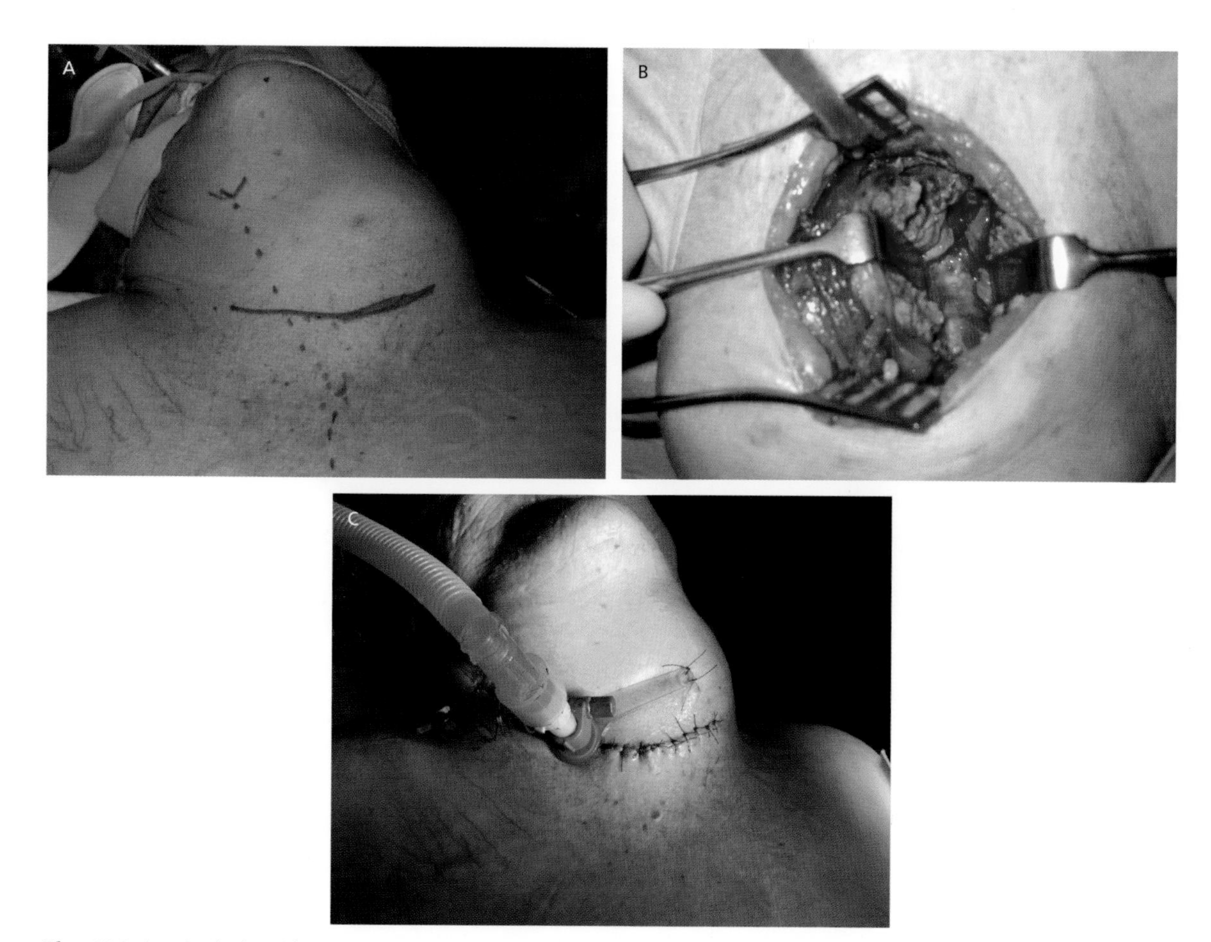

Plate 11.3 Anaplastic thyroid cancer presents as a rapidly enlarging neck mass (A). Establishing a surgical airway can be challenging due to significant tracheal deviation (B). An adjustable flange tracheostomy tube may be required (C).

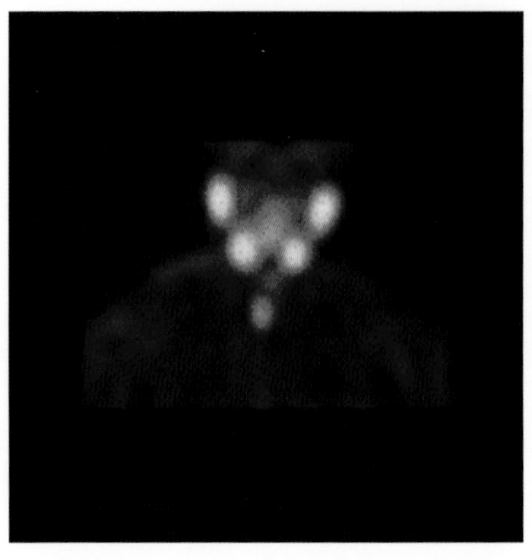

Plate 14.1 A SPECT image from a patient with a right inferior parathyroid adenoma. http://www.endocrineweb.com/viewspect.html.

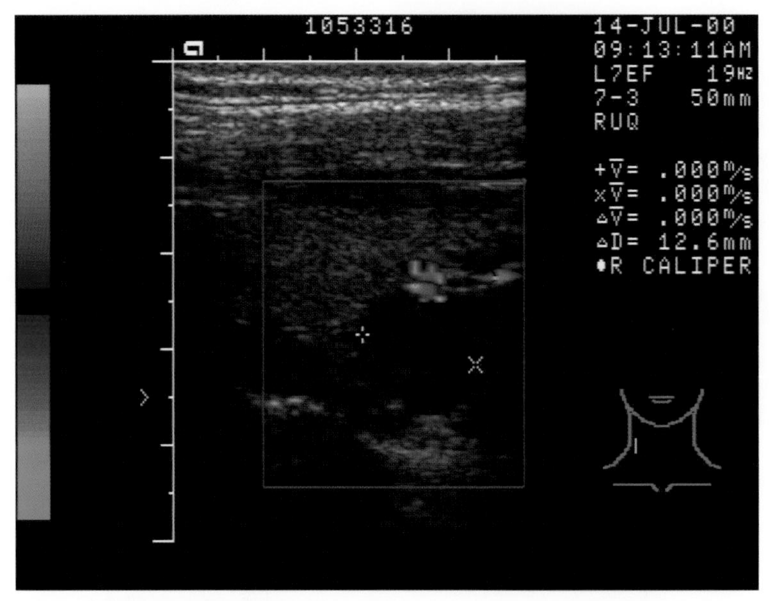

Plate 14.2 Ultrasound. There is is a right upper quadrant, hypoechoic lesion underneath the thyroid with a rim of colour flow Doppler activity. This is classic for a parathyroid adenoma. (Courtesy of Jon Meilstrup, MD.)

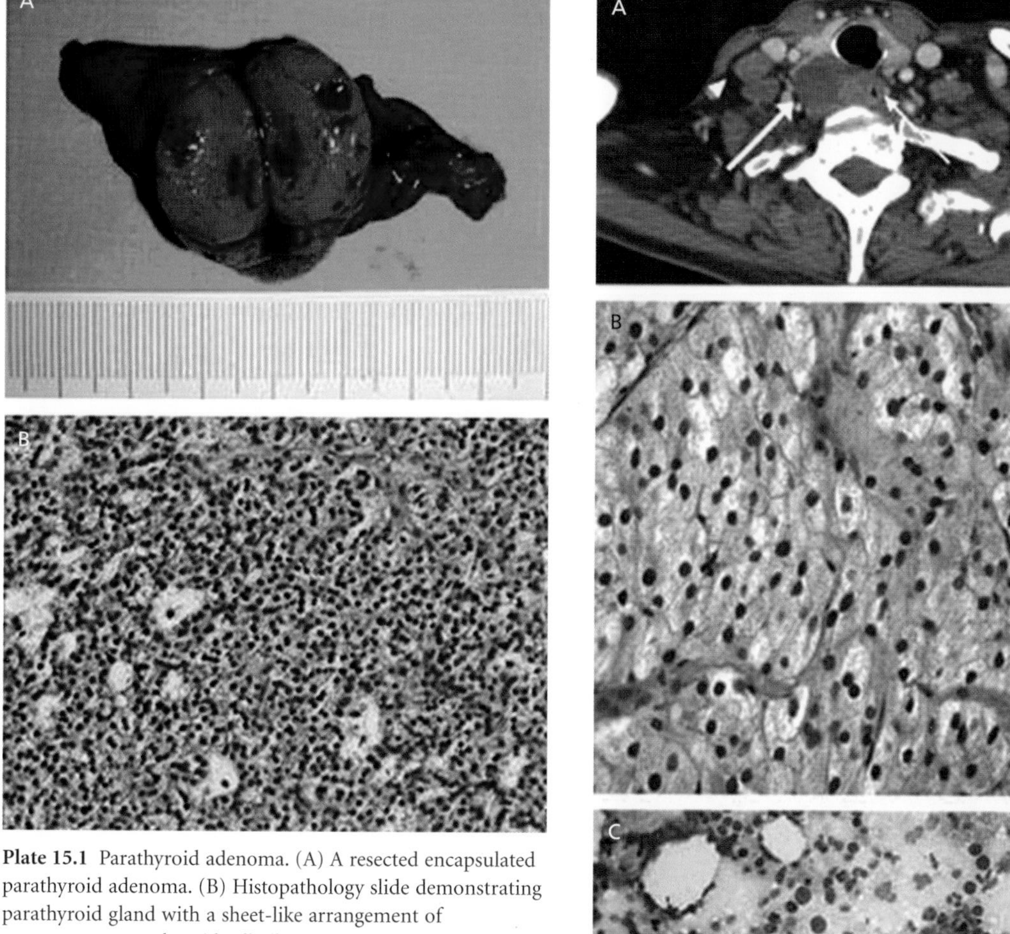

Plate 15.1 Parathyroid adenoma. (A) A resected encapsulated parathyroid adenoma. (B) Histopathology slide demonstrating parathyroid gland with a sheet-like arrangement of monotonous parathyroid cells (haematoxylin and eosin ×200).

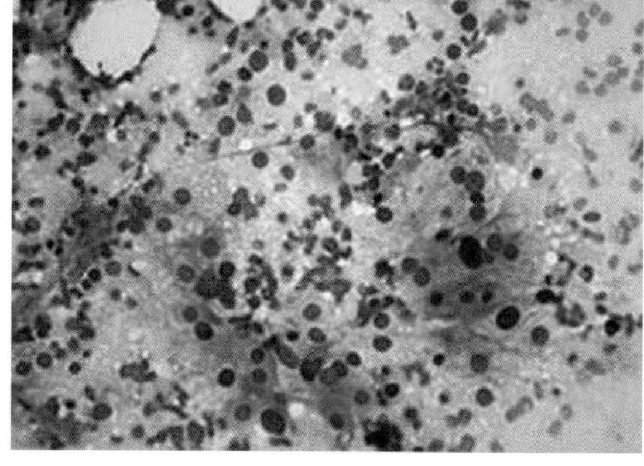

Plate 15.2 CT image of the neck, histology of the liver biopsy and cytology of the neck mass in the patient with parathyroid carcinoma. (A) CT scan of the neck of the patient showing a mass behind the right lobe of the thyroid (thick arrow). The thin arrow indicates the oesophagus, and the arrowhead indicates the enlarged cervical lymph node. (B) Liver biopsy showing the neuroendocrine tumour (stained with haematoxylin and eosin, magnification ×400). (C) Fine needle aspiration of the neck mass showing cells similar to those from the liver (stained with Papanicolaou stain, magnification ×400). Reprinted by permission from Macmillan Publishers Ltd: Nature Clinical Practice Endocrinology & Metabolism (2, 291–296), copyright (2006).

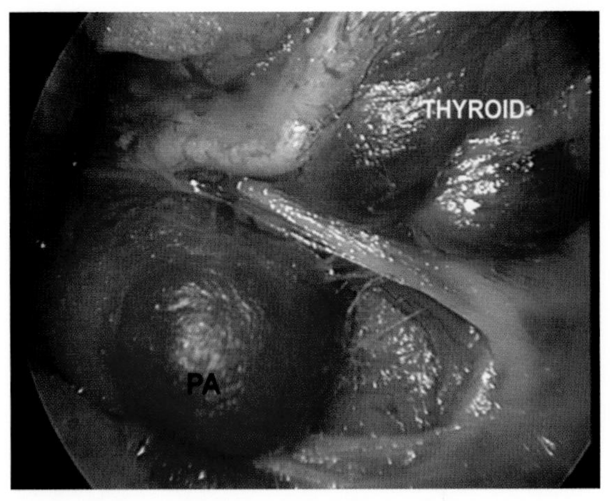

Plate 17.1 Endoscopic view during video-assisted parathyroidetomy. The parathyroid adenoma (PA) is well visualized due to excellent optical magnification afforded by the 30° endoscope.

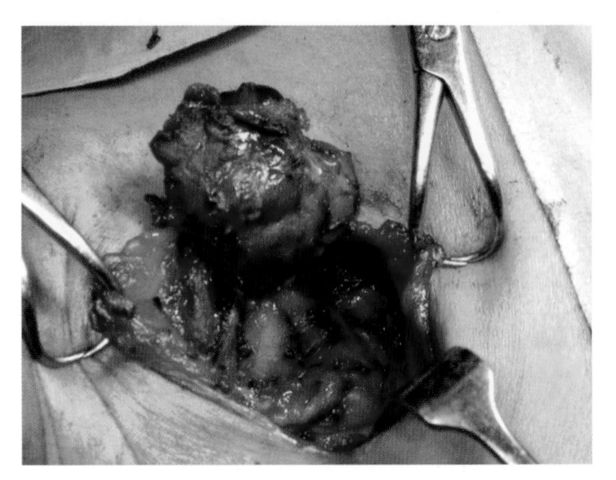

Plate 17.2 Parathyroid carcinoma.

11 Surgical management of thyroid cancer

Neil S. Tolley[1], Asit Arora[1] & Christos Georgalas[2]

[1] St Mary's Hospital, Imperial College Healthcare NHS Trust, London, UK
[2] Department of Otorhinolaryngology, Academic Medical Centre, Amsterdam, The Netherlands

KEY POINTS

- Mortality from differentiated thyroid cancer (DTC) is invariably due to Stage IV disease
- 80% of patients do extremely well regardless of the surgical strategy employed. In contrast, 5% of patients do very badly and will die of their cancer. In 15% of patients the surgical management employed will directly impact on their survival
- All patients should be discussed with an appropriate multidisciplinary team before surgery. The team should comprise a surgeon, endocrinologist, oncologist, radiologist, cytopathologist and histopathologist
- Medullary thyroid carcinoma (MTC) has a worse prognosis than DTC, with 10-year survival of approximately 75%. In contrast to DTC, the presence of nodal metastasis does significantly impact on disease-specific survival
- Genetic testing of family members of patients with multiple endocrine neoplasia (MEN) syndromes or familial MTC provides the opportunity for prophylactic surgical intervention

INTRODUCTION

Thyroid cancer is unique because it exhibits an extremely wide variance in clinical outcome. This ranges from 100% survival in patients with early-differentiated tumours to 100% mortality in patients with advanced anaplastic cancer. No other cancer exhibits such diverse clinical behaviour. This wide variability in outcome is largely a reflection of biological factors outlined in Chapters 9 and 10. In addition, there is convincing evidence to suggest that clinical management impacts on the long-term outcome of patients diagnosed with the disease.[1–3]

Despite a plethora of guidelines, management remains suboptimal in the UK, with survival rates 8% (male) and 5% (female) lower than the European average.[4] This finding, in the context of a disease which usually has a favourable outcome, has provoked criticism in the UK literature.[5–7] This concern is substantiated by the results of a national surgical audit which have highlighted inconsistent surgical management.[8] This finding raises questions about the operational organization and effectiveness of how thyroid malignancy is discussed and managed within the UK. A lack of multidisciplinary team (MDT) input is undoubtedly an important factor. Encouragingly, the recently published second national British Association of Endocrine and Thyroid Surgeons audit does suggest an increased trend to practise within a thyroid MDT in the UK.[9]

This chapter intends to provide a concise synopsis and practical guide on how to manage thyroid cancer. It is evidence based where possible and grades of recommendation have been annotated where appropriate.

DIFFERENTIATED THYROID CANCER (DTC)

Epidemiology

DTC is an incidental finding in 37% of post-mortem specimens. This 'biological cancer' has no clinical significance, in contrast to its rare 'clinical' counterpart. DTC is twice as common in women and commonly presents in the third and fourth decades. The incidence of DTC is 2/100 000, and this figure is rising due to higher surveillance and early detection. Eighty-seven percent of tumours are less than 2 cm.[10] In the UK, there are approximately 900 new cases diagnosed and 250 deaths per annum.[11] Locoregional recurrence occurs in 5–20% and distant metastases in 5–15% of patients.

SEER (Surveillance, Epidemiology and End Results) data from the USA have shown that survival rates for DTC are approximately 94%.[12] The detection of an increasing number of early cancers will favourably bias survival figures. Indeed, an analysis of the number of

A Practical Manual of Thyroid and Parathyroid Disease, 1st Edition.
Edited by Asit Arora, Neil Tolley & R. Michael Tuttle.

Table 11.1 American Joint Committee on Cancer (AJCC) stage groupings

Papillary or follicular thyroid cancer	
Younger than 45 years	
Stage I:	any T, any N, M0
Stage II:	any T, any N, M1
Age 45 years and older	
Stage I:	T1, N0, M0
Stage II:	T2, N0, M0
Stage III:	T3, N0, M0
	T1–3, N1a, M0
Stage IVA:	T4a, N0, M0
	T4a, N1a, M0
	T1–3, N1b, M0
	T4a, N1b, M0
Stage IVB:	T4b, any N, M0
Stage IVC:	any T, any N, M1
Medullary thyroid cancer	
Stage I:	T1, N0, M0
Stage II:	T2, N0, M0
Stage III:	T3, N0, M0
	T1–3, N1a, M0
Stage IVA:	T4a, N0, M0
	T4a, N1a, M0
	T1–3, N1b, M0
	T4a, N1b, M0
Stage IVB:	T4b, any N, M0
Stage IVC:	any T, any N, M1
Anaplastic thyroid cancer	
Automatically Stage IV T4a: intrathyroidal anaplastic carcinoma—surgically resectable	
T4b: extrathyroidal anaplastic carcinoma—surgically unresectable	

patients who succumb to thyroid cancer reveals that this figure has remained constant. National Cancer Data Base (NCDB) data from the USA have shown that mortality from DTC is invariably due to Stage IV disease (see Table 11.1).[13]

Aetiology

The only factor which definitely predisposes to thyroid cancer is radiation.[14] Iodine deficiency, whilst not increasing the incidence of cancer, is associated with a higher incidence of follicular tumours. This trend is reversed when iodine replete. Genetic factors are rarely associated, such as in Gardener's and Cowden's syndromes, and rare hereditary forms of DTC also exist.

Staging

There are a plethora of staging systems, all of which have their merits (see Chapter 10). Although they provide a guide to prognosis, patient management and literature analysis, none at present includes an assessment of inherent biological tumour behaviour. In general, 80% of patients do extremely well regardless of the surgical strategy employed. Indeed there is sufficient evidence in the literature to support any surgical paradigm of treatment for this group. In stark contrast, 5% of patients do very badly and will die of their cancer. Although biological factors are inherently responsible for this poor outcome, in 15% of patients the surgical management employed does impact on their survival.

There have been significant advances in our understanding of thyroid cancer at a molecular and genetic level (see Chapter 9). However, we are still some way from a combined biological and clinical staging system which will depict survival outcomes and guide patient management more accurately than the present systems employed. The TNM (Union Internationale Contre le Cancer (UICC)) classification is probably the most widely used system. In 2002 this was updated to a 6th edition. One area of great contention is the re-classification of T1 and T2 disease. In the 5th edition, tumours less than 1 cm were classified as T1 and placed within a microcarcinoma category. In the 6th edition, T1 classification includes all tumours up to 2 cm. Several authorities have significant reservations regarding this change because the propensity for nodal metastasis increases quite sharply once a tumour reaches 1 cm. Although this has not been proven to impact on survival, there may be an increased risk of recurrence. Nevertheless, the 6th edition is established and used as the point of reference for this chapter (Table 11.2).

Presentation and investigation

The vast majority of DTC is papillary (PTC) in nature while a smaller percentage are follicular (FTC). This includes all histological subtypes such as the follicular variant, tall cell, insular, etc. Eighty-seven percent of tumours are less than 2 cm and they usually present as a unilateral thyroid swelling.

Advanced cancers which exhibit extracapsular breach may involve the recurrent laryngeal nerves, resulting in hoarseness and swallowing dysfunction. Cervical node metastases are palpable in 33% of patients, and the incidence of impalpable micrometastases in PTC is even

Table 11.2 TNM classification (UICC 6th edition)

Primary tumour (T)
All categories may be subdivided into (a) solitary tumour or (b) multifocal tumour (the largest determines the classification).

TX:	Primary tumour cannot be assessed
T0:	No evidence of primary tumour
T1:	Tumour 2 cm or less in greatest dimension, limited to the thyroid
T2:	Tumour larger than 2 cm but 4 cm or smaller in greatest dimension, limited to the thyroid
T3:	Tumor larger than 4 cm in greatest dimension limited to the thyroid or any tumour with minimal extrathyroid extension (e.g. extension to sternothyroid muscle or perithyroid soft tissues)
T4a:	Tumour of any size extending beyond the thyroid capsule to invade subcutaneous soft tissues, larynx, trachea, oesophagus or recurrent laryngeal nerve
T4b:	Tumour invades prevertebral fascia or encases carotid artery or mediastinal vessels

Regional lymph nodes (N)
Regional lymph nodes are the central compartment, lateral cervical and upper mediastinal lymph nodes.

NX:	Regional lymph nodes cannot be assessed
N0:	No regional lymph node metastasis
N1:	Regional lymph node metastasis
N1a:	Metastasis to level VI (pre-tracheal, paratracheal and pre-laryngeal/Delphian lymph nodes)
N1b:	Metastasis to unilateral or bilateral cervical or superior mediastinal lymph nodes

Distant metastases (M)

MX:	Distant metastasis cannot be assessed
M0:	No distant metastasis
M1:	Distant metastasis

higher, ranging from 55 to 70% at presentation[15–17] (Plate 11.1).

Clinically, a hard, non-tender thyroid swelling is a typical finding. Haemoptysis signifies tracheal invasion and is an extremely rare presenting symptom of advanced cancer. In the vast majority of patients, it is possible to make a pre-operative diagnosis of thyroid cancer. All patients should have a fine needle aspiration cytology (FNAC) and ultrasound (US) scan of the thyroid gland and neck as a minimum. Vocal cord examination is mandatory. All patients should be discussed at an appropriate MDT meeting prior to surgical management. The MDT usually comprises a surgeon, endocrinologist, oncologist, radiologist, cytopathologist and histopathologist, as well as support staff such as specialist nurse and MDT coordinator.

Management

Surgical management is dependent upon a number of factors. Tumour size, presence of nodal metastases, family history, history of radiation exposure and age are the most important considerations. In younger patients, thyroid cancer is more likely to be multifocal and associated with nodal metastases. The same applies on the rare occasions when there is a familial history of PTC or radiation exposure. Total thyroidectomy and central level VI dissection is the most appropriate surgical management in these rare instances.

The literature supports a hemithyroidectomy as being sufficient management for the young patient below the age of 45 years and for tumours less than 1 cm. The authors advocate inclusion of a unilateral level VI dissection whenever a pre-operative diagnosis has been made. Some authorities may consider this a controversial management policy. Our rationale is that it allows us to stage the rare instances of microcarcinoma that have nodal metastases and avoids re-operation within this area when the eventual clinical course determines that completion thyroidectomy is necessary.

For tumours larger than 1 cm, a policy of total thyroidectomy with bilateral level VI dissection should be employed. Similarly, a total thyroidectomy should be performed in all patients presenting with nodal metastasis because these patients will require radioiodine ablation following surgical treatment. Total thyroidectomy is also advisable for histological subtypes associated with less favourable outcome such as insular and tall cell tumours. Likewise, a total thyroidectomy and central level VI dissection should be the minimum surgery performed in Hurthle cell cancer due to its lack of radioiodine avidity.

Follicular tumours require a different treatment strategy because FTC cannot be diagnosed cytologically. In our unit, approximately 25% of follicular neoplasms (Thy 3) will turn out to be FTC. FTC has a propensity for angioinvasion rather than lymph node metastasis. Central level VI dissection should not be routinely performed with a diagnostic thyroid lobectomy. In tumours less than 1 cm with no angioinvasion, thyroid lobectomy is sufficient treatment provided it is supplemented with moderate TSH suppression. In tumours larger than 1 cm or those exhibiting angioinvasion, a completion thyroidectomy is recommended. This should be followed by radioiodine ablation and TSH suppression.

Lateral compartment disease

A less aggressive approach can be adopted for the lateral compartment compared with medullary cancer. Disease within this compartment can be mapped by high resolution US and surgery planned accordingly. Nodal disease rarely occurs in level I and therefore its routine dissection is not indicated. Nodal metastasis anywhere in the deep jugular system warrants a level II–IV dissection as a minimum. Level V dissection should only be included when this is radiologically, cytologically or clinically indicated.

Lateral neck disease is not associated with increased patient mortality and does not impact on prognosis except, perhaps, in the elderly male. It is imperative that experienced, high volume surgeons perform these procedures when indicated so that morbidity and complications are kept to a minimum.[18]

ADVANCED DISEASE

Recurrent laryngeal nerve

Vocal cord palsy is a sign of extracapsular extension of tumour and an advanced stage. The site of infiltration is usually just below the cricoid cartilage. A clinically involved, non-functioning nerve should be resected with tumour. A functioning nerve requires sacrifice in exceptional circumstances only. It may be impossible to clear microscopic disease on a functioning nerve. However, gross disease on the nerve should never be left behind in the frequent but mistaken belief that post-operative radioiodine will eradicate the disease remnant.

Trachea

Advanced invasion of the trachea should be identified prior to surgery by a non-contrast computed tomography (CT) scan. Tracheal resection is indicated when tumour breaches the trachea wall and is intraluminal. Tracheal shave excision is usually sufficient when lesser degrees of invasion are present.[19]

Laryngeal cartilages

Cartilage is a poor barrier to the spread of thyroid cancer. The lamina of the thyroid cartilage can be resected in a plane outside hypopharyngeal mucosa. Similarly, cricoid cartilage can be shaved, resected and reconstructed with costal cartilage if required.

Oesophagus

Unlike cartilage, the oesophageal mucosa is a good barrier. When muscle is involved, this can be resected as a cuff in a submucosal plane, usually with minimal morbidity.

MEDULLARY CARCINOMA

Medullary carcinoma of the thyroid (MTC) accounts for 5–10% of thyroid cancer. It was initially described as a type of malignant goitre with amyloid deposition by Jaquet in 1906.[20] In 1959 it was formally recognized as a distinct thyroid tumour by Hazard,[21] and in 1965 Williams[22] described its hereditary form and parafollicular cell origin. This relatively late description is surprising because MTC differs from DTC and anaplastic carcinoma in several fundamental ways. These include its histology, epidemiology, risk factors, genetics, clinical manifestations, natural course and management.

Histology

Unlike DTC which arises from the thyroid follicular cell, medullary tumours originate from the parafollicular cells (C cells) of the thyroid gland. These are neural crest-derived cells which produce a variety of hormones and vasoactive amines including adrenocorticotropic hormone (ACTH), melatonin, histaminase, prostaglandins and, most importantly, calcitonin. As a result, medullary carcinoma (as well as C-cell hyperplasia) is associated with raised calcitonin levels. Calcitonin is a very sensitive and moderately specific tumour marker. Parafollicular cells are not involved in iodine metabolism and thyroid hormone production. This explains why MTC is not associated with iodine deficiency and does not respond to radioiodine or thyroid-stimulating hormone (TSH) suppression with thyroxine. MTC (especially the hereditary variant) frequently arises from C-cell hyperplasia. C cells are spread in islets within the gland, which accounts for the multicentric tendency of MTC.

Aetiology, genetics and epidemiology

Seventy-five percent of MTC is sporadic, while in 25% of patients it is genetically determined. The latter arises either in isolation as familial medullary thyroid carcinoma (FMTC) or as part of multiple endocrine neoplasia (MEN) syndromes 2A and less frequently 2B. Transmission is autosomal dominant with high penetrance and variable expression. The genetic anomaly results in a mutation in the *RET* proto-oncogene, encoding a receptor protein tyrosine kinase on chromosome 10.[23] The mean age of presentation is the fifth and sixth decades for the sporadic variety and the second or third decade for the genetically determined variants. There is no gender predilection.

Clinical manifestations

Patients with the familial or MEN syndrome variant are frequently asymptomatic and are identified by genetic and biochemical screening tests. In the sporadic variety, clinical signs and symptoms are indistinguishable from other thyroid tumours although metastatic lymph nodes tend to occur more frequently. In advanced or metastatic disease, patients occasionally present with paraneoplastic manifestations related to excessive secretion of ACTH (Cushing's syndrome), calcitonin (bone pain) and prostaglandin (diarrhoea—carcinoid syndrome).[24] Thirty percent of patients with MEN2A have concurrent hyperparathyroidism and 50% have pheochromocytomas. In the MEN2B syndrome, presentation with pheochromocytoma, mucosal neuromas, ganglioneuromas and a characteristic marfanoid phenotype are classical but do not invariably occur.

Investigations

For any thyroid mass, the investigation of choice is FNA with US. Almost without exception, diagnosis should be made in the pre-operative setting. Selective calcitonin measurement may result in an earlier diagnosis, particularly in the sporadic variety, which may improve patient outcome.[25,26] Measurement of calcitonin following pentagastrin stimulation is helpful in differentiating C-cell hyperplasia and medullary carcinoma in patients with raised calcitonin levels. All patients with a provisional diagnosis of medullary carcinoma should undergo genetic testing for *RET* proto-oncogene. When this is positive, the test should be extended to first-degree relatives. Exclusion of concurrent pheochromocytoma in a patient diagnosed with medullary carcinoma in the context of MEN2A or 2B syndrome is essential. This is achieved by measurement of urinary catecholamines.

Prognosis—staging

Medullary carcinoma has a worse prognosis than DTC, with 10-year survival of approximately 75%.[13] Sporadic tumours appear to have a worse prognosis than the hereditary variant, although this may be a reflection of lead time bias rather than an inherently more aggressive biological behaviour.[27] Amongst the hereditary variants, patients with MEN2A and FMTC have a better prognosis than patients with MEN2B syndrome. TNM staging (Table 11.2) and the EORTC (European Organization for Research and Treatment of Cancer) prognostic criteria are accurate predictors of survival. The importance of age is controversial.[5]

Treatment

Prophylactic

Advances in molecular biology and our understanding of MTC genetics provides a paradigm of applied genetic screening. Testing the family members of patients with MEN syndromes or FMTC for codon mutations will identify those who will subsequently develop MTC. This provides the opportunity for prophylactic intervention as opposed to therapeutic treatment. Patients with MEN2A and FMTC should undergo total thyroidectomy (with or without central neck dissection) before the age of 6 years.[28,29] Patients identified with MEN2B and/or *RET* codon 883, 918 or 922 mutation should undergo the same treatment during their first year of life. Prophylactic central neck dissection in older children or those with raised calcitonin (consistent with either C-cell hyperplasia or subclinical MTC) is warranted because nodal metastasis is common.

Therapeutic

MTC does not take up radioiodine or respond to TSH suppression because it is derived from the C cell. Radiotherapy has a limited role in locoregional control or the treatment of isolated metastases, and is not curative. Surgery offers the only cure, with total thyroidectomy justified due to its bilateral and multifocal nature. This also permits the earlier detection of recurrent disease through serial calcitonin assay.[30] In a small minority of selected T1 N0 tumours where a hereditary component has been excluded with *RET* mutational analysis, some authorities advocate hemithyroidectomy and isthmusectomy.[31] In our opinion, aggressive surgical management is almost always warranted.

Neck disease

Subclinical neck disease is very common in MTC, with an incidence ranging from 30% in T1 tumours to almost

100% in T4 tumours. In contrast to DTC, the presence of nodal metastasis does significantly impact on disease-specific survival. Metastatic spread follows a pattern from the central neck (level VI) compartment to the lateral and upper mediastinal (level VII) compartments. As a result, a policy of level VI dissection in all clinically apparent tumours is mandatory.[12] Any case with clinically positive nodes (either palpable, detected on ultrasound or discovered intra-operatively) warrants a complete central and lateral compartment neck dissection.[32] When there is nodal involvement, the authors advocate routine bilateral level I–VII selective neck dissection (Plate 11.2). Some authorities argue that as in DTC, level I dissection is unnecessary.

Residual, recurrent and metastatic disease

Follow-up is life-long, with serial measurement of serum calcitonin. This provides the most accurate indication of residual or recurrent disease. Twenty percent of patients with MTC have serological evidence of residual disease following surgical treatment. When a patient presents with nodal metastasis, it is rarely possible to achieve an acalcitonaemic patient with surgical treatment. Patients with elevated but stable calcitonin levels can be observed. However, a progressive rise in calcitonin levels necessitates a search for recurrent disease. Unfortunately, the vast majority of recurrent disease is systemic and therefore microscopic in nature. A diligent search for recurrence with US, magnetic resonance imaging (MRI), CT and nuclear scans often yields disappointing results initially. However, the site(s) and nature of recurrence invariably becomes evident over time. Once again, surgery offers the only chance of cure in these patients. Unfortunately, this is usually not appropriate as many patients are incurable at this stage. Nevertheless, patients survive for many years, so conservative and tailored surgery is appropriate in many patients, particularly when it improves their quality of life and prolongs survival.

ANAPLASTIC THYROID CANCER (ATC)

Patients with ATC are usually elderly and present with a rapidly enlarging neck mass and clinical signs of local invasion of adjacent structures. This includes hoarseness, stridor and progressive dysphagia. Regional lymph node involvement is common, and pulmonary metastases are present in approximately half of patients at the time of initial diagnosis. ATC is thought to arise by de-differentiation of well-differentiated neoplasms and therefore demonstrates little or no radioiodine avidity. It is an extremely aggressive tumour associated with a dismal prognosis. This is reflected by the AJCC staging of this disease which classifies all anaplastic tumours, regardless of size, as Stage IV disease. Most patients die within months of diagnosis from local disease.

Initial investigation with FNA to establish the diagnosis may prove unhelpful, necessitating core needle or open biopsy. Surgical management of most patients is limited to establishing a surgical airway to prevent death due to impending airway obstruction (Plate 11.3). Some authorities advocate aggressive surgical management for selected cases. This may be considered in patients with small volume disease and no evidence of distant metastasis. Surgery should only be undertaken if complete tumour excision can be achieved with limited morbidity. Unfortunately this is rarely possible. Non-surgical treatment options are outlined in Chapter 12. ATC is not very radiosensitive, although combined chemotherapy and hyperfractionated radiotherapy regimes have demonstrated some benefit for disease palliation.

MISCELLANEOUS

Rare cancers such as squamous cell, mucoepidermoid and secondaries from breast, lung and kidney should all be managed by a total thyroidectomy.

EVIDENCE APPRAISAL

The literature and references within this chapter are based on Level III/IV evidence at best.

REFERENCES

1. Mazzaferri EL. An overview of the management of papillary and follicular thyroid cancer. Thyroid 1999;9:421–7.
2. Mazzaferri EL, Jhiang SM. Long-term impact of initial surgical and medical therapy on papillary and follicular thyroid cancer. Am J Med 1994;97:418–28.
3. Mazzaferri EL, Kloos RT. Current approaches to primary therapy for papillary and follicular thyroid cancer. J Clin Endocrinol Metab 2001;86:1447–63.
4. Teppo L, Hakulinen T, Eurocare Working Group. Variation in survival of adult patients with thyroid cancer in Europe. Eur J Cancer 1998;34:2238–52.
5. Kendall-Taylor P. Managing differentiated thyroid cancer. BMJ 2002;324:988–9.

6. Vanderpump MPJ, Alexander L, Scarpello JHB, *et al.* An audit of management of thyroid cancer in a district general hospital. Clin Endocrinol 1998;48:419–24.
7. Kumar H, Daykin J, Holder R, *et al.* An audit of the management of differentiated thyroid cancer in specialist and non-specialist clinic settings. Clin Endocrinol 2001;54:719–23.
8. The British Association of Endocrine and Thyroid Surgeons (BAETS) First National Thyroid/Parathyroid Database Report 2003.
9. The British Association of Endocrine and Thyroid Surgeons (BAETS) Second National Thyroid/Parathyroid Database Report 2007.
10. Shah JP. Sir Felix Semon Lecture. Personal communication Royal Society of Medicine Meeting November 2006.
11. Coleman PM, Babb P, Damiecki P, *et al.* Cancer survival trends in England and Wales 1971–1995: deprivation and NHS region. London: Stationery Office, 1999, series SMPS No 61:471–8.
12. SEER Cancer Statistics Review, 1975–2005. 2008. (Accessed 1 July 2008, at http://seer.cancer.gov/csr/1975_2005.)
13. Hundahl SA, Fleming ID, Fremgen AM, *et al.* A National Cancer Data Base report on 53,856 cases of thyroid carcinoma treated in the US, 1985–1995. Cancer 1998;83:2638–48.
14. Ron E, Lubin JH, Shore RE, *et al.* Thyroid cancer after exposure to external radiation: a pooled analysis of seven studies. Radiat Res 1995;141:259–77.
15. Noguchi M, Kumoki T, Tariya T, *et al.* Bilateral cervical lymph node metastases in well differentiated thyroid carcinoma. Arch Surg 1990;125:804–6.
16. Shaha AR, Shah JP, Loree TR. Patterns of nodal and distant metastasis based on histological varieties in differentiated carcinoma of the thyroid. Am J Surg 1996;172:692–4.
17. Grebe SK, Hay ID. Thyroid cancer nodal metastases: biological significance and therapeutic considerations. Surg Oncol Clin North Am 1996;5:43–63.
18. Sosa JA, Bowman HM, Tielsch MD, *et al.* The importance of surgeon experience for clinical and economic outcomes from thyroidectomy. Ann Surg 1998;228:320–30.
19. McCaffrey JC. Aerodigestive tract invasion by well-differentiated thyroid carcinoma: diagnosis, management, prognosis and biology. Laryngoscope 2006;116:1–11.
20. Jaquet AJ. Ein Fall von metastaserenden amyloidtumouren (lymphosarcoma). Virchow's Arch A Pathol Anat 1906;185: 251–67.
21. Hazard JB, Hawk WA, Crile G Jr. Medullary (solid) carcinoma of the thyroid; a clinicopathologic entity. J Clin Endocrinol Metab 1959;19:152–6.
22. Williams ED. Histogenesis of medullary carcinoma of the thyroid. J Clin Pathol 1966;19:114–8.
23. Mulligan LM, Kwok JB, Healey CS, *et al.* Germ-line mutations of the RET proto-oncogene in multiple endocrine neoplasia type 2A. Nature 1993;363:458–60.
24. Kebebew E, Ituarte PH, Siperstein AE, *et al.* Medullary thyroid carcinoma: clinical characteristics, treatment, prognostic factors, and a comparison of staging systems. Cancer 2000;88:1139–48.
25. Pacini F, Fontanelli M, Fugazzola L, *et al.* Routine measurement of serum calcitonin in nodular thyroid diseases allows the preoperative diagnosis of unsuspected sporadic medullary thyroid carcinoma. J Clin Endocrinol Metab 1994; 78:826–9.
26. Elisei R, Bottici V, Luchetti F, *et al.* Impact of routine measurement of serum calcitonin on the diagnosis and outcome of medullary thyroid cancer: experience in 10,864 patients with nodular thyroid disorders. J Clin Endocrinol Metab 2004;89:163–8.
27. Samaan NA, Schultz PN, Hickey RC. Medullary thyroid carcinoma: prognosis of familial versus sporadic disease and the role of radiotherapy. J Clin Endocrinol Metab 1988;67:801–5.
28. Brandi ML, Gagel RF, Angeli A, *et al.* Guidelines for diagnosis and therapy of MEN type 1 and type 2. J Clin Endocrinol Metab 2001;86:5658–71.
29. Skinner MA, Moley JA, Dilley WG, *et al.* Prophylactic thyroidectomy in multiple endocrine neoplasia type 2A. N Engl J Med 2005;353:1105–13.
30. British Thyroid Association, Guidelines for the management of thyroid cancer in adults, March 2002. http://www.british-thyroid-association.org/complete%20guidelines.pdf (Accessed August 2007).
31. Miyauchi A, Matsuzuka F, Hirai K, *et al.* Prospective trial of unilateral surgery for nonhereditary medullary thyroid carcinoma in patients without germline RET mutations. World J Surg 2002;26:1023–8.
32. Dralle H, Damm I, Scheumann GF, *et al.* Compartment-oriented microdissection of regional lymph nodes in medullary thyroid carcinoma. Surg Today 1994;24:112–21.

MULTIPLE CHOICE QUESTIONS

Select the single most appropriate option.

1. Regarding the 5th edition TNM staging of differentiated thyroid cancer (DTC):
A. T1 classification includes all tumours up to 2 cm in maximum dimension
B. T2 classification includes tumours >4 cm in maximum dimension limited to the thyroid gland
C. T3 classification only includes tumours limited to the thyroid gland
D. N1a classification has a negative impact on disease-specific survival

2. Regarding the management of DTC:
A. Hurthle cell carcinoma is usually radioiodine avid
B. In patients below the age of 45 years with tumours less than 1 cm, hemithyroidectomy represents the optimal surgical management

C. Patients should routinely have a level VI dissection when undergoing a diagnostic thyroid lobectomy for a Thy 3 follicular tumour
D. A more aggressive surgical approach is adopted for the lateral neck compartment compared with medullary cancer

3. Regarding the management of advanced DTC:
A. Advanced invasion of the trachea should be identified prior to surgery with a contrast CT scan
B. External beam radiotherapy is usually warranted for patients with T3 disease
C. The recurrent laryngeal nerve usually needs to be sacrificed in patients presenting with a hoarse voice
D. A clinically involved, non-functioning nerve should be resected with tumour

4. Regarding medullary thyroid cancer (MTC):
A. Patients with the hereditary variants have a worse prognosis than the sporadic form of MTC
B. Amongst the hereditary variants, patients with MEN2A and familial MTC have a worse prognosis than those with MEN2B
C. A policy of level VI dissection in all clinically apparent tumours is mandatory
D. The mean age of presentation is the second or third decades for the sporadic variety

5. Regarding follow-up in patients with MTC:
A. 30% of patients with MTC have serological evidence of residual disease following surgical treatment
B. Most patients respond to radioiodine
C. Calcitonin is a very sensitive and moderately specific tumour marker
D. Patients with elevated but stable calcitonin levels usually require further investigation to search for recurrent disease

Answers

1. A
2. B
3. D
4. C
5. C

12 Medical management of thyroid cancer

Masud Haq & Clive Harmer
Thyroid Unit, Royal Marsden Hospital, Fulham Road, London, UK

KEY POINTS

- Remnant ^{131}I ablation post-thyroidectomy reduces the risk of locoregional recurrence and cause-specific mortality in differentiated thyroid cancer (DTC)
- Radioiodine therapy is the mainstay of treatment for metastatic DTC: a significant proportion of patients can be cured and, in others, durable palliation achieved
- In anaplastic carcinoma, multimodality treatment comprising high dose radiotherapy, chemotherapy and radical surgery offer the possibility of prolonging survival
- An elevated serum calcitonin level following surgery for medullary thyroid carcinoma demands investigation to identify potential sites of residual tumour for which further surgery should be considered
- Genetic testing should be performed soon after birth in offspring of patients with familial medullary thyroid carcinoma, MEN2A and MEN2B

DIFFERENTIATED THYROID CANCER

Ablation of residual thyroid tissue with radioactive iodine

The value of post-operative radioiodine (^{131}I) to ablate residual thyroid is still debated. Arguments in favour of remnant ablation are that it permits subsequent identification of residual or metastatic carcinoma by whole-body scan (WBS) and increases the sensitivity of serum thyroglobulin (Tg) measurement for follow-up.[1] Several retrospective studies have documented that it decreases tumour recurrence and death[2,3] (Fig. 12.1). The beneficial effect of ^{131}I ablation is mainly in patients at high risk of recurrence such as those with larger tumours, extra-thyroid extension, lymph node involvement and residual disease.[4] In low risk patient groups, prognosis is sufficiently good following surgery alone such that little further improvement is possible with ^{131}I ablation.[5]

The optimal activity of ^{131}I required to achieve successful ablation is controversial, with doses ranging between 1.1 and 3.7 GBq. Higher initial iodine doses were thought to be more effective in achieving complete ablation with a single administration. This is based on the observation that a high dose ablates remnant disease in addition to potential micrometastatic deposits.[6] Delivering a maximal radiation dose from the first iodine administration is important as the biological half-life of subsequent administrations falls, thereby reducing the radiation dose delivered. Other advantages include patient convenience, lower cost and a reduced risk of treatment-related complications associated with lower whole-body radiation exposure.

The only prospective randomized clinical trial to evaluate the optimal ^{131}I ablation dose (involving 149 patients) showed that increasing the administered activity beyond 1.85 GBq resulted in plateauing of the dose–response curve. A radiation absorbed dose to the thyroid remnant greater than 300 Gy did not result in a higher ablation rate.[7] Successful ablation was achieved in 77% of thyroid remnants with the lower dose of 1.85 GBq. Maxon *et al.* used dosimetry to individualize administered activity to deliver a radiation dose of 300 Gy to the thyroid remnant.[8] They reported an 81% successful ablation rate with no advantage associated with administration of a dose greater than 300 Gy. However, one meta-analysis found that a single administered activity of 1110 MBq was less likely to ablate thyroid remnants successfully compared with higher activities of 2775–3700 MBq.[9] A recent comprehensive systematic review of all published literature concluded it was not possible to determine reliably whether ablation success rates using 1.1 GBq were similar to that using 3.7 GBq.[10] The HiLo trial (Cancer Research UK) is the first prospective multicentre randomized trial of thyroid cancer to be conducted in the UK. It compares ablation success between 1.1 and 3.7 GBq of ^{131}I. The trial

A Practical Manual of Thyroid and Parathyroid Disease, 1st Edition. Edited by Asit Arora, Neil Tolley & R. Michael Tuttle.

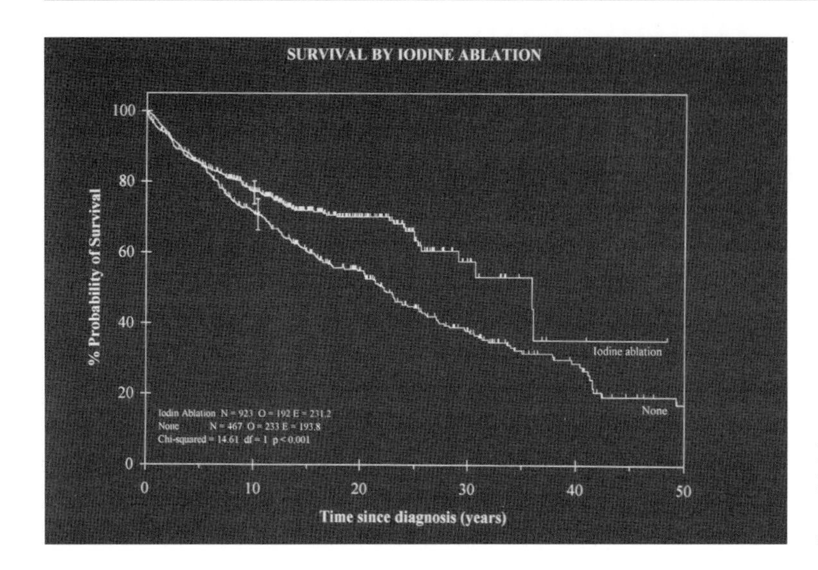

Fig. 12.1 Differentiated thyroid cancer: Royal Marsden Hospital experience 1929–1999 (1390 patients). Survival in relation to radioiodine ablation.

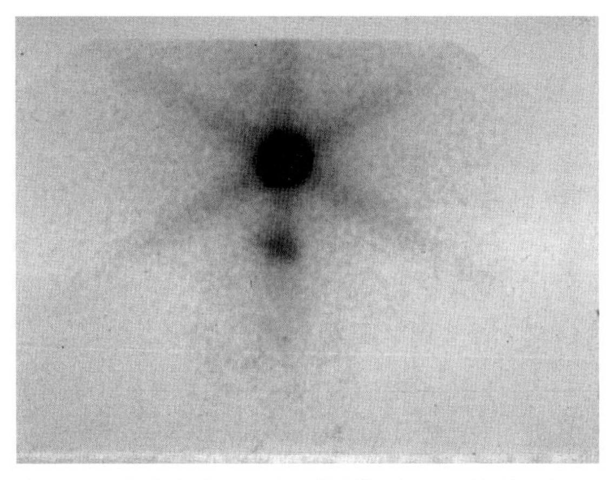

Fig. 12.2 Whole-body scan (neck) following an ablation dose of 3 GBq of ^{131}I, showing intense uptake in the thyroid bed.

will also determine whether standard thyroid hormone withdrawal versus administration of recombinant human thyroid-stimulating hormone (rhTSH) has any impact on success. Patient recruitment commenced in early 2007.

Four weeks after total thyroidectomy, by which time the TSH level should be >30 mU/l,[11] we recommend administering an ablation dose of 3 GBq of ^{131}I to the vast majority of patients with DTC. Exceptions include children over the age of 10 with small node-negative tumours and patients in whom carcinoma is an incidental microscopic histological finding. This ablates 75% of remnants and delivers a mean radiation dose of 410 Gy.[12] Following radioiodine scans of the neck and whole body obtained on the third day (Fig. 12.2), the patient is usually discharged subject to an acceptable total body radioactivity level. Replacement thyroid hormone (tri-iodothyronine 20 µg three times a day) is commenced and on day 6 the protein-bound ^{131}I blood level (PBI) is measured.[13]

Updated British Thyroid Association Guidelines for Thyroid Cancer were published in 2007. Similar guidelines for children have been published by the British Society of Paediatric Endocrinology and Diabetes.[14] The British Thyroid Foundation has published information leaflets for adult patients outlining key aspects of thyroid cancer and its diagnosis, including surgical treatment and radioiodine ablation.[15]

Historically, ablation success was determined by a diagnostic scan performed with 74–185 MBq of ^{131}I at 6–12 months.[16] Success was defined as no visible uptake in the thyroid bed (or uptake of <0.1% above background) together with an undetectable serum Tg. This is no longer universally practised except in patients with anti-Tg antibodies, which renders Tg measurement invalid. The current recommended criteria for successful ablation are an undetectable serum Tg (<1 µg/l) following rhTSH stimulation in association with a negative neck ultrasound (US) at 9–12 months.[17] Provided these criteria are met and there are no adverse features, no further treatment is required (Fig. 12.3). The patient is switched to life-long thyroxine at an average daily dose of 200 µg in order to suppress TSH to an undetectable

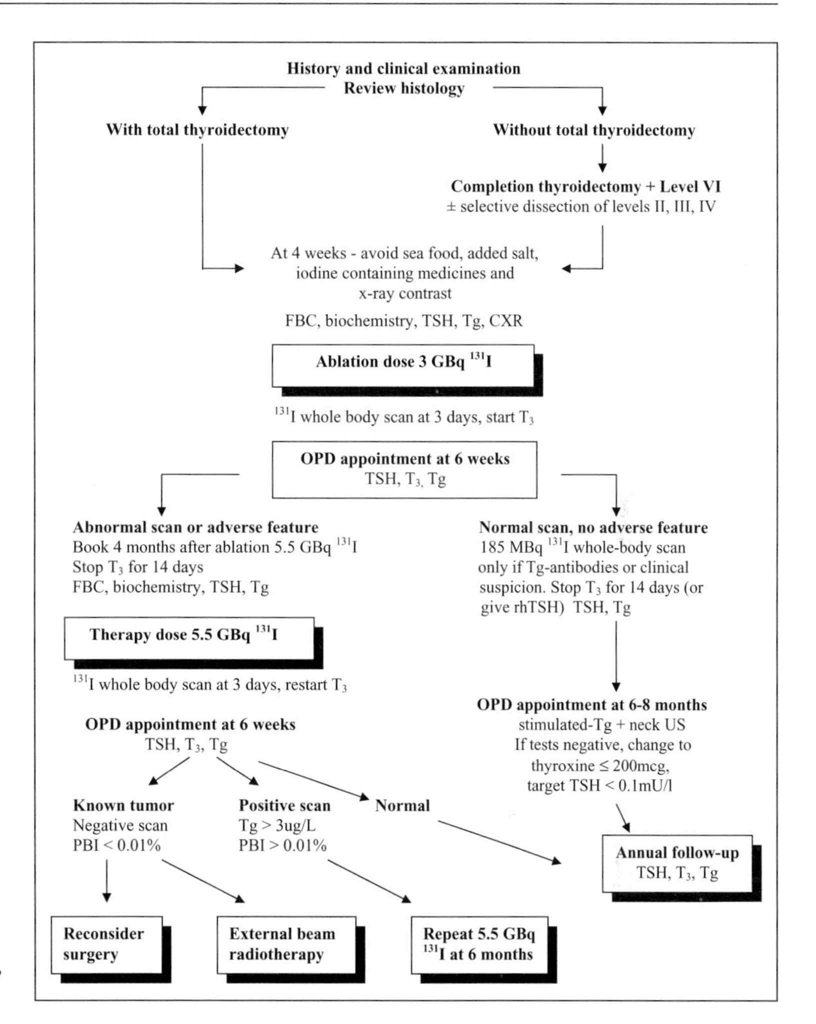

Fig. 12.3 New patient referred with differentiated thyroid cancer. T3, Lio-thyronine; FBC, full blood count; TSH, thyroid-stimulating hormone; CXR, chest radiograph; US, ultrasound; Tg, thyroglobulin; PBI, protein-bound radioactive iodine concentration; rhTSH, recombinant human TSH.

level. If the Tg becomes elevated, further imaging and treatment are required. If therapeutic radioiodine is indicated, this should be repeated at 6–12 monthly intervals until uptake disappears and the Tg again becomes undetectable.

Recombinant TSH

To optimize iodine uptake by both residual normal thyroid and cancer cells, TSH stimulation is necessary and therefore patients should be hypothyroid at the time of ^{131}I administration. Adequate preparation is achieved by a low iodine diet, avoidance of iodine-rich contrast media and discontinuation of tri-iodothyronine for 14 days (or 28 days for thyroxine) prior to ablation. As an alternative to hormone withdrawal, patients may be prepared for ablation with rhTSH while remaining on thyroid hormone replacement. The uncertainty over whether ablation rates differ between patients given rhTSH and those prepared with standard hormone withdrawal has largely been resolved. A recent prospective study following ablation with 3.7 GBq confirmed comparable ablation rates (each of 100%),[18] and a further study confirmed comparable ablation success rates with 1.85 and 3.7 GBq of ^{131}I.[19]

Until recently, rhTSH was available in the UK only for diagnostic ^{131}I scans and stimulated Tg measurement. This has now changed, with rhTSH licensed in the UK for ablation with an activity of 3.7 GBq. At the time of writing, it remains unlicensed for low dose ablation therapy.[20] It markedly improves the quality of life in patients, which is otherwise severely impaired during prolonged periods of hypothyroidism. We recommend its routine use for diagnostic purposes and for ablation or therapy, especially in patients unable to produce TSH and those in whom thyroid hormone withdrawal is medically contraindicated. This includes patients with cardiac disease, psychiatric disorders, hypopituitarism and patients who are post-partum or unable to tolerate prolonged hypothyroidism. Its expense currently limits wider use in the UK, although this does not seem to be the case in the rest of Europe or North America.

TSH suppression

The beneficial effect of TSH suppression has not been assessed in prospective studies. However, available data suggest that TSH-suppressive doses of thyroxine reduce the risk of recurrence, tumour progression and death from thyroid cancer.[21] It is generally accepted that a TSH level below 0.1 mU/l is desirable,[22] but there is no evidence that an undetectable TSH level offers any advantage over low but detectable levels. In low risk patients it may be adequate to keep the serum TSH at the lower level of the normal reference range. Monitoring the free thyroxine (T4) level in the athyroid patient receiving thyroxine often gives a false high value; therefore, we prefer to measure the free tri-iodothyronine (T3) level and maintain this in the normal range.[23] Although permanently low TSH levels are associated with accelerated bone turnover, this does not appear to translate into an increased fracture risk.[24,25] Nevertheless, post-menopausal women will benefit from adequate dietary calcium intake, biphosphonates or hormone replacement therapy.

Annual follow-up

Annual follow-up, comprising clinical examination and estimation of free T3, TSH and Tg, is essential to ensure normal thyroid function with TSH suppression and to detect recurrent tumour. Early discovery of recurrence is of paramount prognostic significance for both cure and survival.[26] Local or regional relapse develops in 5–20% of patients with DTC. Most relapses occur during the early years but may be detected even after 40 years, so follow-up should be life-long. The risk of locoregional failure relates to tumour aggressiveness, being higher with certain histological subtypes (tall cell, columnar cell and diffuse sclerosing papillary variants). Other factors include poorly differentiated carcinomas, large tumours, lymph node involvement at presentation, and the extent of initial treatment. Limited thyroidectomy results in a higher recurrence rate than complete thyroidectomy.[21]

Recurrence in the thyroid bed or cervical lymph nodes may be discovered by palpation. US or magnetic resonance imaging (MRI) are useful to delineate the extent of disease. Serum Tg is usually elevated, although it may be undetectable in 20% of patients on thyroxine who have isolated lymph node metastasis.[27] WBS following administration of ^{131}I reveals uptake in 60–80% of patients with lymph node disease.

Surgery is the treatment for locoregional recurrence, and complete resection should be attempted in all patients. Even if disease cannot be completely removed, surgical debulking facilitates subsequent radioiodine therapy. If surgical removal is not feasible or is incomplete, radioiodine treatment and external beam radiotherapy (EBRT) can be administered.[28,29] The outcome of patients with locoregional recurrence is closely related to its site, initial prognostic factors and response to treatment. Mortality after local recurrence is quite high in most series: a 10-year survival rate of only 60% has been reported.[30]

Management of metastatic disease

Distant metastases develop in 5–23% of patients with DTC, mainly in lung and bone. In any individual patient, an interplay between patient and tumour characteristics seems to determine outcome. Multivariate analysis has highlighted the adverse prognostic effect of older age at the time of discovery of metastases on survival.[26,31] Treatment comprises repeated doses of radioiodine. Activities ranging from 3.7 to 11.1 GBq at 3–9 month intervals have been employed. Many centres use a dose of 5.5 GBq at 6-monthly intervals (Fig. 12.4). There is no maximum limit to the cumulative ^{131}I dose given to patients with persistent disease provided that individual doses do not exceed 2 Gy total body exposure, progressive improvement can be documented and each pre-treatment blood count confirms absence of bone marrow damage.

A WBS 3 days after iodine administration provides scintigraphic assessment of disease, and serial scanning documents response to treatment. Diagnostic scanning using a tracer dose of iodine is not necessary prior to therapy. Indeed, this may have an adverse impact since tumour stunning by the diagnostic dose may reduce uptake of therapeutic ^{131}I.[32] A significant proportion of patients with residual tumour, as evidenced by an elevated Tg, demonstrate a negative diagnostic scan, but uptake can be documented in the post-therapy scan.[33,34]

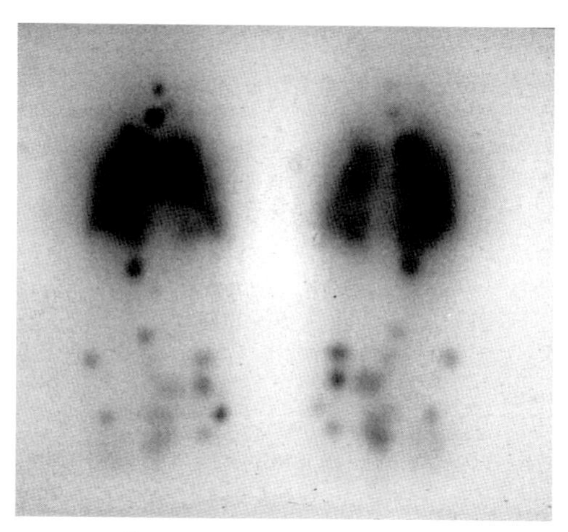

Fig. 12.4 Post-^{131}I therapy whole-body scan (anterior and posterior views) demonstrating multiple metastases in the neck, mediastinum, lungs, pelvis and lower limbs.

The value of ^{123}I as a scanning agent to prevent stunning has been confirmed, although this is expensive and not widely available in the UK.[35]

At least one large study has clearly demonstrated that iodine treatment exerts an independent prognostic benefit on survival. Younger patients with limited volume disease, mainly in the lungs, achieved a complete response to radioiodine treatment with a 15-year survival of 89%.[26] In contrast, older patients and those with large metastases or bone involvement are less likely to respond.[36] Microscopic foci appear to be more radiosensitive. Complete response is reported in 82% of patients with lung metastases not detected by chest radiography compared with 15% of those with radiologically visible micro- or macronodules.[37] Bone lesions demonstrate a low response rate to radioiodine. Surgical excision should be performed whenever possible, with EBRT reserved for cases not amenable to resection.[38,39] Surgical resection with curative intent for patients with a solitary non-avid deposit and with bulky disease resistant to iodine has achieved 46% (post-metastasectomy) 5-year survival.[40] Although distant metastases, particularly in lung, may remain stable for years, there is evidence that early treatment improves outcome. In a retrospective review of 400 patients, [^{18}F]fluorodeoxyglucose positron emission tomography (FDG-PET) positivity was a strong adverse predictor of survival on multivariate analysis (in addition to age), suggesting that these patients should be treated more aggressively.[44]

Sometimes metastases persist despite administration of substantial ^{131}I therapy doses.[41] This may be due to rapid turnover of radioiodine in the tumour (short effective half-life). The effective half-life in metastases which respond to therapy is more than double that of non responding lesions.[42] Lithium carbonate can prolong the biological half-life without increasing whole-body radiation exposure.[43] Blood levels need to be closely monitored to avoid toxicity, and the need for readily available psychiatric expertise limits routine use.

A fundamental problem for patients with metastatic disease is the decreased expression of the sodium–iodide symporter. At least a quarter of patients become iodine negative following repeated ^{131}I therapy. Treatment options are limited in these patients. Initial reports of re-differentiation to enhance the efficacy of iodine uptake have not been substantiated.[45] However, studies using selective agonists of retinoic X receptors have demonstrated enhanced sodium–iodide symporter gene expression in vitro.[46] An alternative approach is the administration of peptide receptor-targeted therapy with ^{90}Y lanreotide, based on the premise that non-iodine-avid tumours may express somatostain receptors. Initial results have been promising and clinical trials are ongoing. Further novel molecular targeted therapies are described in Chapter 9.

^{131}I dosimetry

Historically, use of radioiodine has been empirical, with fixed activities of 1–3.7 GBq administered for remnant ablation and 3.7–7.5 GBq for therapy. Measurement of the absorbed dose (Gy) has several advantages.[47,48] One is that patients are not overtreated and their overall radiation exposure is kept as low as possible. Secondly, it is the only way to determine whether further ^{131}I therapy will be effective so that alternative treatment can be considered in unsuccessful cases. The most important reason for administering iodine therapy based on lesion dosimetry is the resultant dose optimization which represents the best chance of completely eradicating disease.[49] Current information suggests that a stunning effect occurs with incomplete or inadequate therapy which may be permanent. Therefore, the most effective management strategy is to eradicate tumour with as few treatments as possible.

Analysis of 25 dosimetry studies in patients with metastatic disease showed a wide variation in radiation absorbed dose (5–621 Gy) from an administered ^{131}I activity of 5.5 GBq.[50] There was evidence of a dose–response relationship which explains the spectrum of clinical response. MIRD (medical internal radiation dose) dosimetry calculations are based on two assumptions: radioactivity is uniformly distributed throughout the tumour and ^{131}I washout is governed by a single exponential function. If either assumption is inaccurate, error will be introduced into the dosimetry estimates. Research is now focused on sequential registered three-dimensional single photon emission computed tomography (SPECT) images and dose–volume histograms of therapy distributions.[51] This will lead to greater accuracy and should improve the effectiveness of treatment.

Side effects of radioiodine treatment

Radioiodine therapy is well tolerated, with few patients experiencing mild nausea within the first 24 hours post-administration. Radiation thyroiditis may occur in the first week following ablation. This is characterized by pain, swelling and localized tenderness in the neck. Symptoms may be severe if there is a large thyroid remnant but generally respond well to steroid treatment. Acute sialadenitis affecting the parotid or submandibular glands occasionally occurs within 48 hours of administration and may last a few days.[52] A liberal fluid intake and frequent use of lozenges reduces salivary uptake and limits this reaction. Sialadenitis may persist into a chronic phase, with episodes recurring over years. Decreased salivary function can result in xerostomia and is dose related.[53]

Most patients demonstrate a mild transient reduction in platelet and white cell counts (lymphopenia) following ^{131}I therapy which is of no clinical significance. These effects reach a nadir 4–6 weeks after therapy with subsequent recovery within 6 months in most patients. Myelodysplasia leading to aplastic anaemia is rare and only likely to occur in patients with extensive bone metastases who have received a high cumulative dose in excess of 2 Gy per treatment.[54] Acute radiation pneumonitis and chronic pulmonary fibrosis have been reported in patients with diffuse lung metastases following single therapeutic activities exceeding 9 GBq.[55] If serial lung function tests indicate early damage, future doses can be fractionated. An interval of 6–12 months between iodine doses also reduces the risk of this complication.

A temporary increase in follicule-stimulating hormone (FSH) levels has been noted following ^{131}I treatment in both sexes, indicating temporary gonadal dysfunction. A positive correlation between FSH levels and the cumulative activity of iodine has been also reported.[56] In a small prospective study using thermoluminescent dosimetry, the radiation absorbed dose to the testes was found to be relatively low: 5.4–9.8 and 12–19.2 cGy following administration of 3 and 5.5 GBq, respectively.[57] Sperm banking should be offered if more than two therapeutic doses are contemplated. Regarding female patients, no significant difference was observed in fertility rates, birth rates or prematurity among women treated with radioiodine and those not treated.[58,59]

A recent multicentre study involving 6841 thyroid cancer patients has quantified the risk of subsequent second primary malignancy.[60] Compared with the general population, an increased risk of 27% was seen. It is estimated that 3.7 GBq of ^{131}I results in 53 solid malignant tumours and three leukaemias per 10,000 patients followed over 10 years. There is also a strong correlation between the cumulative radioiodine activity and the risk of bone, soft tissue, colorectal and salivary gland cancers. These findings highlight the need to restrict radioiodine treatment only to those likely to benefit.

External beam radiotherapy and chemotherapy

Indications for EBRT include macroscopic unresectable residual tumour, microscopic disease and positive excision margins. EBRT does not preclude simultaneous administration of radioiodine. ^{131}I should be given first whenever possible as its uptake may be diminished after radiotherapy. If radioiodine uptake is good, EBRT may not even be necessary. However, 20% of tumours fail to concentrate iodine effectively. Radiotherapy is not indicated in patients with favourable prognostic features or in young patients with residual disease which demonstrates avid iodine uptake.[61] Factors associated with a higher risk of persistent disease or locoregional recurrence include a large number of lymph node metastases (>10) at presentation, nodes demonstrating extracapsular extension (>3), involvement of central lymph nodes and tumour size greater than 4 cm.[62]

Farahati *et al.* suggested that adjuvant EBRT should be restricted to patients older than 40 years with locally advanced tumours which are non-iodine avid.[63] Observing these criteria, EBRT improved local control from 22 to 90% at 10 years ($P = 0.01$) in patients with invasive papillary cancer and lymph node involvement. Patients with follicular cancer did not show any significant benefit. Locoregional recurrence is infrequent in patients without lymph node disease, such that EBRT is rarely indicated. Tsang *et al.* have since reported on 207 patients (155 papillary, 52 follicular) with post-operative residual microscopic disease.[64] In papillary carcinoma, irradiated patients had a 10-year cause-specific survival of 100% and a local relapse-free rate of 93%. This was significantly better than the non-irradiated group which showed 95% survival and 78% local relapse-free rates. EBRT had no significant effect on follicular carcinoma.

Inoperable macroscopic disease is a clear indication for EBRT. In our retrospective study, complete regression was achieved in 37.5% and partial regression in 25%.[29] Similarly, Chow *et al.*[65] reported an improvement in local control from 24 to 56% at 10 years ($P < 0.001$). Irradiation is also effective for advanced and recurrent inoperable Hurthle cell carcinoma. It represents an important treatment option for patients with this tumour which is frequently non-iodine avid.[66]

Despite the small study size, the 5-year local recurrence rates from Birmingham (UK) indicate a possible dose response.[67] These were 63% following a dose of less than 50 Gy but only 15 and 18% for doses of 50–54 Gy and more than 54 Gy, respectively.

Our policy is to use EBRT infrequently because side effects, particularly oesophagitis, are unavoidable. The phase I target volume comprises both sides of the neck, thyroid bed and superior mediastinum from the level of the hyoid down to the carina, with shielding of the subapical portions of the lungs (Fig. 12.5). Anterior and undercouched fields ensure comprehensive coverage. Lead protection of the submandibular gland is required when the treatment volume extends proximally to the mastoid tip. A perspex shell is fashioned for the phase II volume which includes sites of micro- or macroscopic tumour. We recommend three-dimensional planning and conformal beam shaping assisted by a multileaf collimator. The aim is to deliver 60 Gy in 30 daily fractions over 6 weeks using 4–6 MV photons. The phase I prescription should be a mid-plane dose of 46 Gy in 2 Gy daily fractions (maximum spinal cord tolerance) with phase II delivering 14 Gy in seven fractions. Residual tumour in the thyroid bed or neck nodes may be treated with a small phase III volume, adding 6 Gy in three fractions, provided there is no additional dose to the spinal cord. Intensity-modulated radiotherapy (IMRT) improves dose distribution by minimizing the dose to the spinal cord, thus enabling dose escalation.[68]

A brisk cutaneous eythema occurs with radiation oesophagitis. Treatment includes liquid analgesia, liberal hydration and adequate dietary intake. Symptoms usually resolve within 2 weeks, as does acute laryngitis and dysphonia. Late effects include dysphagia, which occurs months or years later due to oesophageal stricture or motility changes. Limiting the oesophagus in the phase II volume minimizes such risks. Apical lung fibrosis may be visible on chest radiograph but is of no clinical significance.

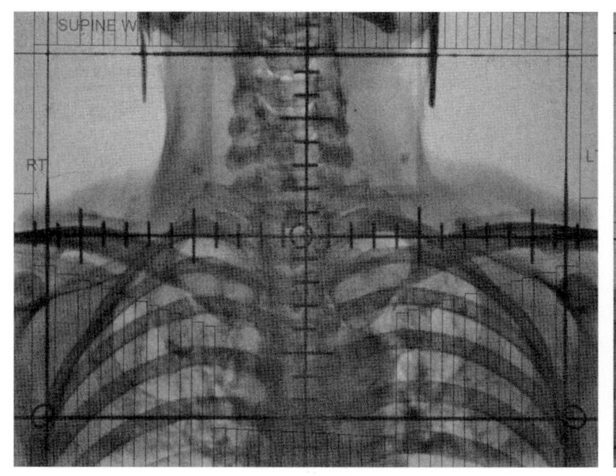

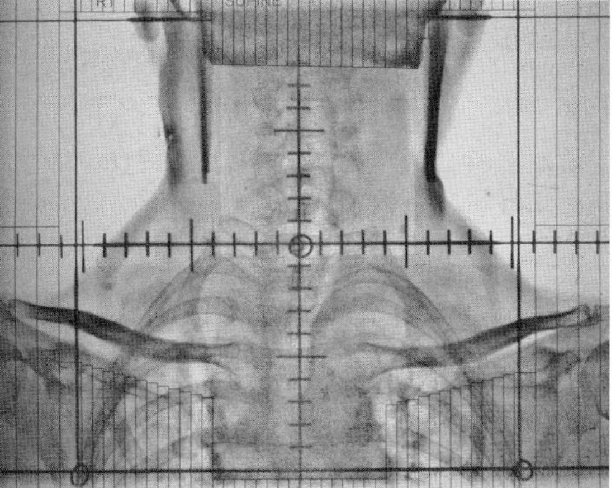

Fig. 12.5 EBRT phase I volume: comprises anterior and undercouched fields extending from the hyoid to carina excluding parotid and submandibular salivary glands. A multileaf collimator protects the infraclavicular portions of lungs. Chin strap immobilization is associated with less skin toxicity than a perspex shell. When the level II cervical nodes must be treated, the beam extends to the mastoid tips. The mandible and submandibular salivary glands still warrant protection.

Palliative radiotherapy is indicated for fungating nodes, bleeding, stridor, dysphagia and superior vena caval obstruction due to progressive inoperable disease. Further indications include painful bone metastases, vertebral involvement threatening the spinal cord, long bone involvement when there is a risk of fracture, and brain metastases. A dose of 35 Gy in 15 fractions is required or 6 Gy once weekly for up to four fractions when the central nervous system is not in field.

Experience with chemotherapy in differentiated thyroid cancer is limited because the vast majority of tumours are controlled by surgery, radioiodine and EBRT. The chemotherapy agents presently available are of limited benefit and cause significant morbidity. Indications for treatment include patients with inoperable, progressive, symptomatic disease that fails to concentrate radioiodine.[69] Of the several agents investigated, doxorubicin is the most effective, with response rates of 30–40%. Combination with cisplatin has produced similar response rates but with greater toxicity. Responses are usually partial and of short duration, although worthwhile palliation has been reported.[70] Phase II studies are in progress evaluating tyrosine kinase inhibitors for non-iodine-avid tumours and metastatic medullary thyroid carcinoma (further details are outlined in Chapter 9).

TREATMENT OF ANAPLASTIC CARCINOMA

Patients with anaplastic carcinoma present with rapidly progressive local disease and regional lymph node involvement. Surgery is rarely possible and prognosis is dismal, with a median survival of only 6 months. Local growth results in upper airway and oesophageal obstruction.[71]

Anaplastic cancer is the least radiosensitive of all thyroid tumours. Experience with 50–60 Gy administered over 5–6 weeks achieved local response in less than 45% of patients, and 75% still died from local progression.[72] There is little effect on survival, and the majority of patients spend a significant period of their remaining life undergoing treatment and recovering from its toxicity.

Better response rates are reported with combined chemotherapy and radiotherapy, particularly if the latter is delivered in a hyperfractionated schedule, although this is at the cost of increased morbidity.[73] Doxorubicin is the most effective agent, and its combination with radiation appears to produce a synergistic effect. In a study from Sweden, 22 patients were treated with hyperfractionated accelerated radiotherapy concurrently with doxorubicin followed by debulking surgery. Despite the patients' advanced age (>60 years) and locally extensive disease, this aggressive treatment modality achieved local control in 77% of patients. None of the patients who underwent surgery demonstrated local failure, and 9% survived for more than 2 years.[74]

Control of local disease is important for palliation and prolonging survival. Improvements in radiotherapy fractionation schedules and conformal beam shaping may improve local control whilst reducing toxicity. However, even when local control is achieved, patients still die from metastatic disease. No response was observed in distant metastases in either the Swedish study[74] or the French study[73] which employed doxorubicin (60 mg/m^2), cisplatin (90 mg/m^2) and local radiation. Our management approach is shown in Fig. 12.6.

MEDULLARY THYROID CANCER (MTC)

Total thyroidectomy with dissection of lymph nodes in the central compartment of the neck and lateral jugular nodes is the optimal surgery for MTC (see Chapter 11). A modified neck dissection is indicated if metastatic nodes are found during sampling.[75] Bilateral neck dissection has been recommended[76] because adequacy of the initial operation is a prerequisite for cure. Excision of mediastinal lymph nodes should also be performed if they are involved. Ideally, the post-operative calcitonin will fall to an undetectable level. Measurement of serum calcitonin should be repeated annually together with clinical evaluation. Life-long thyroxine is necessary, although this can be given at a physiological dose because there is no advantage in achieving complete TSH suppression.

Elevated post-operative calcitonin levels often persist and may be detected in up to 70% of patients with nodal involvement.[77] The most frequent sites of disease are nodes in the neck and mediastinum, while distant metastases may involve the liver, lungs and bones. The frequent identification of liver metastases by angiography[82] explains the low efficacy of a neck dissection to render a high calcitonin level undetectable post-operatively. Non-invasive imaging methods for detecting occult disease include US, CT, MRI and radionuclide scanning using ^{99m}Tc-pentavalent dimercaptosuccinic acid (V-DMSA), [^{123}I]metaiodobenzylguanidine (mIBG) or [^{111}In]octreotide. These isotope techniques are not particularly specific or sensitive. In our experience, the sensitivity only reaches 30%.[78] Other methods for investigating recurrent MTC include selective venous catheterization to assay

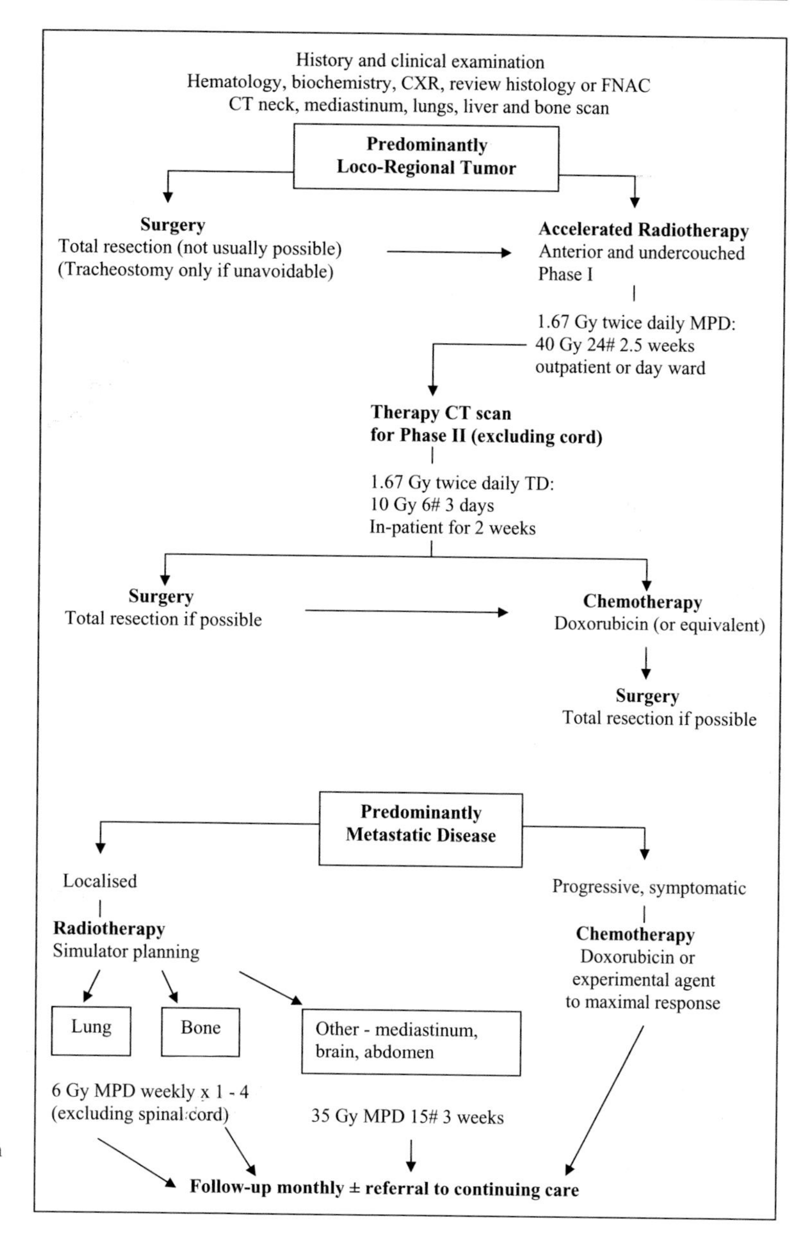

Fig. 12.6 New patient referred with anaplastic thyroid cancer. CXR, chest radiograph; FNAC, fine needle aspiration cytology; CT, computed tomography; MPD, mid-plane dose; TD, total dose.

calcitonin levels[79] and radioimmunoscintigraphy with monoclonal antibodies such as [^{131}I]anti-carcinoembryonic antigen (CEA).[80] PET is probably the investigation of choice at the present time.[81]

Residual MTC is usually progressive and is reflected by a rise in calcitonin levels over time. An average annual increase of 117% of the initial value was demonstrated in 35 of 40 patients.[83] Progressive increases may continue following the first post-operative measurement or may occur after a long period of stability. In a series from the Mayo Clinic, only 11 of 31 patients with raised calcitonin and negative imaging developed overt recurrent disease over a mean follow-up period of 12 years. Re-operation for clinically documented local recurrence did not result in calcitonin levels returning to normal. However, overall survival at 5 and 10 years was 90 and 86%, respectively.[84] Analysis of calcitonin doubling times in patients with abnormal calcitonin levels after total thyroidectomy and bilateral lymph node dissection showed that the majority of patients with a doubling time of more than 2 years were alive at the end of the study (3–30 years). On univariate analysis, TNM stage and doubling time were significant predictors of survival, but only the latter was significant on multivariate analysis ($P = 0.002$).[85]

An aggressive approach to treating residual disease was adopted by Tisell who performed meticulous 12 hour neck dissections often removing 40–60 cervical lymph nodes.[86] In a series of 11 patients, the calcitonin normalized in four patients (36%) and dramatically improved in four patients. However, follow-up was short (2–4.5 years) and there is no evidence that biochemical improvements translate into a survival advantage.[87] This aggressive policy is associated with higher complication rates than conventional surgery. In view of these findings, we advocate close follow-up, with surgery reserved for clinically recurrent disease.[88]

The role of post-operative radiotherapy is controversial due to lack of prospective studies. Retrospective series comparing surgery alone with surgery and radiotherapy are subject to selection bias. A favourable response in terms of tumour reduction and local control has been reported.[89,90] At the Institut Gustave-Roussy, the survival of 68 patients treated with surgery alone was similar to that of 59 patients who received post-operative radiotherapy. However, in patients with involved lymph nodes, 5-year survival improved significantly with post-operative radiotherapy from 36 to 81%.[91] In contrast, an adverse effect of radiotherapy was reported from the M.D. Anderson Cancer Center, Houston. Survival was significantly worse for 24 patients given post-operative radiotherapy compared with 39 age- and disease-matched patients treated with surgery alone.[92] We recommend the use of adjuvant radiotherapy in patients with locally advanced disease at presentation, multiple involved lymph nodes and patients with persistently elevated post-operative calcitonin levels (the latter indicating microscopic residual disease) (Fig. 12.7).[93] Radiotherapy should also be considered in patients with bulky inoperable disease. Significant palliation may be achieved with doses of 60 Gy in 6 weeks, and occasionally subsequent surgery becomes possible. Palliative radiotherapy can also be used to treat inoperable mediastinal disease and painful bone metastases.

Many patients with metastatic medullary cancer survive for years with minimal symptoms and, apart from medication to control diarrhoea, do not require any other treatment. Chemotherapy should be reserved for those with inoperable, progressive and symptomatic disease. Doxorubicin produces a symptomatic response in approximately 30% of patients, but this is usually partial and of short duration.[69] Similar response rates are obtained when doxorubicin is used alone or in combination with other drugs.[94] The selective uptake of [^{131}I] mIBG and [^{111}In]octreotide by 30–50% of medullary cancers has generated interest in their potential use for targeted radiotherapy, although treatment is relatively ineffective.[95] Treatment with unlabelled somatostatin analogues may be helpful to control severe diarrhoea, although side effects can be troublesome. Recombinant interferon α-2a has not demonstrated worthwhile benefit.

The clinical course of MTC varies widely. In our series, overall survival was 72% at 5 years, 56% at 10 years, 40% at 15 years and 30% at 20 years.[96] Patients with MEN2B have the most aggressive tumours, often with early development of metastases and high mortality rate. Multivariate analysis confirms that older age at diagnosis, lymph node involvement, metastases at presentation and incompleteness of initial surgical resection are all significant adverse prognostic factors.[96] In some retrospective series, patients with familial cancer survived longer than patients with the sporadic form.[92] However, when patients were matched for age, gender, extent of disease and treatment, this difference disappeared.

Familial medullary thyroid cancer: FMTC, MEN2A and 2B

The *RET* proto-oncogene is a 21-exon gene located on chromosome 10q 11–2 which encodes a tyrosine kinase transmembrane receptor. The aim of screening for MEN2 is to identify gene carriers early in an attempt to modify the outcome of the disease. The two life-threatening manifestations are MTC and phaeochromocytoma. There is compelling evidence that early intervention in both conditions improves outcome.[97]

Genetic testing by *RET* mutation analysis is the most cost-effective approach to detect affected individuals and should be performed soon after birth.[98] Family members who are not gene carriers do not require further testing, and the same also applies to their descendants. Adults who are gene carriers are at high risk of developing MTC. Therefore, total thyroidectomy with central lymph node dissection should be performed following exclusion of phaeochromocytoma. In children who are gene carriers, annual pentagastrin stimulation of calcitonin is performed.[99] However, pentagastrin testing sometimes fails to identify early stage C-cell abnormalities. In one study, approximately 50% of children had microscopic MTC rather than C-cell hyperplasia.[100] Thus in MEN2B, total

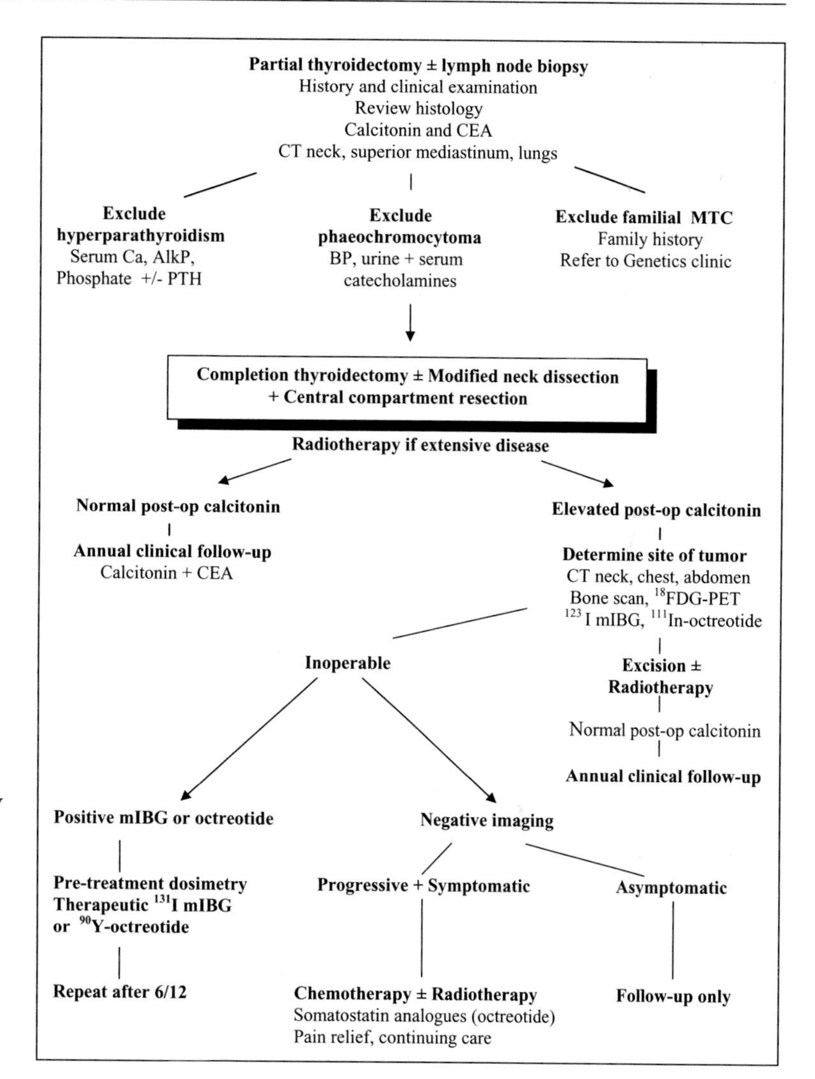

Fig. 12.7 New patient referred with medullary thyroid carcinoma. CEA, carcinoembryonic antigen; CT, computed tomography; MTC, medullary thyroid cancer; Ca, serum calcium; AlkP, serum alkaline phosphatase; PTH, parathyroid hormone; ^{99m}Tc-DMSA, ^{99m}Technetium pentavalent dimercaptosuccinic acid; ^{18}FDG-PET, [^{18}F]fluorodeoxyglucose positron emission tomography; mIBG, meta-iodobenzylguanidine; ^{111}In, 111-Indium; ^{90}Y, 90-Yttrium.

thyroidectomy should be performed as soon as possible under 2 years of age.[101] Surgery is well tolerated and the risk of recurrent laryngeal nerve damage or hypoparathyroidism is no greater than in older children.[97] In MEN2A, total thyroidectomy should be performed at 10 years of age or at a younger age if the pentagastrin stimulation test is positive. In FMTC, annual follow-up should be undertaken together with a pentagastrin stimulation test. Surgery is indicated at the first positive test.

Annual measurement of 24 hour urinary catecholamines and metanephrines provides a reliable outpatient screening tool to detect phaeochromocytoma. Elevated epinephrine or an elevated epinephrine/norepinephrine ratio is the most commonly observed pattern. Basal or exercise-stimulated plasma catecholamine is an alternative method of screening. MRI is used to confirm phaeochromocytoma or an enlarged adrenal medulla. In most cases, abnormalities involve both adrenals, and bilateral adrenalectomy is recommended.[88]

Serum calcium should be measured annually in MEN2A gene carriers to screen for hyperparathyroidism. When hypercalcaemia is detected, serum intact parathyroid hormone (PTH) should be measured to confirm the diagnosis. The majority of patients with hyperparathyroidism will have diffuse but unequal multiglandular hyperplasia. Only a small proportion (10–15%) demonstrate a single adenoma. There is controversy regarding optimal surgical management which incorporates either total parathyroidectomy with immediate autotransplantation or subtotal parathyroidectomy. This is outlined in further detail in Chapters 13 and 17.

TREATMENT OF THYROID LYMPHOMA

Patients with primary thyroid lymphoma usually present with confluent cervical/mediastinal lymphadenopathy (stage IIE). In about one-third of patients, tumour is confined to the thyroid gland (IE). Haematology, biochemistry, staging CT scan (neck, thorax and abdomen) and bone marrow aspirate and trephine are essential for accurate staging. These patients are often elderly and may require urgent intervention to relieve airway obstruction, which invariably delays staging investigations.

Aggressive surgery to debulk tumour is unnecessary. For localized disease, EBRT was the standard treatment for several decades, resulting in 5-year survival rates of approximately 35%. Local bulky disease and gross mediastinal involvement are associated with treatment failure

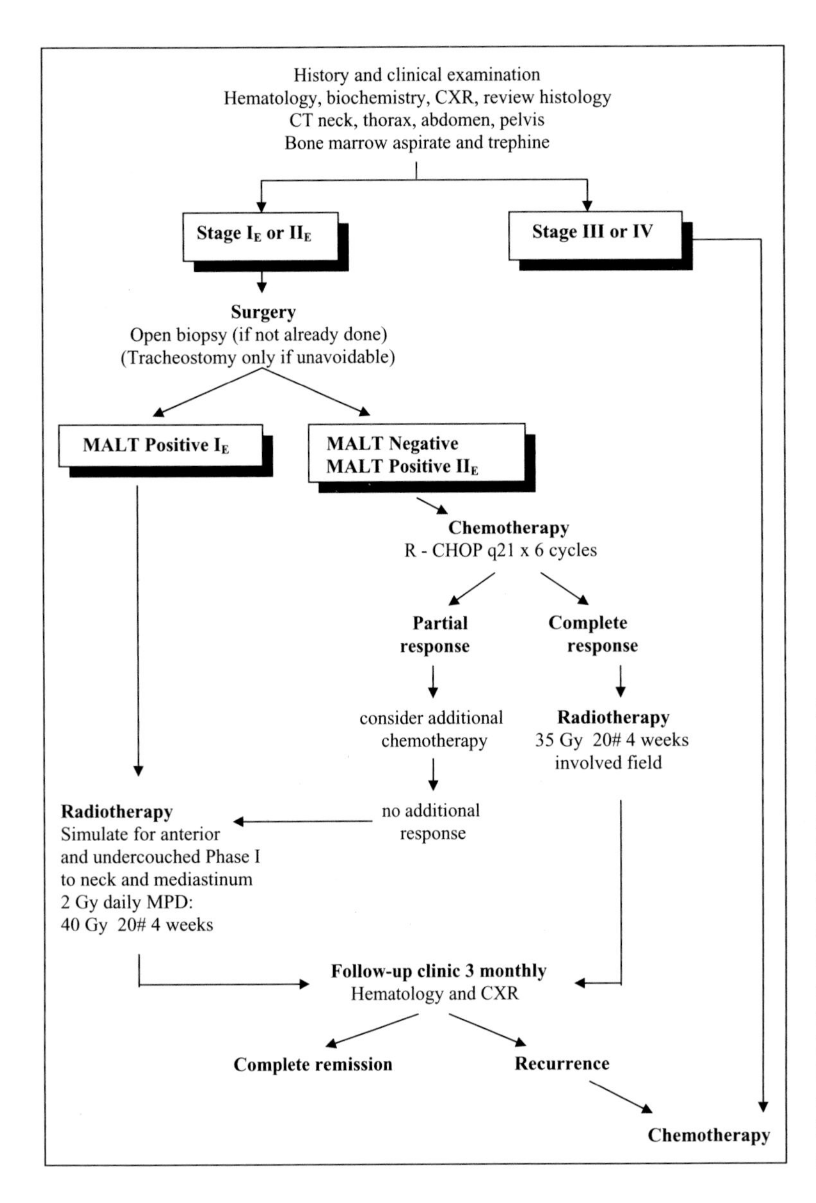

Fig. 12.8 New patient referred with primary lymphoma of the thyroid. CXR, chest radiograph; MALT, mucosa-associated lymphoid tissue; R-CHOP, rituximab, cyclophosphamide, hydroxydaunomycin (doxorubicin), vincristine (oncovin) and prednisone; MPD, mid-plane dose. Ann Arbor Classification: Stage IE, disease in a single lymph node region; Stage IIE, disease in two or more lymph regions on the same side of the diaphragm; Stage III, disease in lymph node regions on both sides of the diaphragm; Stage IV, widespread disease with multiple involvement at one or more extranodal sites such as bone marrow.

which occurs distant from the irradiated volume.[102] Chemotherapy for high grade lymphoma has demonstrated better local and distant disease control, with overall long-term disease-free survival of about 50%. Combination treatment of radiotherapy preceded by chemotherapy is now the standard practice, with 5-year survival rates of 65–90%.[103] Six cycles of rituximab plus cyclophosphamide, doxorubicin, vincristine and prednisolone (R-CHOP) given over 4 months is the recommended regime.[104]

Lymphoma with mucosa-associated lymphoid tissue (MALT) usually presents as localized extranodal tumour which follows an indolent course.[105] Radiotherapy, as a single modality treatment, produces complete response rates of almost 100%. The relapse rate is around 30%, the salvage rate is over 50% and overall cause-specific survival is almost 90% at 5 and 10 years.[106] Our policy is to treat stage IEA MALT-positive lymphoma with radiotherapy and to use combination treatment for all other tumours (Fig. 12.8). Treatment volume includes the neck and superior mediastinum irradiated by a pair of anterior and undercouched fields to 35–40 Gy in 20 fractions over 4 weeks. Primary Hodgkin's disease of the thyroid is very rare and is treated in a similar fashion to extranodal Hodgkin's disease found at any other site in the body.

EVIDENCE APPRAISAL

The British Thyroid Association in collaboration with the Royal College of Physicians (RCP) has published guidelines for thyroid cancer with recommendations for the management of differentiated thyroid cancer and medullary carcinoma. Data are based on published series and expert opinion; Level III and IV.[22]

The activity selected for remnant ablation remains controversial. The majority of publications present Level III or IV evidence, although Bal *et al.*[7] performed a prospective randomized study increasing administered activities for remnant thyroid ablation; Level II. The publication by Hackshaw *et al.*[10] was a meta-analysis of published literature comparing low and high dose ablation; Level I.

Several studies have assessed the role of rhTSH in remnant thyroid ablation. Most of these studies are Level III.[18–20] At the time of writing, rhTSH is licensed in the UK for remnant ablation with 3.7 GBq ^{131}I only.

The role of TSH suppression in the management of DTC is based on Level IV evidence.

The role of radioiodine dosimetry in DTC is based on a small number of studies; Levels III and IV.

REFERENCES

1. Schlumberger M, Fragu P, Parmentier C, *et al.* Thyroglobulin assay in the follow-up of patients with differentiated thyroid carcinomas: comparison of its value in patients with or without normal residual tissue. Acta Endocrinol 1981;98:215–21.
2. Mazzaferri EL, Jhiang SM. Long-term impact of initial surgical and medical therapy on papillary and follicular thyroid cancer. Am J Med 1994;97:418–28.
3. Vini L, Harmer C. Radioiodine treatment for differentiated thyroid cancer. Clin Oncol (R Coll Radiol) 2000; 12:365–72.
4. Taylor T, Specker B, Robbins J, *et al.* Outcome after treatment of high-risk papillary and non-Hurthle-cell follicular thyroid carcinoma. Ann Intern Med 1998;129:622–7.
5. Hay ID, Grant CS, van Heerden JA, *et al.* Papillary thyroid microcarcinoma: a study of 535 cases observed in a 50-year period. Surgery 1992;112:1139–46.
6. Beierwaltes WH, Rabbani R, Dmuchowski C, *et al.* An analysis of 'ablation of thyroid remnants' with I-131 in 511 patients from 1947–1984: experience at University of Michigan. J Nucl Med 1984;25:1287–93.
7. Bal C, Padhy AK, Jana S, *et al.* Prospective randomized clinical trial to evaluate the optimal dose of 131 I for remnant ablation in patients with differentiated thyroid carcinoma. Cancer 1996;77:2574–80.
8. Maxon HR III, Englaro EE, Thomas SR, *et al.* Radioiodine-131 therapy for well-differentiated thyroid cancer—a quantitative radiation dosimetric approach: outcome and validation in 85 patients. J Nucl Med 1992;33:1132–6.
9. Doi SA, Woodhouse NJ. Ablation of the thyroid remnant and 131I dose in differentiated thyroid cancer. Clin Endocrinol (Oxf) 2000;52:765–73.
10. Hackshaw A, Harmer C, Mallick U, *et al.* 131I activity for remnant ablation in patients with differentiated thyroid cancer: a systematic review. J Clin Endocrinol Metab 2007; 92:28–38.
11. Harmer CL, McCready VR. Thyroid cancer: differentiated carcinoma. Cancer Treat Rev 1996;22:161–77.
12. O'Connell ME, Flower MA, Hinton PJ, *et al.* Radiation dose assessment in radioiodine therapy. Dose–response relationships in differentiated thyroid carcinoma using quantitative scanning and PET. Radiother Oncol 1993; 28:16–26.
13. Hammersley PA, Al Saadi A, Chittenden S, *et al.* Value of protein-bound radioactive iodine measurements in the management of differentiated thyroid cancer treated with 131I. Br J Radiol 2001;74:429–33.
14. www.bsped.org.uk. 2007.
15. www.btf-thyroid.org. 2007.
16. Taylor H, Hyer S, Vini L, Pratt B, Cook G, Harmer C. Diagnostic 131I whole body scanning after thyroidectomy and ablation for differentiated thyroid cancer. Eur J Endocrinol 2004;150:649–53.

17. Pacini F, Schlumberger M, Harmer C, *et al.* Post-surgical use of radioiodine (131I) in patients with papillary and follicular thyroid cancer and the issue of remnant ablation: a consensus report. Eur J Endocrinol 2005;153:651–9.
18. Pacini F, Ladenson PW, Schlumberger M, *et al.* Radioiodine ablation of thyroid remnants after preparation with recombinant human thyrotropin in differentiated thyroid carcinoma: results of an international, randomized, controlled study. J Clin Endocrinol Metab 2006;91:926–32.
19. Pilli T, Brianzoni E, Capoccetti F, *et al.* A comparison of 1850 (50 mCi) and 3700 MBq (100 mCi) 131-iodine administered doses for recombinant thyrotropin-stimulated postoperative thyroid remnant ablation in differentiated thyroid cancer. J Clin Endocrinol Metab 2007;92: 3542–6.
20. Barbaro D, Boni G. Radioiodine ablation of post-surgical thyroid remnants after preparation with recombinant human TSH: why, how and when. Eur J Surg Oncol 2007;33:535–40.
21. Mazzaferri EL. Papillary thyroid carcinoma: factors influencing prognosis and current therapy. Semin Oncol 1987;14:315–32.
22. British Thyroid Association. Guidelines for the management of thyroid cancer in adults. London: Royal College of Physicians, 2002.
23. Liewendahl K, Helenius T, Lamberg BA, *et al.* Free thyroxine, free triiodothyronine, and thyrotropin concentrations in hypothyroid and thyroid carcinoma patients receiving thyroxine therapy. Acta Endocrinol 1987;116:418–24.
24. Giannini S, Nobile M, Sartori L, *et al.* Bone density and mineral metabolism in thyroidectomized patients treated with long-term l-thyroxine. Clin Sci 1994;87:593–7.
25. Leese GP, Jung RT, Guthrie C, *et al.* Morbidity in patients on l-thyroxine: a comparison of those with a normal TSH to those with a suppressed TSH. Clin Endocrinol 1992; 37:500–3.
26. Schlumberger M, Challeton C, de Vathaire F, *et al.* Radioactive iodine treatment and external radiotherapy for lung and bone metastases from thyroid carcinoma. J Nucl Med 1996;37:598–605.
27. Schlumberger M, Baudin E. Serum thyroglobulin determination in the follow-up of patients with differentiated thyroid carcinoma. Eur J Endocrinol 1998;138:249–52.
28. Haq M, Harmer C. Non-surgical management of differentiated thyroid cancer. In: Mazzaferri E, Harmer C, Mallick U, *et al.*, eds. Practical management of thyroid cancer. London: Springer, 2006: 171–92.
29. O'Connell ME, A'Hern RP, Harmer CL. Results of external beam radiotherapy in differentiated thyroid carcinoma: a retrospective study from the Royal Marsden Hospital. Eur J Cancer 1994;30A:733–9.
30. Mazzaferri EL. An overview of the management of papillary and follicular thyroid carcinoma. Thyroid 1999;9: 421–7.
31. Haq M, Harmer C. Differentiated thyroid carcinoma with distant metastases at presentation: prognostic factors and outcome. Clin Endocrinol 2005;63:87–93.
32. Park HM, Perkins OW, Edmondson JW, *et al.* Influence of diagnostic radioiodines on the uptake of ablative dose of iodine-131. Thyroid 1994;4:49–54.
33. Fatourechi V, Hay ID, Mullan BP, *et al.* Are posttherapy radioiodine scans informative and do they influence subsequent therapy of patients with differentiated thyroid cancer? Thyroid 2000;10:573–7.
34. Pineda JD, Lee T, Ain K, *et al.* Iodine-131 therapy for thyroid cancer patients with elevated thyroglobulin and negative diagnostic scan. J Clin Endocrinol Metab 1995; 80:1488–92.
35. Siddiqi A, Foley RR, Britton KE, *et al.* The role of 123I-diagnostic imaging in the follow-up of patients with differentiated thyroid carcinoma as compared to 131I-scanning: avoidance of negative therapeutic uptake due to stunning. Clin Endocrinol 2001;55:515–21.
36. Haq M, McCready R, Harmer C. Treatment of advanced differentiated thyroid carcinoma with high activity radioiodine therapy. Nucl Med Commun 2004;25:799–805.
37. Maxon HR, Thomas SR, Samaratunga RC. Dosimetric considerations in the radioiodine treatment of macrometastases and micrometastases from differentiated thyroid cancer. Thyroid 1997;7:183–7.
38. Marcocci C, Pacini F, Elisei R, *et al.* Clinical and biologic behavior of bone metastases from differentiated thyroid carcinoma. Surgery 1989;106:960–6.
39. Niederle B, Roka R, Schemper M, *et al.* Surgical treatment of distant metastases in differentiated thyroid cancer: indication and results. Surgery 1986;100:1088–97.
40. Vini L, Harmer C, Goldstraw P. The role of metastasectomy in differentiated thyroid cancer. Eur J Surg Oncol 1998;24:348.
41. Wechalekar K, Haq M, Harmer C, *et al.* Metastatic thyroid carcinoma causing superior vena caval obstruction diagnosed on I-131 scan. Clin Nucl Med 2005;30:548–9.
42. Maxon HR, Thomas SR, Hertzberg VS, *et al.* Relation between effective radiation dose and outcome of radioiodine therapy for thyroid cancer. N Engl J Med 1983; 309:937–41.
43. Koong SS, Reynolds JC, Movius EG, *et al.* Lithium as a potential adjuvant to 131I therapy of metastatic, well differentiated thyroid carcinoma. J Clin Endocrinol Metab 1999;84:912–6.
44. Robbins RJ, Wan Q, Grewal RK, *et al.* Real-time prognosis for metastatic thyroid carcinoma based on 2-[18F]fluoro-2-deoxy-d-glucose-positron emission tomography scanning. J Clin Endocrinol Metab 2006;91:498–505.
45. Short SC, Suovuori A, Cook G, *et al.* A phase II study using retinoids as redifferentiation agents to increase iodine uptake in metastatic thyroid cancer. Clin Oncol (R Coll Radiol) 2004;16:569–74.

46. Haugen BR, Larson LL, Pugazhenthi U, *et al.* Retinoic acid and retinoid X receptors are differentially expressed in thyroid cancer and thyroid carcinoma cell lines and predict response to treatment with retinoids. J Clin Endocrinol Metab 2004;89:272–80.
47. Haq M, Pratt B, Harmer C, *et al.* Whole-body, blood and patient-specific dosimetry of radioiodine in the treatment of differentiated thyroid cancer. Eur J Nucl Med 2004;31:P877.
48. Haq M, Gear J, Flux G, Harmer C. Whole-body and blood dosimetry for radioiodine treatment of differentiated thyroid cancer. Nucl Med Commun 2004;25:314.
49. Haq M, Hyer S, Flux G, *et al.* Differentiated thyroid cancer presenting with thyrotoxicosis due to functioning metastases. Br J Radiol 2007;80:e38–43.
50. Vini L, Chittenden S, Pratt B, *et al.* In vivo dosimetry of radioiodine in patients with metastatic differentiated thyroid cancer. J Nucl Med 1998;25:904.
51. Haq M. Radioiodine dosimetry in differentiated thyroid cancer. MD thesis (University of London), 2007.
52. Hyer S, Kong A, Pratt B, *et al.* Salivary gland toxicity after radioiodine therapy for thyroid cancer. Clin Oncol (R Coll Radiol) 2007;19:83–6.
53. Bohuslavizki KH, Brenner W, Lassmann S, *et al.* Quantitative salivary gland scintigraphy in the diagnosis of parenchymal damage after treatment with radioiodine. Nucl Med Commun 1996;17:681–6.
54. Benua R, Cicale NR, Sonenberg M, *et al.* The relation of radioiodine dosimetry to results and complications in the treatment of metastatic thyroid cancer. Am J Roentgenol Radium Ther Nucl Med 1962;87:171–82.
55. Rall JE, Alpers JB, Lewallen CG, *et al.* Radiation pneumonitis and fibrosis: a complication of radioiodine treatment of pulmonary metastases from cancer of the thyroid. J Clin Endocrinol Metab 1957;17:1263–76.
56. Pacini F, Gasperi M, Fugazzola L, *et al.* Testicular function in patients with differentiated thyroid carcinoma treated with radioiodine. J Nucl Med 1994;35:1418–22.
57. Hyer S, Vini L, O'Connell M, *et al.* Testicular dose and fertility in men following I(131) therapy for thyroid cancer. Clin Endocrinol 2002;56:755–8.
58. Schlumberger M, de Vathaire F, Ceccarelli C, *et al.* Exposure to radioactive iodine-131 for scintigraphy or therapy does not preclude pregnancy in thyroid cancer patients. J Nucl Med 1996;37:606–12.
59. Vini L, Hyer S, Al Saadi A, *et al.* Prognosis for fertility and ovarian function after treatment with radioiodine for thyroid cancer. Postgrad Med J 2002;78:92–3.
60. Rubino C, de Vathaire F, Dottorini ME, *et al.* Second primary malignancies in thyroid cancer patients. Br J Cancer 2003;89:1638–44.
61. Harmer C, Bidmead M, Shepherd S, *et al.* Radiotherapy planning techniques for thyroid cancer. Br J Radiol 1998;71:1069–75.
62. Leboulleux S, Rubino C, Baudin E, *et al.* Prognostic factors for persistent or recurrent disease of papillary thyroid carcinoma with neck lymph node metastases and/or tumor extension beyond the thyroid capsule at initial diagnosis. J Clin Endocrinol Metab 2005;90:5723–9.
63. Farahati J, Reiners C, Stuschke M, *et al.* Differentiated thyroid cancer. Impact of adjuvant external radiotherapy in patients with perithyroidal tumor infiltration (stage pT4). Cancer 1996;77:172–80.
64. Tsang RW, Brierley JD, Simpson WJ, *et al.* The effects of surgery, radioiodine, and external radiation therapy on the clinical outcome of patients with differentiated thyroid carcinoma. Cancer 1998;82:375–88.
65. Chow SM, Law SC, Mendenhall WM, *et al.* Papillary thyroid carcinoma: prognostic factors and the role of radioiodine and external radiotherapy. Int J Radiat Oncol Biol Phys 2002;52:784–95.
66. Mills S, Haq M, Smellie W, Harmer C. Hurthle cell carcinoma of the thyroid: Retrospective review of 62 patients treated at the Royal Marsden Hospital. Eu J Surg Onc 2009; 35:230–4.
67. Ford D, Giridharan S, McConkey C, *et al.* External beam radiotherapy in the management of differentiated thyroid cancer. Clin Oncol (R Coll Radiol) 2003;15:337–41.
68. Nutting CM, Convery DJ, Cosgrove VP, *et al.* Improvements in target coverage and reduced spinal cord irradiation using intensity-modulated radiotherapy (IMRT) in patients with carcinoma of the thyroid gland. Radiother Oncol 2001;60:173–80.
69. Hoskin PJ, Harmer C. Chemotherapy for thyroid cancer. Radiother Oncol 1987;10:187–94.
70. Ahuja S, Ernst H. Chemotherapy of thyroid carcinoma. J Endocrinol Invest 1987;10:303–10.
71. McIver B, Hay ID, Giuffrida DF, *et al.* Anaplastic thyroid carcinoma: a 50-year experience at a single institution. Surgery 2001;130:1028–34.
72. Levendag PC, De Porre PM, van Putten WL. Anaplastic carcinoma of the thyroid gland treated by radiation therapy. Int J Radiat Oncol Biol Phys 1993;26:125–8.
73. Schlumberger M, Parmentier C, Delisle MJ, *et al.* Combination therapy for anaplastic giant cell thyroid carcinoma. Cancer 1991;67:564–6.
74. Tennvall J, Lundell G, Wahlberg P, *et al.* Anaplastic thyroid carcinoma: three protocols combining doxorubicin, hyperfractionated radiotherapy and surgery. Br J Cancer 2002;86:1848–3.
75. Dralle H, Scheumann GF, Proye C, *et al.* The value of lymph node dissection in hereditary medullary thyroid carcinoma: a retrospective, European, multicentre study. J Intern Med 1995;238:357–61.
76. Scollo C, Baudin E, Travagli JP, *et al.* Rationale for central and bilateral lymph node dissection in sporadic and hereditary medullary thyroid cancer. J Clin Endocrinol Metab 2003;88:2070–5.
77. Block MA, Jackson CE, Tashjian AH Jr. Management of occult medullary thyroid carcinoma: evidenced only by serum calcitonin level elevations after apparently adequate neck operations. Arch Surg 1978;113:368–72.

78. Vini L, Al-Saadi A, Pratt B, *et al.* The role of radionuclide imaging (V-DMSA, 131I-mIBG, 111In-Octreotide) in medullary thyroid cancer. Nucl Med Commun 1998;19: 384.
79. Medina-Franco H, Herrera MF, Lopez G, *et al.* Persistent hypercalcitoninemia in patients with medullary thyroid cancer: a therapeutic approach based on selective venous sampling for calcitonin. Rev Invest Clin 2001;53:212–7.
80. Juweid M, Sharkey RM, Swayne LC, *et al.* Improved selection of patients for reoperation for medullary thyroid cancer by imaging with radiolabeled anticarcinoembryonic antigen antibodies. Surgery 1997;122:1156–65.
81. Diehl M, Risse JH, Brandt-Mainz K, *et al.* Fluorine-18 fluorodeoxyglucose positron emission tomography in medullary thyroid cancer: results of a multicentre study. Eur J Nucl Med 2001;28:1671–6.
82. Szavcsur P, Godeny M, Bajzik G, *et al.* Angiography-proven liver metastases explain low efficacy of lymph node dissections in medullary thyroid cancer patients. Eur J Surg Oncol 2005;31:183–90.
83. Tisell LE, Dilley WG, Wells SA Jr. Progression of postoperative residual medullary thyroid carcinoma as monitored by plasma calcitonin levels. Surgery 1996;119:34–9.
84. van Heerden JA, Grant CS, Gharib H, *et al.* Long-term course of patients with persistent hypercalcitoninemia after apparent curative primary surgery for medullary thyroid carcinoma. Ann Surg 1990;212:395–400.
85. Barbet J, Campion L, Kraeber-Bodere F, *et al.* Prognostic impact of serum calcitonin and carcinoembryonic antigen doubling-times in patients with medullary thyroid carcinoma. J Clin Endocrinol Metab 2005;90:6077–84.
86. Tisell LE, Hansson G, Jansson S, *et al.* Reoperation in the treatment of asymptomatic metastasizing medullary thyroid carcinoma. Surgery 1986;99:60–6.
87. Moley JF, Wells SA, Dilley WG, *et al.* Reoperation for recurrent or persistent medullary thyroid cancer. Surgery 1993;114:1090–5.
88. Heshmati HM, Gharib H, van Heerden JA, *et al.* Advances and controversies in the diagnosis and management of medullary thyroid carcinoma. Am J Med 1997;103: 60–9.
89. Fife KM, Bower M, Harmer CL. Medullary thyroid cancer: the role of radiotherapy in local control. Eur J Surg Oncol 1996;22:588–91.
90. Simpson WJ. Radioiodine and radiotherapy in the management of thyroid cancers. Otolaryngol Clin North Am 1990;23:509–21.
91. Schlumberger M, Gardet P, de Vathaire F. External radiotherapy and chemotherapy in MTC patients. In: Calmettes C, Guliana J, eds. Medullary thyroid carcinoma. Paris: INSERM, 1991:213–20.
92. Samaan NA, Schultz PN, Hickey RC. Medullary thyroid carcinoma: prognosis of familial versus sporadic disease and the role of radiotherapy. J Clin Endocrinol Metab 1988;67:801–5.
93. Fersht N, Vini L, A'Hern R, *et al.* The role of radiotherapy in the management of elevated calcitonin after surgery for medullary thyroid cancer. Thyroid 2001;11:1161–8.
94. Nocera M, Baudin E, Pellegriti G, *et al.* Treatment of advanced medullary thyroid cancer with an alternating combination of doxorubicin–streptozocin and 5 FU–dacarbazine. Groupe d'Etude des Tumeurs a Calcitonine (GETC). Br J Cancer 2000;83:715–8.
95. Kaltsas G, Rockall A, Papadogias D, *et al.* Recent advances in radiological and radionuclide imaging and therapy of neuroendocrine tumours. Eur J Endocrinol 2004;151: 15–27.
96. Hyer SL, Vini L, A'Hern R, *et al.* Medullary thyroid cancer: multivariate analysis of prognostic factors influencing survival. Eur J Surg Oncol 2000;26:686–90.
97. Wells SA Jr, Chi DD, Toshima K, *et al.* Predictive DNA testing and prophylactic thyroidectomy in patients at risk for multiple endocrine neoplasia type 2A. Ann Surg 1994;220:237–47.
98. Ponder BA. Genetic screening for multiple endocrine neoplasia type 2. Exp Clin Endocrinol 1993;101:53–6.
99. Brandi ML, Gagel RF, Angeli A, *et al.* Guidelines for diagnosis and therapy of MEN type 1 and type 2. J Clin Endocrinol Metab 2001;86:5658–71.
100. Gagel RF, Tashjian AH Jr, Cummings T, *et al.* The clinical outcome of prospective screening for multiple endocrine neoplasia type 2a. An 18-year experience. N Engl J Med 1988;318:478–84.
101. Pinchera A, Elisei R. Medullary thyroid cancer: diagnosis and management. In: Mazzaferri E, Harmer C, Mallick U, *et al.*, eds. Practical management of thyroid cancer. London: Springer-Verlag, 2006:255–79.
102. Tupchong L, Hughes F, Harmer CL. Primary lymphoma of the thyroid: clinical features, prognostic factors, and results of treatment. Int J Radiat Oncol Biol Phys 1986; 12:1813–1821.
103. Matsuzuka F, Miyauchi A, Katayama S, *et al.* Clinical aspects of primary thyroid lymphoma: diagnosis and treatment based on our experience of 119 cases. Thyroid 1993; 3:93–9.
104. Haq M, Harmer C. Rare thyroid cancers. In: Mazzaferri E, Harmer C, Mallick U, *et al.*, eds. Practical management of thyroid cancer. London: Springer-Verlag, 2006:393–402.
105. Thieblemont C, Mayer A, Dumontet C, *et al.* Primary thyroid lymphoma is a heterogeneous disease. J Clin Endocrinol Metab 2002;87:105–11.
106. Laing RW, Hoskin P, Hudson BV, *et al.* The significance of MALT histology in thyroid lymphoma: a review of patients from the BNLI and Royal Marsden Hospital. Clin Oncol (R Coll Radiol) 1994;6:300–4.

MULTIPLE CHOICE QUESTIONS

Select more than one option where appropriate.

1. Except for low risk patient groups, post-thyroidectomy TSH suppression reduces the risk of:

A. Recurrence
B. Tumour progression
C. Osteoporosis
D. Tumour-related death.

2. Except for low risk patient groups, ^{131}I ablation:

A. Permits subsequent identification by whole-body scanning of any residual or metastatic carcinoma
B. Increases the sensitivity of Tg measurement for follow-up
C. Decreases tumour recurrence
D. Increases cause-specific survival

3. In sporadic medullary carcinoma, tumour is multifocal in:

A. 10%
B. 20%
C. 30%
D. 40%
E. 50%

4. In MEN2B, thyroidectomy should be performed:

A. Under the age of 2 years
B. Between the ages of 2 and 5 years
C. Between the ages of 5 and 10 years
D. Between the ages of 10 and 15 years

5. Patients with stage IIE thyroid lymphoma should be treated with:

A. Surgery only
B. Radiotherapy only
C. Chemotherapy only
D. Surgery + radiotherapy
E. Surgery + chemotherapy
F. Radiotherapy + chemotherapy

Answers

1. A, B, D
2. A, B, C, D
3. B
4. A
5. F

Section 2 Parathyroid disease

13 Symptoms, differential diagnosis and management

Jeremy Cox[1] & Mike Stearns[2]

[1] St Mary's Hospital, Imperial College Healthcare NHS Trust, London, UK
[2] Royal Free Hospital, London, UK

KEY POINTS

- Primary hyperparathyroidism (HPT) is the most common cause of hypercalcaemia in the outpatient setting. Symptoms may be relatively non-specific and therefore a low index of suspicion is essential. Screening is indicated when there is a history of renal stones or osteoporosis
- Surgical trauma to the parathyroid glands is the most common cause of hypoparathyroidism. Involvement of other endocrine glands should be considered in all non-surgical cases
- Primary HPT should be distinguished from familial hypocalciuric hypercalcaemia, where the serum calcium level is elevated along with serum PTH but 24 hour urinary calcium excretion is low. Renal hyperparathyroidism is characterized by hyperphosphataemia and low calcitriol levels driving secondary HPT
- Genetic causes of HPT should be considered in young-onset, recurrent or multigland disease, and in cases of parathyroid cancer
- Surgery is the only definitive treatment for primary HPT. It is sometimes indicated even when cases do not fulfil current surgical guidelines. Recent data on asymptomatic patients with primary HPT support surgical management because the bone mineral density may decline even after prolonged periods of stability.

INTRODUCTION

Parathyroid hormone (PTH) has been identified in teleost fish, so dating its origin to around 500 million years ago. Its role in fish remains poorly understood and they do not possess discrete parathyroid glands. However, in humans, it is recognized as being fundamental to calcium homeostasis. PTH is responsible for the minute by minute regulation of serum calcium levels. It does this by releasing calcium from bone via bone resorption, increasing renal calcium reabsorption and increasing renal 1,25-dihydroxyvitamin D production which increases gut calcium absorption.

Abnormalities of parathyroid function therefore cause abnormalities in serum calcium. By far the most common is *hyper*calcaemia, a diagnosis which has become more prevalent following the advent of multichannel biochemical analysers in the 1970s. Since this time there has been a marked shift in the emphasis of research towards the effects of asymptomatic HPT. Simultaneous advances in genetics have increased our understanding of the pathophysiology of parathyroid disorders. These combined advances have led to the recognition of rare familial forms which cause both hyper- and hypofunction. The current epidemic of osteoporosis has stimulated interest in normocalcaemic HPT and the conflicting actions of PTH on bone.

BASIC CALCIUM PHYSIOLOGY

Calcium ions are the most ubiquitous and pluripotent cellular signalling molecules in man, responsible for the control of a wide range of cellular processes. These include cell differentiation, apoptosis, muscular contraction and hormonal secretion. Calcium is involved in both extracellular and intracellular processes. Both rely on constant, tightly controlled concentrations of ionized calcium. Intracellular cytosolic calcium levels are 1000 times lower than extracellular fluid (ECF) levels, so its flux into the cell can be used as a signalling system. The system is controlled by a limited number of conserved transporters/channels which allow calcium ions to move across cell membranes.[1]

Extracellular calcium levels are monitored by the calcium-sensing receptor (CaSR), a G-protein-coupled receptor discovered by Brown in 1993.[2] In the parathyroid gland this receptor resides within invaginations of the plasma membrane (calveolae). It associates with several important scaffold proteins which allow the

A Practical Manual of Thyroid and Parathyroid Disease, 1st Edition. Edited by Asit Arora, Neil Tolley & R. Michael Tuttle.

receptor to interact with signalling proteins. Activation by extracellular calcium causes suppression of PTH synthesis and its release. There is a steep inverse sigmoidal relationship between the calcium concentration and PTH release such that a small change in calcium leads to a large change in PTH secretion (see Chapter 16, Fig. 16.4). The presence of several calcium-binding sites on the extracellular domain accounts for this via the mechanism of 'positive co-operativity'.[3] A baseline level of PTH secretion is always present, protecting against hypocalcaemia. The CaSR is resistant to desensitization from continued exposure to high extracellular calcium concentrations, so that PTH remains suppressed when there is non-PTH-related hypercalcaemia.[4]

The role of the CaSR has been well demonstrated in familial hypocalciuric hypercalcaemia (FHH) and autosomal dominant hypoparathyroidism (ADH), which are discussed later.[5] Both disorders exhibit CaSR involvement which is limited to the parathyroids and kidneys. The CaSR does, however, demonstrate a much wider tissue distribution and is present in the other organs involved with calcium homeostasis including bone, cartilage, intestine and thyroid C cells. It has also been identified in the brain, pituitary, pancreas and skin, where its role is less clear.[4]

Approximately 45% of serum calcium is protein bound, mainly to albumin. Ten percent is complexed with anions such as citrate and phosphate and the remainder is free as ionized calcium. The normal range of serum calcium reported by our laboratory is 2.15–2.6 mmol/l; this is a total concentration and a correction is made for protein levels:

$$\text{Corrected calcium} = [\text{calcium}]_{\text{total}} + 0.02\,(45 - [\text{albumin}])$$

When there is acid–base disturbance only the ionized calcium level is accurate.

The major regulatory organs in calcium homeostasis are bone, kidneys and intestine[6] (Fig. 13.1).

- Bone contains 99% of the body's calcium which is approximately 1 kilogram. PTH stimulation of osteoblasts enhances bone resorption by osteoclasts to release calcium. Daily bone turnover causes a flux of about 500 milligrams with the extracellular compartment.
- Intestinal absorption of calcium occurs throughout the gut, with 90% occurring in the duodenum and jejunum. Two mechanisms have been described. Active transport occurs via the epithelial calcium channel TRPV6, stimulated by 1,25-dihydroxyvitamin D. This is a saturable process which accounts for 10–15% of dietary input. It is activated in conditions of high calcium demand such as pregnancy, lactation and growth. Passive transport occurs via a paracellular, diffusional process which exhibits a linear relationship with intraluminal calcium concentration. Efficiency of overall net calcium absorption declines with age, and there is a fixed loss of about 200 mg/day due to intestinal secretions.
- The kidney acts as a regulator of plasma calcium. The majority of filtered calcium is reabsorbed by mass

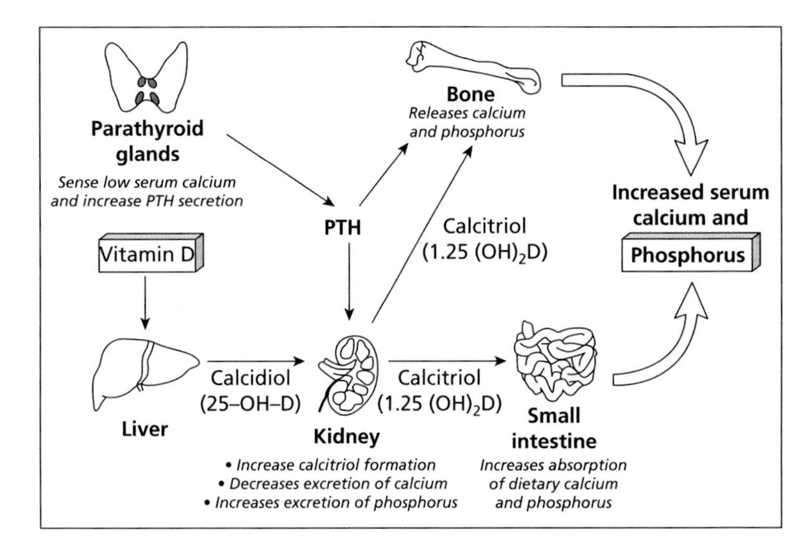

Fig. 13.1 Overview of calcium homeostasis.

transport coupled to sodium in the proximal tubule (PT). This process is not under PTH control. Factors such as ECF volume depletion enhance sodium reabsorption, thereby increasing calcium reabsorption. PTH exerts its main action in the cortical thick ascending limb (CTAL) of the loop of Henle and distal convoluted tubule (DCT) where 20 and 15% of filtered calcium is reabsorbed, respectively. In the CTAL, PTH increases the activity of the Na/K/2Cl co-transporter which increases the transepithelial potential difference driving paracellular calcium uptake. This is antagonized by the CaSR (see 'Hypercalcaemia' section below). In the DCT, PTH stimulates active transcellular calcium uptake by upregulating the basolateral Na^+/Ca^{2+} exchanger which is enhanced by 1,25-dihydroxyvitamin D.

PARATHYROID HORMONE

PTH is an 84 amino acid polypeptide produced by the chief cells of the parathyroid glands. The major regulator of PTH secretion is ionized calcium. A decrease in serum calcium causes inhibition of the CaSR and stimulates PTH secretion acutely and parathyroid cell growth chronically.

PTH causes an increase in serum calcium by:

- signalling to osteoblasts which increase osteoclastic activity via the RANK pathway, thus releasing calcium into the ECF
- directly increasing calcium absorption from the CTAL and DCT of the kidney
- stimulating renal 1α-hydroxylase activity, so increasing synthesis of 1,25-dihydroxyvitamin D which increases intestinal absorption of calcium.

PTH secretion is stimulated by:

- hypocalcaemia
- hyperphosphataemia
- reduced 1,25-dihydroxyvitamin D levels.

PTH secretion is inhibited by:

- hypercalcaemia
- 1,25-dihydroxyvitamin D
- fibroblast growth factor 23 (FGF23).

A further outline of calcium homeostasis and parathyroid physiology can be found in Chapter 16.

HYPERCALCAEMIA

Hypercalcaemia is defined as a total serum calcium greater than 2 standard deviations above the normal mean when corrected for serum albumin levels. Typically this means a calcium level greater than 2.6 mmol/l. Abnormalities of parathyroid function are the most common cause, and therefore hypercalcaemia may be broadly categorized as PTH- or non-PTH-related (Table 13.1). Although this is a useful clinical approach, it is something of an understatement. For instance, PTH-like action accounts for the majority of hypercalcaemia arising in malignancy. This includes systemic PTH-related protein (PTHrP) action in humoral hypercalcaemia of malignancy (HHM) and local PTHrP action in local osteolytic hypercalcaemia (LOH).

Table 13.1 Causes of hypercalcaemia

Causes
PTH-related
Primary hyperparathyroidism
Sporadic
Familial
Familial isolated (FIHP)
MEN 1
MEN2A
MEN4
HPT-JT
Tertiary hyperparathyroidism
CaSR disorders
Familial hypocalciuric hypercalcaemia
Neonatal severe hyperparathyroidism
Ectopic PTH production
Lithium
PTH-independent
Malignant disease
Humoral hypercalcaemia of malignancy
Local osteolytic hypercalcaemia
Excess calcitriol related
Granulomatous diseases
Medications
Milk–alkali syndrome
Vitamins A and D
Thiazides
Endocrine
Thyrotoxicosis
Addisons
Phaeochromocytoma
Immobilization
Post-rhabdomyolysis acute renal failure

Symptoms

Historically, the symptoms and signs of hypercalcaemia have been described by the adage 'Moans, bones, groans and renal stones'. These are not specific to either hypercalcaemia or hyperparathyroidism, but describe a combination of their manifestations. Although the full complex is rarely seen now, there is an increased understanding of their significance.

- **Gastrointestinal symptoms** ***(moans)***: peptic ulceration, nausea, vomiting, constipation, pancreatitis.
- **Skeletal** ***(bones)***: bone pain, arthralgia, osteitis fibrosa cystica (von Recklinghausen's disease of the bone), osteoporosis.
- **Neuromuscular** ***(groans)***: depression, fatigue, confusional state, muscle weakness, corneal calcification, lethargy.
- **Renal** ***(renal stones)***: nephrocalcinosis, polyuria, polydipsia, nephrogenic diabetes insipidus.
- **Cardiovascular**: hypertension, arrthymias, vascular calcification.

The effects of hypercalcaemia are partly mediated by the action of the CaSR in different tissues rather than by the high calcium level *per se*. The CaSR may account for the renal- and gut-related symptoms mentioned. Animal studies have shown that CaSR is present in particularly high concentrations on the basolateral membrane of tubular cells in the CTAL where PTH is known to act. In the CTAL, paracellular calcium resorption is driven by the generation of a lumen positive transepithelial potential gradient by the furosemide-sensitive Na/K/2Cl co-transporter. Resorption here is suppressed by high calcium and the CaSR may mediate this by directly inhibiting the co-transporter, causing a loop diuresis of sodium, calcium and magnesium.[7]

The CaSR is also found in the medullary thick ascending limb (MTAL) and intramedullary collecting duct (IMCD). Both play an important role in urinary concentration. In the MTAL, CaSR-mediated reduction of NaCl absorption leads to a reduced medullary concentration gradient for urinary concentration. In the IMCD, it is postulated that during hypercalcaemia the CaSR mediates the inhibition of vasopressin-stimulated aquaporin-2 water channel expression. Thus, the CaSR causes a desired aquaresis which dilutes the calcium-rich tubular fluid and affords protection from calcium stone formation. The CaSR is also found in the hypothalamic thirst centre where it may counteract dehydration by stimulating thirst.[7]

Apart from non-specific features such as mild anorexia, gastrointestinal symptoms of hypercalcaemia are relatively rare. Peptic ulceration can be explained by the presence of the CaSR in the stomach. In rat models, the CaSR is found in gastric glands, and stimulation by hypercalcaemia increases acid secretion from parietal cells. A direct stimulatory effect on the parietal cell H^+ ATPase may account for this. Alternatively, modulation of the hormonal control of parietal cell H^+ ATPase activity may be responsible. The CaSR, identified in G cells in the human stomach, increases gastrin secretion in response to stimulation, which would account for this.[8] The marked peptic ulceration seen in multiple endocrine neoplasia type 1 (MEN1) is more directly explainable by the occurrence of gastrinomas.

Pancreatitis is generally only seen in severe hypercalcaemia, although some families with FHH may suffer from recurrent pancreatitis. Constipation occurs as a result of decreased activity of the enteric nervous system and is also due to CaSR-mediated reduction of fluid secreted in the colon.[8]

Skeletal manifestations of hypercalcaemia are secondary to the underlying disease pathology and are discussed in the relevant sections below.

Neuromuscular problems arise because hypercalcaemia increases the resting membrane potential in excitable cells, so raising their depolarization threshold. Muscle cells become refractory to activation, causing weakness, fatigue and myopathy. Neurological sequalae range from generalized fatigue and mild cognitive impairment to gross obtundation. The latter appears to be age dependent as the young tolerate marked hypercalcaemia well. Neuropsychological symptoms have been extensively studied in primary hyperparathyroidism (PHPT) and will be discussed later in the chapter.

PTH-RELATED CAUSES OF HYPERCALCAEMIA

Primary hyperparathyroidism

This is the most common cause of hypercalcaemia in the general population. It has an annual incidence of about 0.1% in the USA and is more common in females, particularly in the first decade after the menopause.[9] The condition is characterized by hypersecretion of PTH causing hypercalcaemia associated with hypophosphataemia. Individuals may be normocalcaemic when there is coexisting vitamin D deficiency. A solitary adenoma in one gland is responsible for 80% of cases, 15% have chief cell hyperplasia affecting all four glands, 2% are due to adenomas in multiple glands and in 1% of cases there is parathyroid carcinoma.

Clinical features

The clinical profile of PHPT has transformed from an overtly symptomatic presentation to one that is less

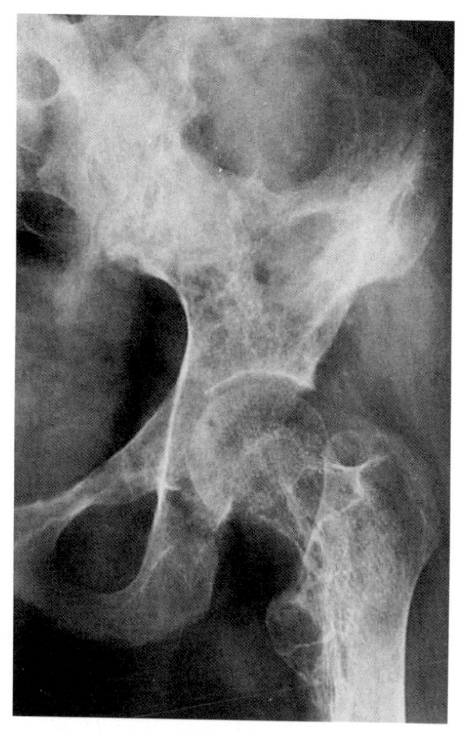

Fig. 13.2 Extensive bone changes of the pelvis and femur secondary to primary hyperparathyroidism.

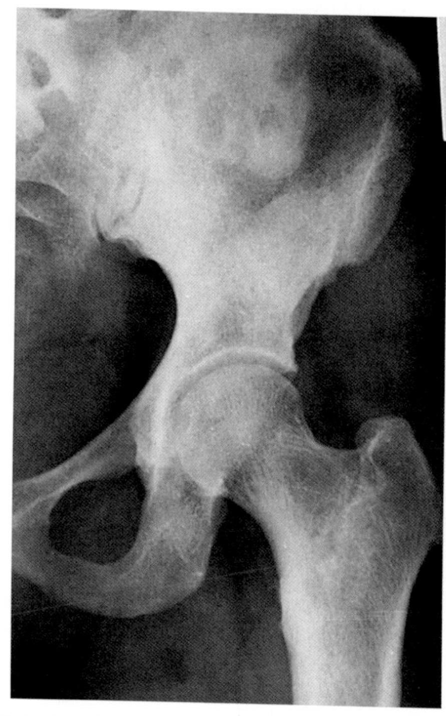

Fig. 13.3 Complete resolution of bone changes in the same patient as shown in Fig. 13.2 following treatment of primary hyperparathyroidism.

obvious. Difficulty in diagnosis arises because symptoms may be relatively non-specific and are present to some degree in the normal population. Patients tend to present with vague symptoms and often complain of feeling generally unwell and tired. They may also complain of depression and polyuria.[10]

Bone problems used to be a common finding with classical PHPT. These included generalized and focal bone pain, fragility fractures and Brown tumours with localized swelling. Radiological changes such as subperiosteal bone resorption were not infrequent (Figs 13.2 and 13.3). Osteolytic lesions with 'salt and pepper' appearances in the skull and Brown tumours in the long bones occurred in severe forms of the disease (Von Recklinghausen's disease of bone). Although 80% of patients with PHPT do not exhibit these classical features, the catabolic effect of continuously elevated PTH levels on cortical bone is evident in bone histomorphometry and bone mineral density (BMD) studies.[11] Bone histomorphometry demonstrates cortical thinning, increased cortical porosity and endosteal resorption, although trabecular volume and connectivity are well preserved.[12] The Columbia University prospective cohort study of mild PHPT showed that although lumbar spine BMD remains unchanged with time, the distal radius BMD falls by 35% and femoral neck BMD by 10% over 15 years.[13] Despite the observations relating to lumbar spine BMD, there is good evidence that trabecular bone changes are clinically significant. There appears to be a subset of patients with a very low lumbar spine BMD,[14] and the risk of vertebral fracture is increased in PHPT.[15] Furthermore, the BMD at vertebral sites increases markedly post-parathyroidectomy.[13,16,17]

All patients with a history of calcium-containing renal stones should be investigated for PHPT. Although the incidence of renal stones has almost halved in the last 50 years, it nevertheless remains a significant clinical issue. Parathyroidectomy reduces the risk of stone formation both in asymptomatic disease and in patients with a prior history of stone formation.[10,18] Although renal function (assessed by serum creatinine) remains unchanged, surgery improves renal concentrating ability and hypercalciuria.[13,19] The clinical impact of the latter is uncertain; interestingly, hypercalciuria does not appear to predict renal stone formation in PHPT.[20]

Cardiovascular sequelae are an increasingly important consideration, particularly in view of the high incidence of asymptomatic PHPT.[20] Severe PHPT is associated with hypertension, left ventricular hypertrophy (LVH), myocardial and valvular calcification, diastolic dysfunction and, ultimately, increased cardiovascular mortality.[21,22] Although it reduces with time, an increase in mortality persists post-parathyroidectomy, and hypertension remains irreversible.[23,24] Asymptomatic PHPT with mean serum calcium levels around 2.8 mmol/l has not been shown to adversely impact on mortality.[25,26] However, other clinical sequelae do occur, such as hypertension (which persists post-parathyroidectomy), LVH and diastolic dysfunction.[20,27] Population studies suggest that the serum calcium level is an independent risk factor for myocardial infarction.

Neuropsychological issues are prominent in severe HPT. Symptoms include fatigue, cognitive impairment, sleep disturbance, anxiety, depression and somatization. Observational studies in mild PHPT have suggested there may be an improvement in global health-related quality of life (physical, psychological and social functioning) or cognition post-parathyroidectomy, but results have been variable.[28] Recently, two randomized controlled trials (RCTs) compared parathyroidectomy against no surgical treatment using similar quality of life outcome measures. Both studies found little difference at baseline from a normal control population, although specific areas were identified where neuropsychological functioning improved following surgery.[16,29] A third RCT showed worse scores in all measured psychological areas, but no clear improvement was seen post-surgery.[30] In summary, there was insufficient evidence for its inclusion as an indication for surgery in the most recent 2009 guidelines.[20]

Diagnosis

The conventional diagnosis of PHPT is based upon a high total or ionized serum calcium level in the presence of a PTH level which is either frankly elevated or inappropriately in the upper half of the normal range. The expected physiological effect of an elevated serum calcium is to decrease serum PTH via negative feedback through the CaSR. Therefore, autonomous PTH production is suggested if PTH levels are not appropriately suppressed by the hypercalcaemia.

There may be additional clues in the basic biochemistry which aid the diagnosis. The serum phosphate tends to be low-normal, or frankly low in 30% of cases due to the phosphaturic effect of PTH in the PT. The serum bicarbonate may be low due to bicarbonate wasting in the PT, with a small increase in serum chloride concentration. Elevated alkaline phosphatase and urine NTX (cross-linked N-telopeptide of type 1 collagen) levels may be present, reflecting increased bone formation and resorption.

The most common confounder to the diagnosis is vitamin D deficiency. This may hide the true level of serum calcium and therefore cause confusion with secondary hyperparathyroidism. The situation is further complicated by the fact that PHPT is associated with low serum 25-hydroxyvitamin D levels, probably due to enhanced catabolism. Vitamin D deficiency exacerbates several features of PHPT such as adenoma size, bone disease, post-operative hypocalcaemia and hungry bone syndrome. Patients must therefore be rendered vitamin D replete as part of the formal work-up. Studies show this to be safe. Replacement with 800 U/day of vitamin D3 if the 25-hydroxy vitamin D level is <50 nmol/l is reasonable.[31]

PHPT must be differentiated from FHH as surgery is rarely indicated in the latter and is generally inappropriate. This can be done by measuring the 24 hour urine calcium/creatinine clearance ratio. Spot urine calcium/creatinine ratios and simple 24 hour urine calciums are less sensitive and specific. The 24 hour urinary calcium excretion is typically raised in PHPT. The clearance ratio is >0.01. Conversely, in FHH the presence of an inactivated renal CaSR allows the kidney to conserve calcium, which results in a low calcium/creatinine clearance ratio, typically <0.01.[32] However, these ratios have been developed with patients on a fixed calcium diet, and recent studies of FHH families on a free diet suggest the overlap in ratios is much greater than initially appreciated. Indeed, many FHH individuals demonstrate a ratio >0.01. Furthermore, several confounding factors cause falsely low urine calcium excretion in patients with PHPT. These include vitamin D deficiency, hypomagnesaemia and medications such as thiazides or lithium. Therefore, if hypocalciuria exists in a patient with suspected PHPT, we advocate the following safeguards to differentiate between PHPT and FHH.

- Correct confounders: vitamin D deficiency and hypomagnesaemia.
- Stop interfering medications: thiazides, lithium.
- Obtain a good family history with serum and urine calciums obtained from three relatives if possible.
- Obtain results of earlier blood tests; these may be invaluable as hypercalcaemia in FHH is evident from infancy.

Mutational analysis of the CaSR gene on chromosome 3q is widely available but has a high false-negative rate because 30% of cases show no mutation with current techniques. In addition, other loci (chromosome 19p and 19q) are sometimes implicated. CaSR gene testing is indicated in the following instances:[31]

- hypocalciuric hypercalcaemia where no family cases are available for evaluation
- familial isolated hyperparathyroidism (FIHP) in the absence of low urine calcium, as 10% have CaSR mutations.[33]

Having confirmed the biochemical diagnosis, the next step is to consider the special situations that may cause PHPT such as familial disease and parathyroid carcinoma. The presence of either condition alters the pre-operative work-up and the extent of surgery to be performed.

In MEN1, PHPT has an extremely high penetrance of 95% by the age of 50 years. MEN1 should be suspected and screened for in:

- familial disease
- patients under the age of 30
- true recurrent disease
- dual or multiple concurrent adenomas
- specific MEN1-related tumours outside the parathyroids.

In such cases *MENIN* gene analysis is recommended,[31,34] which has a sensitivity of about 70% in familial cases. It is also reasonable to screen simultaneously with prolactin, insulin-like growth factor-1 (IGF-1) and a fasting gut hormone profile.

In contrast to MEN1, it is very unusual for MEN2A to present with primary hyperparathyroidism. Penetrance is mutation specific, averaging about 30%, and the diagnosis is usually already evident.

Hyperparathyroidism–jaw tumour (HPT-JT) syndrome should be suspected if there is an early aggressive onset with multiple asynchronous adenomas or a history of parathyroid cancer in the patient or family. *HPRT2* gene analysis should be performed, which has 70% sensitivity. Other indications for gene analysis include:[31]

- sporadic cases of parathyroid carcinoma
- FIHP, although mutations are rare.[35]

An orthopantomogram is indicated to assess the mandible for ossifying fibromas, and a renal ultrasound to assess for cysts or tumours.

The current standard for *in vivo* PTH measurement is the second-generation intact PTH immunoradiometric assay which was first developed by Nichols. This is a two-site test, using a capture antibody against hPTH 39–84 and a revealing antibody against hPTH 1–34. The latter also detects N-terminal-deficient fragments of 'intact' PTH (particularly 7–84 and 15–84) which accounts for 20% of activity seen in normal individuals and up to 50% activity in patients with renal impairment. Apart from this caveat, they offer good sensitivity of about 90%. Because there is no cross-reactivity with PTHrP, the second-generation assay reliably distinguishes between various causes of hypercalcaemia.[31] Third-generation assays which also avoid this problem are being introduced and have a similar sensitivity.[36] PTH assay is discussed in further detail in Chapter 14.

Further evaluation of PHPT involves tests to determine any additional manifestations. Investigations include serum creatinine, three-site BMD scanning and renal ultrasound. The latest guidelines are discussed in the following sections.

Primary hyperparathyroidism: 2009 guidelines for surgical intervention

In 1990, the National Institute for Health in the USA produced guidelines for surgical intervention in primary hyperparathyroidism. These were based on recommendations of the Consensus Development Conference on the Management of Asymptomatic Hyperparathyroidism. The group recognized the increasingly asymptomatic nature of the disease and that surgery may not be appropriate in all cases.[37] The guidelines were revised in 2002 and most recently in 2009.[38,39]

Parathyroidectomy is recommended in patients who fulfil the following criteria:

- age <50 years
- serum calcium >0.25 mmol/l above the normal range
- calculated GFR reduced to <60 ml/min
- T-score less than –2.5 at any site and/or previous fragility fracture
- medical surveillance is neither desired nor possible.

Parathyroid surgery is the only definitive treatment for PHPT. Emerging data on the natural history of asymptomatic PHPT increasingly support surgical management because BMD can decline even after many years of stability.[13] This process is both preventable and reversible by surgery. The inclusion of a third BMD site, the distal one-third radius, in the 2002 guidelines underlines the importance of monitoring cortical bone, where bone loss is greatest. In the current guidelines the use of z scores for appropriate age groups has been included, e.g. premenopausal women and men under the age of 50. Fragility fractures are also an indication for surgery because they reflect bone health and factors such as bone quality that may not show up on BMD studies.

Surgery should always be considered an option, even in patients who do not fulfil the surgical guidelines outlined. Thus, it is may also be recommended in patients with organ complications, overt neuromuscular disease or symptoms of hypercalcaemia.[40]

Hypercalciuria is no longer included as an indication, for several reasons. Twenty-four hour urine collection is liable to inaccuracy, and urine calcium excretion is extremely variable between individuals. Stone formation is dependent on many factors other than the urine calcium concentration, such as urine pH, volume, oxalate, citrate and urate concentrations. Thus, hypercalciuria is not predictive of renal stone formation in patients with PHPT.[39]

Chapter 17 outlines the surgical management of PHPT, parathyroid hyperplasia and carcinoma.

Primary hyperparathyroidism: 2009 guidelines for monitoring

Monitoring guidelines have changed in line with the indications for surgical intervention. The following investigations are recommended in medically managed patients:[39]

- annual serum calcium
- annual serum creatinine
- BMD at three sites every 1–2 years.

These guidelines assume adequate repletion of vitamin D, with serum 25-hydroxyvitamin D levels >50 nmol/l and a normal calcium diet.

The major difference compared with guidelines in previous years relates to monitoring for kidney stones. Renal ultrasound and/or abdominal X-ray are no longer recommended unless there is a clinical suspicion of stones. Twenty-four hour urine calcium as a predictor of future stone risk has been discounted, as previously discussed.

Primary hyperparathyroidism: medical treatment

Historically, the mainstay of medical management of PHPT has been hormone replacement therapy (HRT) and more recently bisphosphonates. Each class of agents has a different profile of action.[41] For instance, if the calcium is >2.8 mmol/l but the patient is not a candidate for surgery, oral bisphosphonates will have limited efficacy whereas cinacalcet is extremely effective in reducing the calcium level.[42]

Most of the studies with oral bisphosphonates involve alendronate, and they have demonstrated a significant benefit relating to bone.[43–45] Markers of bone turnover were substantially reduced by 3 months, which was associated with gains in BMD at lumbar spine, total hip and distal one-third radius sites. In one RCT, BMD improved by 8.6% at lumbar spine and 4.8% at total hip over a 2 year period, which compares favourably with patients managed surgically.[43] Some studies have shown that oral bisphosphonates achieve a statistically significant reduction in serum calcium,[44] but this is not a consistent finding.[43] Urine calcium excretion is not altered and PTH levels may temporarily rise.[43]

Intravenous pamidronate has been used to treat acute hypercalcaemia for many years. In most cases it suppresses serum calcium into the normal range, although effects are short-lived and repeat infusion is necessary after 4–6 weeks. There are no data on its use as a long-term treatment in PHPT.

Oestrogen replacement has been used for many years in PHPT.[46] Its effects are similar to those of bisphosphonates. There is only a small change in serum calcium (total) or PTH, but there is a substantial improvement in BMD, which is maintained over time. The decline in urine calcium excretion is not maintained.[47,48] Short-term data on raloxifene, a selective oestrogen receptor modulator (SERM), suggests that it has a similiar but less marked effect than HRT on calcium and bone turnover.[49] Although BMD data are limited to a few cases, its use is consistent with a beneficial effect.

Cinacalcet is the first available medication in the new class of calcimimetics. These agents stimulate the CaSR in parathyroid cells, thereby signalling a high calcium level and reducing PTH secretion. It has been shown to reduce PTH secretion in normal glands, hyperplastic glands secondary to chronic renal impairment, discrete parathyroid adenomas and parathyroid carcinoma. In addition, it reduces parathyroid cell growth and proliferation.

Proof of principle in PHPT was first established in 1997 using the calcimimetic agent R-568. A recent year-long RCT with cinacalcet has demonstrated its efficacy in PHPT.[42] This study showed that serum calcium could be normalized from a mean baseline level of 2.68 ± 0.13 mmol/l in 73% of patients, with a mean reduction of 0.13 mmol/l. In 90% of cases this was achieved with a dose of 30 mg twice daily. Successful reduction of calcium levels was maintained at 1 year and further open-label extension data suggest that the effect persists at 5 years. No change in either bone turnover markers or BMD was observed, although it should be noted that the cohort's baseline bone densities were well preserved. No changes in urine calcium were seen. Cinacalcet has a short duration of action, with peak PTH suppression 2 hours post-dose. Adverse effects include nausea and occasional hypocalcaemia.

Primary hyperparathyroidism: localization studies

Imaging studies play no role in establishing a diagnosis of PHPT. Once the diagnosis is made, and if surgical management is indicated, imaging is useful to localize the site of abnormal parathyroid tissue pre-operatively. This may not be indicated if a bilateral neck exploration is required due to suspected or confirmed familial disease, such as MEN1. The next chapter focuses in detail on the various techniques, the most common of which are briefly outlined below.

Technetium tc 99m sestamibi scanning

This is the most sensitive method of localizing abnormal parathyroid activity. It identifies the anatomical position of an adenoma with an accuracy >80% in some centres. It is able to localize ectopic glands in the mediastinum, although small, multiple adenomas may be difficult to localize. The majority of hyperplastic parathyroids do not demonstrate sestamibi uptake, and nodular thyroid disease may also reduce its accuracy.

Ultrasound scanning

Ultrasound scanning in experienced hands is a very effective method of identifying an enlarged parathyroid gland and localizing the precise anatomical position. Unlike sestamibi scanning, it can also indicate the size of the lesion.

CT scanning

This has a limited role in the identification of a parathyroid gland adenoma as it may be difficult to differentiate parathyroid tissue from other structures such as lymph nodes. With improving techniques and in combination with PET scanning it is increasingly being used in persistent or recurrent disease.

MRI scanning

Contrast-enhanced MRI can sometimes be useful when other modalities fail in persistent or recurrent disease.

Selective venous sampling with arteriography

This is reserved for recurrent disease in specialist centres, but in experienced hands it has a high rate of localization.

Primary hyperparathyroidism: familial disease

Familial hypocalciuric hypercalcaemia (FHH)

This is an autosomal dominant condition characterized by a life-long modest elevation of serum calcium associated with a low 24 hour urinary calcium excretion. It has also been called familial benign hypercalcaemia (FBH), reflecting its generally asymptomatic nature. The condition is due to inactivating mutations in the CaSR on chromosome 3q. In two families, separate linkage to 19p and 19q were also identified.[5]

Clinical features are limited and may include chondrocalcinosis, acute pancreatitis and premature vascular calcification. The typical complications of PHPT do not occur: BMD and fracture rates are normal and there is not an increased incidence of renal stones. Biochemical penetrance of hypercalcaemia is near 100% from infancy. The hypercalcaemia is generally mild, although a few cases have been reported where the serum calcium is >3 mmol/l. PTH levels are usually in the upper end of the normal range. In 20% of cases levels are frankly elevated, and very rarely PTH levels are twice the upper limit of normal. Serum magnesium is high-normal or may be mildly elevated.[5,32,50]

Critical to its differentiation from PHPT has been the 24 hour urine calcium creatinine clearance ratio, as previously mentioned. The presence of the CaSR in the kidneys results in relative hypocalciuria, with 75% of cases showing levels <2.5 mmol in 24 hours. However, recent studies have shown that levels are very variable in members of affected families. Furthermore, certain families have been identified with hypercalciuria and kidney stones.[51]

Subtotal parathyroidectomy is not curative and surgery is only reserved for special circumstances such as relapsing pancreatitis or a serum calcium >3.5 mmol/l. Traditional medical therapy to lower calcium is not generally indicated as it is rarely successful. Cases reports with cinacalcet suggest this may useful in exceptional circumstances.

Neonatal severe primary hyperparathyroidism

This is a very rare neonatal disorder which occurs due to the inheritance of two mutated alleles for the CaSR. It presents with life-threatening hypercalcaemia and multiple bony problems such as fractures and ribcage deformities.[5] Respiratory distress may also occur. All four parathyroid glands are grossly enlarged and urgent total parathyroidectomy is warranted.

MEN syndromes (Table 13.2)

MEN1

MEN1 is defined as the presence of tumours in two of the three most affected tissues:

Table 13.2 MEN syndromes

MEN1
Parathyroid adenomas
Enteropancreatic tumours
Gastrinoma
Insulinoma
Non-functioning tumours
Glucagonoma
VIPoma
Foregut carcinoid tumours
Thymic carcinoid
Bronchial carcinoid
Gastric enterochromaffin-like tumours
Pituitary adenomas
Prolactinoma
GH secreting
ACTH secreting
Adrenal cortical tumours
MEN2
Familial medullary thyroid carcinoma
MEN2A
Medullary thyroid carcinoma
Parathyroid hyperplasia
Phaeochromocytoma
Cutaneous lichen amyloidosis
MEN2B
Medullary thyroid carcinoma
Phaeochromocytoma
Mucosal neuromas, intestinal ganglioneuromas
Marfanoid physique

- parathyroid glands
- pituitary gland
- enteropancreatic tissues.

Familial MEN1 is defined as a proband with MEN1 and a first-degree relative with a tumour in at least one of these tissues.[34] Several other tumours may also be present.

MEN1 is a rare disorder with a prevalence of 2 in 100 000. It is due to inactivating mutations in the tumour suppressor *MENIN* gene located on chromosome 11q13. It has an autosomal dominant inheritance pattern. In addition to the inherited or sporadic germline mutation, a somatic 'second hit' occurs later in life in a tissue-specific pattern. This 'second hit' inactivates the remaining normal *MENIN* allele and initiates tumorigenesis[52]

Parathyroid disease is generally the earliest feature of MEN1. There is an early age of onset (recorded from 8 years old) with 95% penetrance by 50 years. Clinical presentation usually occurs in the second to fourth decades and there is an equal sex distribution.[53] Multi-gland adenomas exhibiting a large size discrepancy are common.

MEN1 accounts for only 2% of all PHPT cases, but it has also been found in a number of families with familial isolated HPT.[54] Gene sequencing should be considered in these cases and also in recurrent PHPT, young-onset disease and when multiple adenomas are found.[34] In the UK, the MEN1 detection rate is >90% for cases of familial parathyroid disease with tumours in two other tissues. However, this figure is as low as 0% in sporadic cases of recurrent or young-onset PHPT.[55]

The optimal timing for surgery in MEN1 is a controversial issue. Pre-symptomatic intervention is not routinely recommended and the indications for surgery are the same as for sporadic HPT. Given the high rate of recurrence, four-gland exploration with removal of three and a half glands followed by marking or autotransplantation of the remaining half gland is recommended. Transcervical near total thymectomy should also be performed to ensure no glands are missed and to reduce the risk of thymic carcinoid.[34,56]

Patients require long-term surveillance with annual biochemical screening and interval imaging for other MEN1 tumours.[34] Unlike MEN2, the specific mutation does not predict tumour specificity or the clinical course of the disease.

MEN2

MEN2 consists of three autosomal dominant clinical syndromes; familial medullary thyroid cancer (FMTC), MEN2A and MEN2B. The common feature in all these syndromes is the development of malignant tumours of the thyroid parafollicular C cells which exhibit high penetrance (>90%).

MEN2A families show other features with lower penetrance including phaeochromocytomas (50%), parathyroid hyperplasia (20%) and cutaneous lichen amyloidosis.

MEN2B is similarly characterized by phaeochromocytomas, but does not include parathyroid disease. Individuals may have mucosal neuromas, intestinal ganglioneuromas and a marfanoid body habitus with a decreased upper/lower body ratio and joint hypermobility[34] (Fig 13.4).

MEN2 is caused by activating mutations in the *RET* gene. This is a proto-oncogene on chromosome 10, which codes for a receptor tyrosine kinase involved in cell growth and differentiation. Overactivity leads to C cell hyperplasia followed by tumorigenesis.[52] Progression

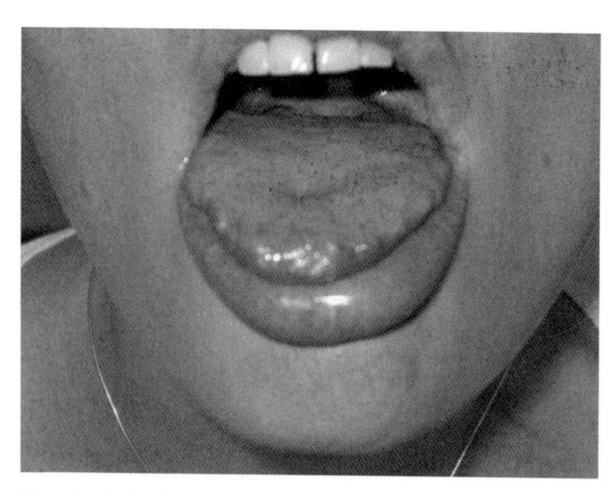

Fig. 13.4 The clinical image demonstrates multiple ganglioneuromas on the tongue of a patient with MEN2B.

rates are mutation specific, which has allowed the development of codon-based intervention strategies for early prophylactic thyroidectomy in affected individuals.[57] Fortunately, because mutational analysis is highly sensitive (95%), annual biochemical screening of at-risk individuals with calcitonin is generally no longer required. Post-operatively, calcitonin monitoring is critical to monitor for recurrence in affected individuals.

Parathyroid disease affects 20–30% of MEN2A cases. This is a multigland hyperplastic process, although not all glands are found to be affected at surgery. Hypercalcaemia tends to be milder than in MEN1. Most patients are asymptomatic and recurrence rates are lower post-operatively.[58,59] Parathyroid disease is particularly associated with mutations in codon 634 which is the most prevalent codon affected in MEN2A.

MTC is the presenting feature in most cases of MEN2A, although it can occasionally present as hypercalcaemia.[58] The diagnosis is usually evident, so most experts do not advocate *RET* screening in cases of early, familial or recurrent PHPT.[31,56]

Indications for surgery are the same as for sporadic PHPT and should include bilateral neck exploration to identify all the parathyroid glands. Due to the excellent outcomes following parathyroid surgery in MEN2, it has been suggested that removal of only the affected glands may be sufficient.[59] Total parathyroidectomy and autotransplantation may not be warranted due to the increased risk of hypoparathyroidism. Most experts advocate treating as multigland disease and favour subtotal parathyroidectomy.[34,56]

Hyperparathyroidism–jaw tumour (HPT-JT) syndrome

This is a rare autosomal dominant familial syndrome characterized by

- primary hyperparathyroidism
- fibro-osseous lesions of the mandible and maxilla
- renal cysts and tumours.

It is caused by mutations in *HRPT-2*, a tumour suppressor gene on chromosome 1q, which codes for parafibromin.[60]

HPT-JT is highly penetrant, affecting 80% of individuals, and the age of onset is as early as the first decade. Hypercalcaemia may be severe enough to cause individuals to present with hypercalcaemic crisis. Parathyroid adenomas develop asynchronously in multiple glands; sometimes only one gland is found to be affected at surgery, but double adenomas are common. Adenomas have an unusual cystic appearance.[61]

HPT-JT is strongly associated with parathyroid carcinoma. Up to 15–20% of individuals are affected and they can present with lung metastases as young as the third decade. Analysis of sporadic parathyroid carcinoma has shown that there is somatic loss of *HRPT-2* in most of the tumours and in many cases there are also germline mutations in *HRPT-2*.[62] This is not the case for sporadic parathyroid adenomas.

Mutational analysis is only 70% sensitive so it does not fully exclude at-risk individuals in some families known to be affected clinically. All at-risk members should be screened for hypercalcaemia from the age of 15 years. An orthopantomogram is advocated every 3 years to look for ossifying fibromas of the jaw, and an abdominal ultrasound is indicated annually. There is no consensus regarding the optimal surgical approach. Given the risks of parathyroid carcinoma, prophylactic surgery has been suggested, but there is no evidence for this. Surgery is usually performed as soon as HPT develops. A bilateral neck exploration removing the affected glands is the minimum approach. Others advocate total parathyroidectomy without autotransplantation.[56,61]

Familial isolated hyperparathyroidism (FIHP)

FIHP has been described in over 100 families, and is defined as hereditary primary hyperparathyroidism without the association of non-parathyroid tumours or features seen in other syndromes.[33,63] As genetic analyses for new syndromes emerge, it is becoming clear that some cases of FIHP represent milder or allelic variants of these other syndromes. For instance, one of the kindreds of FIHP in the largest, well-documented series was found to be have an *HRPT-2* mutation and so was a variant on HPT-JT.[35] Occult FHH[33] and MEN1[54] have also been frequently identified. Syndromes may manifest themselves in FIHP patients with increasing age and as new genetic advances arise. Surgery should follow standard indications and should involve a bilateral neck exploration with removal of affected glands only. All patients should remain under long-term follow-up.

Renal hyperparathyroidism

Renal osteodystrophy refers to the bone disease that develops in chronic renal impairment due to changes in mineral and PTH metabolism. The process involves several organ systems including bone, kidneys and the vasculature. Its importance in contributing to the mortality associated with chronic renal failure has become increasingly apparent. The condition has recently been named chronic kidney disease-mineral bone disorder (CKD-MBD) in recognition of this.[64]

Pathogenesis

Secondary HPT

Secondary HPT develops early in renal impairment, before the GFR drops significantly. This is an adaptive response which helps maintain normal phosphate levels as well as maintaining 1, 25-dihydroxyvitamin D (calcitriol) and calcium levels. It also helps maintain normal osteoblast activity and a low bone turnover state. Unfortunately, more marked PTH hypersecretion becomes damaging, resulting in classic high-turnover bone disease, osteitis fibrosa cystica, hypercalcaemia, and vascular and soft tissue calcification.[65]

As CKD progresses PTH levels rise in tandem. There is diffuse hyperplasia of all the parathyroid glands, with gland size paralleling serum PTH levels. Monoclonal chief cell growth results in superimposed nodule formation. The two main drivers in this process are hyperphosphataemia and low calcitriol levels.[65]

- With reduced nephron mass, there is a reduction in the filtered load of phosphate which results in hyperphosphataemia. This becomes biochemically apparent at GFRs <40 ml/min and stimulates PTH secretion through several mechanisms.[66] It acts directly on the parathyroid glands, stimulating PTH secretion. There are also indirect mechanisms via reduced 1α-hydroxylase enzyme activity in the PT and by lowering serum calcium levels by calcium–phosphate binding.
- Calcitriol deficiency occurs because the reduced nephron mass and hyperphosphataemia lead to reduced 1α-hydroxylase enzyme activity and therefore less conversion of 25-hydroxyvitamin D to 1,25-dihydroxyvitamin D (calcitriol). Levels becomes biochemically abnormal at GFRs <30 ml/min. Mean levels are lower than in the normal population at GFRs <80 ml/min.[66] It stimulates PTH secretion through several mechanisms. First, there is a reduction of the direct negative feedback on PTH cells. Secondly, there is an indirect effect through reduction of calcitriol-stimulated gut calcium absorption. Both processes are influenced by a generalized reduction in vitamin D receptor (VDR) numbers that occurs.

Tertiary HPT

The parathyroid glands remain responsive to calcium in secondary HPT. The hypocalcaemia caused by the above processes acts as a driver to PTH production by reduced signalling through the CaSR on parathyroid cells. In some chronic cases this hypersecretion becomes refractory to feedback by serum calcium levels and tertiary hyperparathyroidism develops with frank hypercalcaemia. This may be explained by the reduced CaSR numbers on parathyroid cells in CKD, which reduces negative feedback when hypercalcaemia occurs. In tertiary HPT there is usually diffuse massive enlargement of the parathyroid glands, although monoclonal adenomas may also be involved.

Bone disease

Bone involvement follows several patterns of disease which may occur in combination.

- Classical osteitis fibrosa cystica: a state of high-turnover hyperparathyroid bone disease.
- Adynamic bone disease: a state of low-turnover disease mainly due to lack of PTH action but also due to the effects of bisphosphonate.
- Osteomalacia: decreased mineralization due to vitamin D deficiency.
- Osteoporosis: decreased bone density due to excess bone resorption in both high- and low-turnover disease, hypogonadism and chronic acidosis.

Clinical features

In early CKD clinical features are minimal. The most common manifestations are vascular, which develop insidiously as the GFR declines. Systolic blood pressure increases and there is a widened pulse pressure. These are the result of multifactorial processes which lead to reduced vascular compliance. Vascular calcification is an important part of this, and widespread arterial medial calcification is common in CKD. A second type of calcification seen in CKD is atherosclerotic neointimal calcification, which correlates with an increased rate of thrombotic events such as myocardial infarction.

Patients with severe CKD are affected by heterotopic calcification and bone problems. Heterotopic calcification affects multiple tissues. This includes band keratopathy in the eye, red eye syndrome, restrictive lung disease with calcific nodules, and myocardial valve and annular calcification. Periarticular calcification is termed tumoral calcinosis and may be associated with severe restriction and painful joint movement.

Bone symptoms are very variable according to the underlying pathology. Fracture rates are markedly increased as a whole in the haemodialysis population. Adynamic bone disease is generally asymptomatic. Osteitis fibrosa cystica and osteomalacia may both cause non-specific deep-seated pain, particularly in the back and legs. Osteomalacia may cause bone pain and typical rickets deformities in children. Slipped femoral, radial and ulnar epiphyses are associated with osteitis fibrosa in growing children.

Medical therapy

Intervention is indicated in stage 3 CKD, when the GFR drops below 60 ml/min.[67] Medical therapy aims to reverse the two main mechanisms involved in driving secondary HPT; hyperphosphataemia and low 1,25-dihydroxyvitamin D (calcitriol) levels. Recent treatments aim to inhibit PTH secretion directly by acting on the parathyroid.

Hyperphosphataemia is reversed by dietary intervention, phosphate-binding agents and dialysis. With close dietary supervision and protein restriction, phosphate levels may be controlled until the GFR reaches 25–40 ml/min.[68] All haemodialysis patients also require phosphate binders as dialysis is inefficient at removing phosphate. Calcium-based phosphate binders (calcium acetate and carbonate) are cheap and effective, but there have been concerns over the associated risks of increased arterial calcification and the incidence of hypercalcaemia. Sevelamer, a cationic ion-exchange polymer, may avoid this. Hypercalcaemia occurs at a much lower rate with sevelamer, and studies have shown reduced progression of coronary and aortic arterial calcification.[69,70] However, a recent meta-analysis showed no difference in all-cause mortality or cardiovascular deaths.[71] Lanthanum carbonate is another new non-calcium-based phosphate binder.

Nutritional vitamin D deficiency is extremely common in CKD patients, even before calcitriol levels drop significantly. If PTH levels are elevated, guidelines suggest treatment in stage 3 and 4 CKD. Ergocalciferol or cholecalciferol can be used in doses up to 10 000 U/week, depending on baseline levels. The active vitamin D analogues, calcitriol and alfacacidol (1α-hydroxyvitamin D) are routinely used in dialysis patients. These may also be indicated pre-dialysis if ergocalciferol supplementation with phosphate binders fails to normalize PTH to target levels (K/DOQI guidelines). The analogues effectively suppress secondary HPT, but there are concerns because they increase serum calcium levels and the serum calcium × phosphate product by increasing gut calcium and phosphate absorption. They therefore tend to be used at low dosage, starting at 0.25 μg per day, or may be used orally or intravenously on dialysis days only. Newer analogues designed to produce fewer hypercalcaemic effects whilst preserving the ability to suppress PTH have been trialled. These include doxercalciferol and paricalcitol (19-Nor-1-α-dihydroxyvitamin D2). Unfortunately, evidence supporting their use is limited.

Calcimimetic agents are allosteric modulators of the CaSR which reduce PTH secretion. They offer a solution to the problem of hypercalcaemia which arises with vitamin D analogues and of PTH becoming refractory to suppression. Cinacalcet, the only available agent, has been shown to be effective in reducing PTH, serum calcium and phosphate levels when added to standard therapy.[72] There is no evidence yet that the natural history of secondary HPT is altered, but initial experience has been very promising and its use is becoming widespread. Dosage starts at 30 mg once a day, increasing to twice daily, to a maximum of 180 mg total per day.

Indications for surgical intervention

Refractory hyperparathyroidism is common. Approximately 3% of CKD patients on dialysis for >10 years are operated on per year, compared with 0.3% with <5 years dialysis duration.[73] Refractory HPT may represent development of a monoclonal adenoma, delayed or insufficient medical treatment or it may simply reflect the natural history of CKD as hyperphosphataemia becomes resistant to treatment and parathyroid glands become resistant to suppression. Once established, parathyroid hyperplasia is difficult to reverse.

There are no RCTs which confirm improved outcomes after parathyroidectomy. Indications for surgery include high PTH levels with:

- persistent hypercalcaemia
- progressive osteitis fibrosa cystica
- progressive heterotopic calcification

- refractory pruritis
- calciphylaxis.

Asymptomatic persistent secondary HPT without complications is not an indication for surgery. However, when the estimated gland weight is >500 mg, nodular hyperplasia is nearly always present. This has been shown to predict refractoriness to medical therapy.[74] Parathyroid hyperplasia is usually very marked and glands >1 g are common. Localization procedures are not indicated. Surgical management involves bilateral neck exploration and either a subtotal parathyroidectomy or total parathyroidectomy with autotransplantation. Success rates are similar with both approaches and roughly one-third of cases recur.[75] The presence of nodular hyperplasia strongly predicts recurrence, and autotransplantation of nodular parathyroid tissue should therefore be avoided.[76]

HYPOPARATHYROIDISM

Parathyroid underactivity is extremely rare unless the cause is iatrogenic following thyroid/parathyroid surgery.

Congenital parathyroid deficiency

Isolated hypoparathyroidism

Familial isolated hypoparathyroidism has several patterns of inheritance. Autosomal dominant and recessive patterns are both caused by mutations in the signal peptide region of the PTH gene. This results in abnormal processing of preproPTH to PTH.[77,78] Autosomal recessive disease has also been seen with a GCMB (glial cells missing homologue B) transcription factor mutation which is necessary for parathyroid development.[79] X-linked recessive disease causing parathyroid aplasia is due to a deletion–insertion of a fragment from chromosome 2p25 into Xq27.[80]

DiGeorge syndrome

This is a congenital condition characterized by lack of development of the third and fourth pharyngeal pouches. Since the parathyroids and thymus are derived from these, hypoparathyroidism and T cell deficiencies arise. It is usually part of a contiguous gene syndrome caused by *de novo* microdeletions in the gene region 22q11, an area particularly prone to deletions in human disease (1 in 6000 births).[81] Clinical features are described by the acronym 'CATCH 22':

Cardiac defects (conotruncal)
Abnormal facies
Thymic hypoplasia
Cleft palate
Hypocalcaemia
22q11 deletions

Hypoparathyroidism is present in about 60% of cases and may resolve during childhood.

Other syndromic hypoparathyroidism

The mitochondrial disorders Kearnes–Sayre syndrome and MELAS syndrome are associated with hypoparathyroidism.

The Sanjad–Sakati syndrome and Kenny–Caffey syndrome type 1 both involve congenital hypoparathyroidism, mental retardation, facial dysmorphism and growth failure caused by mutations in a tubulin folding protein.

Acquired parathyroid deficiency

Surgical hypoparathyroidism

Surgical trauma to the parathyroid glands is the most common cause of hypoparathyroidism. It can arise following total thyroidectomy for tumour, Graves' disease or multinodular goitre. The incidence of permanent post-operative hypoparathyroidism is quite high. Mazzaferri *et al.* reported a 13% incidence in 576 patients whilst Foster reported a lower incidence of 8% in 24 108 thyroid procedures performed.[82,83]

In patients with persistent or symptomatic hypocalcaemia, calcium supplementation should be prescribed (Sandocal, two tablets four times a day) in addition to a reducing calcitriol regime of 1 μg on the first day, 0.5 μg for the next 2 days and 0.25 μg/day thereafter. Chapter 17 outlines in further detail the management of hypocalcaemia.

Autoimmune parathyroid disease

This is the most common cause of hypoparathyroidism excluding surgical damage. It occurs as an isolated phenomenon, with antibodies against the CaSR, or as part of polyglandular autoimmune syndrome type 1 (PAS1). The latter is an autosomal recessive condition most commonly seen in Finland due to mutations in the autoimmune regulatory gene *AIRE* on chromosome 21q. Hypoparathyroidism typically presents in the first decade and is associated with adrenal insufficency which develops in the teenage years. Its clinical features are remembered by the acronym 'HAM':

Hypoparathyroidism
Adrenal insufficiency
Mucocutaneous candidiasis

These features may not all necessarily develop, and other autoimmune conditions are commonly present including hypogonadism, chronic active hepatitis, alopecia and vitiligo. Malabsorption is also frequent.[84,85]

Infiltrative parathyroid disease

Hypoparathyroidism is well recognized in haemachromatosis and Wilson's disease due to iron and copper deposition in the glands, respectively.

HIV infection is associated with markedly reduced PTH levels compared with normals, and the physiological response to induced hypocalcaemia is also reduced.

Parathyroid hormone resistance

Pseudohypoparathyroidism is a rare autosomal dominant condition first recognized by Albright in 1942. Patients have biochemical features consistent with hypoparathyroidism (i.e. hypocalcaemia and hyperphosphataemia) but the PTH levels are elevated. This represents resistance to PTH action.[86]

There are two key elements to the diagnosis. The phenotypic features, termed the Albright hereditary osteodystrophy (AHO) phenotype, consist of:

- somatic features: short stature, brachydactyly, rounded facies
- developmental delay
- heterotopic ossification.

The biochemical features include:

- hypocalcaemia with hyperphophataemia
- elevated PTH levels
- lack of renal cAMP and phosphaturic response to PTH infusion
- reduced tissue response to GHRH, TSH, LH and FSH hormones.

The underlying defect is a mutation in the *GNAS* gene, which codes for the Gs α-subunit. This subunit couples the stimulation of the PTH1 receptor to activation of adenyl cyclase in the cAMP pathway. This coupling process is critical for the cellular response to PTH. The same subunit is used in other hormone signalling pathways which can therefore also be affected. This explains the other features which may occur, such as short stature or goitre.

Several patterns of disease may be recognzed. These depend on from which parent the abnormal allele was inherited. The maternal allele is preferentially expressed in kidney, pituitary, thyroid and gonads, but not in the bone.

Type 1a disease is inherited from the mother; all tissues are affected and the patient shows the AHO phenotype with the above biochemical derangements.

Type 1b disease is also inherited from the mother, but the mutation is essentially a switch of imprinting to a paternal pattern. Thus, tissues have two 'paternal alleles'. In most tissues this is of no consequence as there is no AHO phenotype. However, in the kidneys and specific endocrine tissues there is almost no gene expression, which results in the characteristic biochemical derangements. Interestingly, bone exhibits features of HPT because the paternal alleles are active in bone.

Pseudopseudohypoparathyroidism cases inherit the abnormal gene from the father. They have the AHO phenotype but biochemistry is normal. Occasionally, only severe heterotopic ossification rather than the full AHO phenotype is seen. This is termed progressive osseous heteroplasia (POH) when it affects muscles, joints and connective tissue, or osteoma cutis when it only affects skin.

Type II pseudohypoparathyroidism is very different. Although the basic biochemistry is similar, the renal cAMP response to PTH infusion is normal, other hormone systems are not involved, there is no family history and there is no AHO phenotype. Chronic vitamin D deficiency produces a similar picture.

Calcium-sensing receptor activation

Autosomal dominant hypoparathyroidism is caused by activating mutations in the CaSR.[87] PTH secretion for any given level of serum calcium is reduced,[88] resulting in 'relative' hypoparathyroidism.

Biochemically, patients have low serum calcium with inappropriately low normal PTH levels. The presence of the CaSR in the CTAL of the kidneys means that relative hypercalciuria occurs and magnesium wasting may lead to hypomagnesaemia.

Clinically most patients are asymptomatic. Children may present during intercurrent illnesses with seizures or muscle spasms and tetany. Adults may present with recurrent kidney stones if the hypocalcaemia has been treated.[87,89]

Treatment is best avoided if possible. If it is necessary, the calcium level should just be kept high enough to prevent symptoms, and preferably this level should be within the low/normal range. This can be achieved with low doses of alfacalcidol and calcium supplements. The resulting hypercalciuria can be reduced with a thiazide diuretic. In some cases a thiazide alone succeeds in maintaining serum calcium levels.[90]

EVIDENCE APPRAISAL

In the treatment of primary hyperparathyroidism, both medical and surgical, there have been a number of single RCTs, level Ib evidence (references 16, 29, 30, 42, 43, 44, 45, 47, 48, 49). For an excellent, comprehensive survey of the literature with recommendations, one should refer to the conclusions of the Third International Workshop on the Management of Asymptomatic Hyperparathyroidism: J Clin Endocrinol Metab 94:333–381, whose findings we have summarized.

REFERENCES

1. Berridge MJ, Bootman MD, Roderick HL. Calcium signalling: dynamics, homeostasis and remodelling. Nat Rev Mol Cell Biol 2003;4:517–29.
2. Brown EM, Gamba G, Riccardi D, *et al.* Cloning and characterization of an extracellular Ca(2+)-sensing receptor from bovine parathyroid. Nature 1993;366:575–80.
3. Huang Y, Zhou Y, Castiblanco A, *et al.* Multiple Ca(2+)-binding sites in the extracellular domain of the Ca(2+)-sensing receptor corresponding to cooperative Ca(2+) response. Biochemistry 2009;48:388–98.
4. Brown EM, MacLeod RJ. Extracellular calcium sensing and extracellular calcium signaling. Physiol Rev 2001;81:239–97.
5. Thakker RV. Diseases associated with the extracellular calcium-sensing receptor. Cell Calcium 2004;35:275–82.
6. Favus MJ, Goltzman D. Regulation of calcium and magnesium. In: Rosen CJ, ed. Primer on the metabolic bone diseases and disorders of mineral metabolism, 7th edn. Washington, DC: American Society for Bone and Mineral Research, 2008:104–7.
7. Ba J, Friedman PA. Calcium-sensing receptor regulation of renal mineral ion transport. Cell Calcium 2004;35:229–37.
8. Hebert SC, Cheng S, Geibel J. Functions and roles of the extracellular Ca2+-sensing receptor in the gastrointestinal tract. Cell Calcium 2004;35:239–47.
9. Wermers RA, Khosla S, Atkinson EJ, *et al.* Incidence of primary hyperparathyroidism in Rochester, Minnesota, 1993–2001: an update on the changing epidemiology of the disease. J Bone Miner Res 2006;21:171–7.
10. Silverberg SJ, Shane E, Jacobs TP, *et al.* A 10-year prospective study of primary hyperparathyroidism with or without parathyroid surgery. N Engl J Med 1999;341:1249–55.
11. Parisien M, Silverberg SJ, Shane E, *et al.* Bone disease in primary hyperparathyroidism. Endocrinol Metab Clin North Am 1990;19:19–34.
12. Eriksen EF. Primary hyperparathyroidism: lessons from bone histomorphometry. J Bone Miner Res 2002;17 Suppl 2:N95–7.
13. Rubin MR, Bilezikian JP, McMahon DJ, *et al.* The natural history of primary hyperparathyroidism with or without parathyroid surgery after 15 years. J Clin Endocrinol Metab 2008;93:3462–70.
14. Silverberg SJ, Locker FG, Bilezikian JP. Vertebral osteopenia: a new indication for surgery in primary hyperparathyroidism. J Clin Endocrinol Metab 1996;81:4007–12.
15. Vestergaard P, Mollerup CL, Frokjaer VG, *et al.* Cohort study of risk of fracture before and after surgery for primary hyperparathyroidism. BMJ 2000;321:598–602.
16. Ambrogini E, Cetani F, Cianferotti L, *et al.* Surgery or surveillance for mild asymptomatic primary hyperparathyroidism: a prospective, randomized clinical trial. J Clin Endocrinol Metab 2007;92:3114–21.
17. Tamura Y, Araki A, Chiba Y, *et al.* Remarkable increase in lumbar spine bone mineral density and amelioration in biochemical markers of bone turnover after parathyroidectomy in elderly patients with primary hyperparathyroidism: a 5-year follow-up study. J Bone Miner Metab 2007;25: 226–31.
18. Deaconson TF, Wilson SD, Lemann J Jr. The effect of parathyroidectomy on the recurrence of nephrolithiasis. Surgery 1987;102:910–13.
19. Hedback G, Abrahamsson K, Oden A. The improvement of renal concentration capacity after surgery for primary hyperparathyroidism. Eur J Clin Invest 2001;31:1048–53.
20. Silverberg SJ, Lewiecki EM, Mosekilde L, *et al.* Presentation of asymptomatic primary hyperparathyroidism: Proceedings of the Third International Workshop. J Clin Endocrinol Metab 2009;94:351–65.
21. Stefenelli T, Mayr H, Bergler-Klein J, *et al.* Primary hyperparathyroidism: incidence of cardiac abnormalities and partial reversibility after successful parathyroidectomy. Am J Med 1993;95:197–202.
22. Palmer M, Adami HO, Bergstrom R, *et al.* Mortality after surgery for primary hyperparathyroidism: a follow-up of 441 patients operated on from 1956 to 1979. Surgery 1987;102:1–7.
23. Hedback G, Tisell LE, Bengtsson BA, *et al.* Premature death in patients operated on for primary hyperparathyroidism. World J Surg 1990;14:829–35; discussion 836.
24. Hedback G, Oden A, Tisell LE. The influence of surgery on the risk of death in patients with primary hyperparathyroidism. World J Surg 1991;15:399–405; discussion 406–7.
25. Wermers RA, Khosla S, Atkinson EJ, *et al.* Survival after the diagnosis of hyperparathyroidism: a population-based study. Am J Med 1998;104:115–22.
26. Soreide JA, van Heerden JA, Grant CS, *et al.* Survival after surgical treatment for primary hyperparathyroidism. Surgery 1997;122:1117–23.
27. Lind L, Jacobsson S, Palmer M, *et al.* Cardiovascular risk factors in primary hyperparathyroidism: a 15-year follow-up of operated and unoperated cases. J Intern Med 1991;230:29–35.

28. Coker LH, Rorie K, Cantley L, *et al.* Primary hyperparathyroidism, cognition and health related quality of life. Ann Surg 2005;242:642–8.
29. Rao DS, Philips ER, Divind GW, *et al.* Randomised controlled clinical trial of surgery versus no surgery in patients with mild PHPT. J Clin Endocrinol Metab 2004;89:5415–22.
30. Bollerslev J, Jansson S, Mollerup CL, *et al*, on behalf of the SIPH Study Group. Medical observation, compared with parathyroidectomy, for asymptomatic primary hyperparathyroidism: a prospective, randomised trial. J Clin Endocrinol Metab 2007;92:1687–92.
31. Eastell R, Arnold A, Brandi ML, *et al.* Diagnosis of asymptomatic primary hyperparathyroidism: Proceedings of the Third International Workshop. J Clin Endocrinol Metab 2009;94:340–50.
32. Marx SJ, Attie MF, Levine MA, *et al.* The hypo-calciuric or benign variant of familial hypercalcaemia. Clinical and biochemical features of fifteen families. Medicine (Baltimore) 1981;60:397–412.
33. Simonds WF, James-Newton LA, Agarwal SK, *et al.* Familial isolated hyperparathyroidism: clinical and genetic characteristics of 36 kindreds. Medicine (Baltimore) 2002;81: 1–26.
34. Brandi ML, Gagel RF, Angeli A, *et al.* Guidelines for diagnosis and therapy of MEN type 1 and type 2. J Clin Endocrinol Metab 2001;86:5658–71.
35. Simonds WF, Robbins CM, Agarwal SK, *et al.* Familial isolated hyperparathyroidism is rarely caused by germline mutations in HRPT2, the gene for the hyperparathyroidism–jaw tumour syndrome. J Clin Endocrinol Metab 2004;89:96–102.
36. Souberbielle JC, Bordou P, Cormier C. Lessons from second- and third-generation parathyroid hormone assays in primary hyperparathyroidism. J Endocrinol Invest 2008;31:463–9.
37. 1991 Proceedings of the Consensus Development Conference on the Management of Asymptomatic Primary Hyperparathyroidism. J Bone Miner Metab 1991;Suppl 2:S1–124.
38. Bilezikian JP, Potts JT, Fuleihan Gel-H, *et al.* Summary statement from a workshop on asymptomatic primary hyperparathyroidism: a perspective for the 21st century. J Bone Miner Metab 2002:17(Suppl 12):N2–11 and J Clin Endocrinol Metab 2002;87:5353–61.
39. Bilezikian JP, Khan AA, Potts JT. Guidelines for the management of asymptomatic primary hyperparathyroidism: summary statement from the Third International Workshop. J Clin Endocrinol Metab 2009;94:335–9.
40. Khan AA, Bilezikian JP, Potts JT. The diagnosis and management of asymptomatic primary hyperparathyroidism revisited. J Clin Endocrinol Metab 2009;94:333–4.
41. Khan AA, Grey A, Shoback D. Medical management of asymptomatic hyperparathyroidism: Proceedings of the Third International Workshop. J Clin Endocrinol Metab 2009; 94:373–81.
42. Peacock M, Bilezikian JP, Klassen PS, *et al.* Cinacalcet hydrochloride maintains long-term normocalcaemia in patients with primary hyperparathyroidism. J Clin Endocrinol Metab 2005;90:135–41.
43. Rossini M, Gatti D, Isaia G, *et al.* Effects of oral alendronate in elderly patients with osteoporosis and mild primary hyperparathyroidism. J Bone Miner Metab 2001;16:113–9.
44. Chow CC, Chan WB, Li JK, *et al.* Oral alendronate increases bone mineral density in post-menopausal women with primary hyperparathyroidism. J Clin Endocrinol Metab 2003;88:581–7.
45. Khan AA, Bilezikian JP, Kung AW, *et al.* Alendronate in primary hyperparathyroidism: a double blind, randomised, placebo controlled trial. J Clin Endocrinol Metab 2004;89:3319–5.
46. Selby PL, Peacock M. Ethinyl estradiol and norethindrone in the treatment of primary hyperparathyroidism in postmenopausal women. N Engl J Med 1986;314:1481–5.
47. Grey AB, Stapleton JP, Evans MC, *et al.* Effect of hormone replacement therapy on bone mineral density in postmenopausal women with mild primary hyperparathyroidism. A randomised controlled trial. Ann Intern Med 1996; 125:360–8.
48. Orr-Walker BJ, Evans MC, Clearwater JM, *et al.* Effects of hormone replacement therapy on bone mineral density in postmenopausal women with primary hyperparathyroidism: four year follow-up and comparison with healthy postmenopausal women. Arch Intern Med 2000;160: 2161–6.
49. Rubin MR, Lee KH, McMahon DJ, *et al.* Raloxifene lowers serum calcium and markers of bone turnover in postmenopausal women with primary hyperparathyroidism. J Clin Endocrinol Metab 2003;88:1174–8.
50. Law WM, Heath H. Familial benign hypercalcaemia (hypocalciuric hypercalcaemia). Clinical and pathogenetic study of 21 families. Ann Intern Med 1985;102:511–9.
51. Carling T, Szabo E, Bai M, *et al.* Familial hypercalcaemia and hypercalciuria caused by a novel mutation in the cytoplasmic tail of the calcium receptor. J Clin Endocrinol Metab 2000;85:2042–7.
52. Marx SJ. Molecular genetics of multiple endocrine neoplasia types 1 and 2. Nat Rev Cancer 2005;5:367–75.
53. Trump D, Farren B, Wooding C, *et al.* Clinical studies of multiple endocrine neoplasia type 1 (MEN1). QJM 1996; 89:653–69.
54. Pannett AAJ, Kennedy AM, Turner JJO, *et al.* Multiple endocrine neoplasia type 1 (MEN1) germline mutations in familial isolated primary hyperparathyroidism. Clin Endocrinol (Oxf) 2003;58:639–46.
55. Ellard S, Hattersley AT, Brewer CM, *et al.* Detection of an MEN1 gene mutation depends on clinical features and supports current referral criteria for diagnostic molecular genetic testing. Clin Endocrinol (Oxf) 2005;62:169–75.
56. Marx SJ, Simonds WF, Agarwal SK, *et al.* Hyperparathyroidism in hereditary syndromes: special expressions and

special managements. J Bone Miner Metab 2002;17:S1: N37–43.
57. Machens A, Niccoli-Sire P, Hoegel J, *et al.*, for the European Multiple Endocrine Neoplasia (EUROMEN) Study Group. Early malignant progression of hereditary thyroid cancer. N Engl J Med 2003;349:1517–25.
58. Raue F, Kraimps JL, Dralle H, *et al.* Primary hyperparathyroidism in multiple endocrine neoplasia type 2A. J Intern Med 1995;238:369–73.
59. O'Riordain DS, O'Brien T, Grant CS, *et al.* Surgical management of primary hyperparathyroidism in multiple endocrine neoplasia types 1 and 2. Surgery 1993;114:1031–7.
60. Carpten JD, Robbins CM, Villablanca A, *et al.* HRPT2, encoding parafibromin, is mutated in HPT–jaw tumour syndrome. Nat Genet 2002;32:676–80.
61. Chen JD, Morrison C, Zhang C, *et al.* Hyperparathyroidism–jaw tumour syndrome. J Intern Med 2003;253: 634–42.
62. Shattuck TM, Valimaki S, Obara T, *et al.* Somatic and germline mutations of the HRPT2 gene in sporadic parathyroid carcinoma. N Engl J Med 2003;349:1722–9.
63. Huang S-M, Duh Q-Y, Shaver J, *et al.* Familial hyperparathyroidism without multiple endocrine neoplasia. World J Surg 1997;21:22–9.
64. Moe S, Drueke T, Cunningham J, *et al.* Definition, evaluation and classification of renal osteodystrophy: a position statement from Kidney Disease: Improving Global Outcomes (KDIGO). Kidney Int 2006;69:1945–53.
65. Hruska KA, Mathew S. Chronic kidney disease mineral bone disorder (CKD-MBD). In: Rosen CJ, ed. Primer on the metabolic bone diseases and disorders of mineral metabolism. Washington, DC: American Society for Bone and Mineral Research, 2008:343–9.
66. Levin A, Bakris GL, Molitch M, *et al.* Prevalence of abnormal serum vitamin D, PTH, calcium, and phosphorus in patients with chronic kidney disease: results of the study to evaluate early kidney disease. Kidney Int 2006;71:31–8.
67. Eknoyan G, Levin A, Levin NW. K/DOQI clinical practice guidelines on bone metabolism and disease in chronic kidney disease. Am J Kidney Dis 2003;42:S12–28; S52–7.
68. Delmez JA, Slatopolsky E. Hyperphosphatemia: its consequences and treatment in patients with chronic renal disease. Am J Kidney Dis 1992;19:303–17.
69. Chertow GM, Burke SK, Raggi P. Sevelamer attenuates the progression of coronary and aortic calcification in hemodialysis patients. Kidney Int 2002;62:245–52.
70. Block GA, Spiegel DM, Ehrlich J, *et al.* Effects of sevelamer and calcium on coronary artery calcification in patients new to hemodialysis. Kidney Int 2005;68:1815–24.
71. Tonelli M. Vitamin D in patients with chronic kidney disease: nothing new under the sun. Ann Intern Med 2007;147:880.
72. Moe SM, Chertow GM, Coburn JW, *et al.* Achieving NKF-K/DOQI bone metabolism and disease treatment goals with cinacalcet HCl. Kidney Int 2005;67:760–71.
73. Malberti F, Marcelli D, Conte F, *et al.* Parathyroidectomy in patients on renal replacement therapy: an epidemiologic study. J Am Soc Nephrol 2001;12:1242–8.
74. Tominaga Y, Tanaka Y, Sato K, *et al.* Histopathology, pathophysiology, and indications for surgical treatment of renal hyperparathyroidism. Semin Surg Oncol 1997;13: 78–86.
75. Gagne ER, Urena P, Leite-Silva S, *et al.* Short- and long-term efficacy of total parathyroidectomy with immediate autografting compared with subtotal parathyroidectomy in hemodialysis patients. J Am Soc Nephrol 1992;3: 1008–17.
76. Tominaga Y, Tanaka Y, Sato K, *et al.* Recurrent renal hyperparathyroidism and DNA analysis of autografted parathyroid tissue. World J Surg 1992;16:595–602; discussion 602–3.
77. Arnold A, Horst SA, Gardella TJ, *et al.* Mutation of the signal peptide-encoding region of the preproparathyroid hormone gene in familial isolated hypoparathyroidism. J Clin Invest 1990;86:1084–1087.
78. Parkinson DB, Thakker RV. A donor splice site mutation in the parathyroid hormone gene is associated with autosomal recessive hypoparathyroidism. Nat Genet 1992;1:149–52.
79. Ding C, Buckingham B, Levine MA. Familial isolated hypoparathyroidism caused by a mutation in the gene for the transcription factor GCMB. J Clin Invest 2001;108: 1215–20.
80. Bowl MR, Nesbit MA, Harding B, *et al.* An interstitial deletion–insertion involving chromosomes 2p25.3 and Xq27.1, near SOX3, causes X-linked recessive hypoparathyroidism. J Clin Invest 2005;115:2822–31.
81. Ryan AK, Goodship JA, Wilson DI, *et al.* Spectrum of clinical features associated with interstitial chromosome 22q11 deletions: a European collaborative study. J Med Genet 1997;34:798–804.
82. Mazzaferri EL, Young RL. Papillary thyroid carcinoma: a 10 year follow-up report on the impact of treatment in 576 patients. Am J Med 1981;70:511.
83. Foster RS Jr. Morbidity and mortality after thyroidectomy. Surg Gynecol Obstet 1978;146:423–9.
84. Eisenbarth GS, Gottlieb PA. Autoimmune polyendocrine syndromes. N Engl J Med 2004;350:2068–79.
85. Betterle C, Greggio NA, Volpato M. Clinical review 93. Autoimmune polyglandular syndrome type 1. J Clin Endocrinol Metab 1998;83:1049–55.
86. Bastepe M. The GNAS locus and pseudohypoparathyroidism. Adv Exp Med Biol 2008; 626:27–40.
87. Pearce SH, Williamson C, Kifor O, *et al.* A familial syndrome of hypocalcemia with hypercalciuria due to mutations in the calcium-sensing receptor. N Engl J Med 1996;335:1115–22.
88. Pearce SH, Bai M, Quinn SJ, *et al.* Functional characterization of calcium-sensing receptor mutations expressed in human embryonic kidney cells. J Clin Invest 1996; 98: 1860–6.

89. Brown EM. Clinical lessons from the calcium-sensing receptor. Nat Clin Pract Endocrinol Metab 2007;3:122–133.
90. Sato K, Hasegawa Y, Nakae J, *et al.* Hydrochlorothiazide effectively reduces urinary calcium excretion in two Japanese patients with gain-of-function mutations of the calcium-sensing receptor gene. J Clin Endocrinol Metab 2002;87:3068–73.

MULTIPLE CHOICE QUESTIONS

Select the single most appropriate option.

1. The normal serum calcium range is:
A. 1.5–2.2 mmol/l
B. 2.1–2.5 mmol/l
C. 2.3–3.3 mmol/l
D. 2.6–3.6 mmol/l

2. Parathyroid hormone acts mainly on
A. Bone and kidney
B. Bone, kidney and gut
C. Bone, kidney and liver
D. Bone and liver

3. Primary hyperparathyroidism occurs in
A. 1% of the population
B. 0.1% of the population
C. 4% of the population
D. 0.01% of the population

4. Vitamin D is hydroxylated to form its **active** metabolite in
A. Liver
B. Kidney
C. Parathyroid gland
D. Small intestine

5. Primary hyperparathyroidism commonly presents with
A. Renal stones
B. Chance finding of decreased phosphate level on routine screening
C. Low 24 hour urinary calcium levels
D. Metastatic calcification

Answers

1. B
2. B
3. A
4. B
5. B

14 Investigations

Brendan C. Stack[1] **& Gregory Randolph**[2]

[1] Department of Otolaryngology-HNS, University of Arkansas for Medical Sciences, Little Rock, AR, USA
[2] Division of Thyroid and Parathyroid Surgery, Department of Laryngology and Otology, Harvard Medical School, Massachusetts Eye and Ear Infirmary, Boston, MA, USA

KEY POINTS

- Biochemical tests are required to confirm a diagnosis of hyperparathyroidism. Essential investigations include serum calcium, parathyroid hormone (PTH, 25 OH vitamin D) and 24 hour urinary calcium
- The vast majority of primary hyperparathyroidism is due to single gland disease
- Pre-operative localization is mandatory when surgery involves a directed, single gland approach.
- Sestamibi is the most sensitive and specific single test for localizing parathyroid adenoma. False negatives are more likely to occur with small glands (<100 g), parathyroid hyperplasia and with multigland disease
- Ultrasound augmented by fine needle aspiration and PTH assay can lead to a specificity approaching 100%

INTRODUCTION

Primary hyperparathyroidism (PHPT) affects approximately 1 in 500 women and 1 in 2000 men per year and usually presents in the fifth to seventh decades.[1–3] PHPT is a biochemical diagnosis which is sometimes made in symptomatic individuals presenting with the hypercalcaemic sequelae outlined in Chapter 13. However, the advent of 'routine' serum biochemistry (as part of surveillance and preventative medicine) has resulted in PHPT becoming an increasingly common diagnosis in otherwise healthy, asymptomatic adults.

Up to 97% of PHPT results from single-adenoma disease, with the remaining cases due to four-gland hyperplasia (up to 10%), multiple adenomas (<3%) and carcinoma (<1%).[4,5] The primary role of pre-operative investigations in PHPT is to establish the biochemical diagnosis and locate the abnormal gland(s). Surgical management typically leads to resolution of the hypercalcaemic state, marked improvement in symptoms and disease regression.[6]

BIOCHEMICAL TESTS

Parathyroid hormone (PTH) assay

PHPT is characterized by hypercalcaemia secondary to raised PTH levels. Typically, the diagnosis is made in the ambulatory setting with matched samples which demonstrate hyperparathormonaemia (as defined by the local laboratory) and hypercalcaemia (either total or ionized). Occasionally the calcium level fails to reach the high cut-off but is nevertheless inappropriately elevated in relation to the corresponding elevated PTH level (eucalcaemic hyperparathyroidism). It is well recognized that calcium levels fluctuate in PHPT and that parathyroid autonomy occurs, resulting in a high PTH with normal or high normal calcium. Twenty-four hour urinary calcium differentiates PHPT from benign familial hypercalcaemic hypocaliuria (BFHH), a level >100 mg being diagnostic for PHPT. Checking the 25-hydroxy vitamin D level is important when there is co-existing vitamin D deficiency (see Chapter 13).

The current 'gold standard' for PTH measurement is the second-generation intact PTH assay. This quantifies circulating PTH by using two separate poly monoclonal antibodies which identify antigenic sites on the PTH molecule (1–34 and either 39–84 or 44–84) in a chemiluminescent reaction. It is widely available, well validated and provides a more reliable measurement than first-generation tests. The latter also utilized antibody reactions to measure different ends or the mid region of the PTH molecule. However, PTH degradation resulted in hormone fragments being cleared from the systemic circulation at different rates and therefore inconsistent results. There have also been some concerns about the reliability of the intact assay because it measures circulating N-terminal truncations which exist as degraded PTH in renal failure patients (see Chapter 13). This problem

A Practical Manual of Thyroid and Parathyroid Disease, 1st Edition.
Edited by Asit Arora, Neil Tolley & R. Michael Tuttle.

is overcome by the latest generation 'whole PTH' assay although it is not yet widely available.[7]

Intra-operative PTH assay

The desire for accurate PTH measurement includes 'real-time' intra-operative PTH assay. This is becoming increasingly available and is used to identify the abnormal gland(s) and confirm successful surgical management. It usually takes upto 20–30 minutes, which includes the time for phlebotomy, specimen transport, serum separation, the actual test (12 minutes for incubation with antibodies, the chemiluminescent reaction and a measurement reading) and communication of results to the operating surgeon.[8]

PRE-OPERATIVE VISUALIZATION TECHNIQUES

Pre-operative localization has been the 'holy grail' of parathyroid surgery since the late 19th century.[9] There has not been a practical, reliable imaging modality available until the last two decades. Prior to this time patients underwent non-directed bilateral neck exploration for treatment of their hyperparathyroidism. In recent years there been a proliferation of accessible, reliable and cost-effective modalities to localize the diseased parathyroid gland(s). Sometimes these imaging modalities are performed in the operating room to assist with the identification of abnormal gland(s) prior to excision. The pre-operative ability to localize disease provides the surgeon with an answer to the question 'where should I start?' Intra-operative PTH analysis provides an answer to the question 'can I stop?' and a combination of both modalities allows successful uniglandular parathyroid surgery to be performed.

Although biochemical tests are required to diagnose hyperparathyroidism, imaging tests are useful to confirm the diagnosis. Whenever minimal access surgery treatment is proposed, pre-operative imaging localization is essential and usually the responsibility of the operating surgeon. Failure to localize an adenoma should not deter the physican from making a surgical referral as imaging techniques are liable to false negatives. Pre-operative imaging helps the surgeon to decide the most appropriate surgical approach. It does not determine surgical candidacy.

Nuclear medicine

Nuclear medicine techniques have evolved considerably over the last 70 years. It represents the mainstay of parathyroid imaging, although with the recent proliferation in out-patient ultrasound, this may change.

The ideal modality for pre-operative parathyroid localization should be both sensitive and specific. The accuracy of a test is influenced by:

- Patient factors: cooperation, specimen size, body habitus, positioning
- Physiological factors: radioactive tracer uptake, washout characteristics, mitochondrial content
- Dosimetry: what dose produces the best image
- Imaging technique: camera position, collimator shape, timing of images, image reading skill and post-capture image processing (computed image production).

Radioactive tracers

In the early 1960s several tracer agents were available including Co-57-cyanocobalamine and Se-75-selenomethionine.[10,11] Uptake of these tracers was suboptimal, resulting in poor image quality. In the late 1970s, thallium-201 was incidentally discovered to demonstrate parathyroid adenoma uptake.[11] Thallium-201 parathyroid avidity was targeted using a subtraction technique[12] which reliably localized adenomas >500 mg (at least 10 times the normal size by weight). However, thallium-201 is not an ideal agent because the energy of its radiation is suboptimal and it is associated with a relatively high radiation exposure for the patient.[13]

Technetium-99-sestamibi was discovered to have persistent uptake in both thyroid and parathyroid tissue during myocardial perfusion studies.[14,15] In contrast to precursor radiotracers such as thallium-201, the washout time from parathyroid tissue is longer than from the thyroid gland. This is due to prolonged retention in the richer mitochondrial tissue of parathyroid adenoma/hyperplasia.[16,17] The time differential has been exploited to good effect for parathyroid evaluation. It has a sensitivity reaching 80% (range 50–90%) on planar studies[4,5,18,19] (see Fig. 14.1). The wide range in sensitivity probably reflects interinstitutional variation in imaging technique as well as patient factors.

Sestamibi identifies adenomas ranging from 64 mg to >8000 mg.[20] False-negative results are attributed to small glands (<100 mg), parathyroid hyperplasia (poor tracer uptake), adenomatous features (high concentration of clear cells) and the presence of the multidrug resistance gene.[5,21–26] Technique is also a significant contributor to false-negative results. False-positive findings commonly occur when there is co-existing thyroid pathology.[27] Dual-isotope studies with sestamibi and low-dose Tc-99m-pertechnicate or iodine-123 are reported to improve sensitivity.[18,28,29]

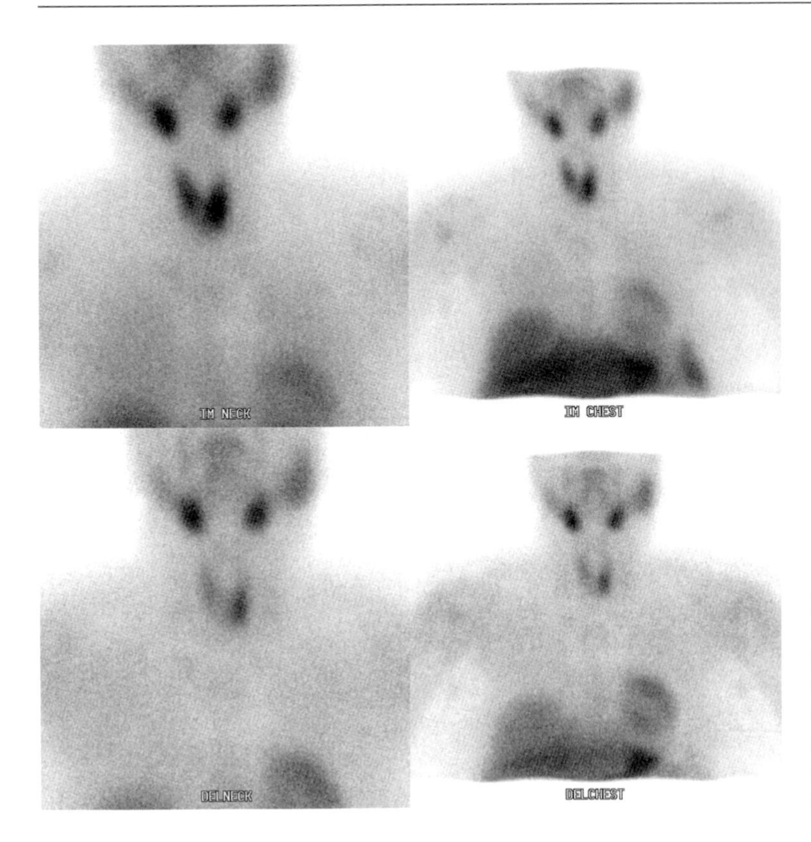

Fig. 14.1 Sestamibi. Four images in clockwise fashion starting from top left: immediate neck view, immediate chest view, 2 hour chest view and 2 hour neck view. This demonstrates the classic appearance of a left inferior parathyroid adenoma which is highly suggestive on the immediate view.

Tc-99m-tetrofosmin is another myocardial perfusion agent which exhibits avid parathyroid uptake, although it tends to clear the parathyroids faster than sestamibi.[30,31] Gallowitsch *et al.*[30] and Ishibashi *et al.*[32] reported a sensitivity comparable with sestamibi. Ishibashi *et al.* achieved 100% sensitivity and specificity with sestamibi and tetrofosmin for detecting adenoma and similar results for hyperplasia. Gallowitsch *et al.*, using less tetrofosmin (10 mCi versus 24 mCi), reported a clearance from parathyroid tissue similar to sestamibi on early images. Delayed studies, several hours after administration, showed greater washout, thereby decreasing its sensitivity to 62%. The use of single photoemission computed tomography (SPECT) with tetrofosmin improves sensitivity for parathyroid adenoma to 94% with a specificity of 85%. Detection of parathyroid adenomas has also been successfully accomplished using lower doses of isotope (5 mCi) administered a short time (1 hour) prior to parathyroidectomy.[33]

Nuclear imaging techniques

Functional imaging requires a radioactive source and camera. More advanced imaging techniques involve multiple camera positions and computer image compilation. A gamma camera consists of a collimator (lens equivalent), a layer of sodium iodide (NaI) crystals positioned under photomultiplier tubes (film equivalent), a position computer and an output monitor/recording device (display). Random X-rays or γ-rays filter through the collimator and strike the NaI crystals, causing a release of photon energy. Photons, captured in the photomultiplier tubes, displace electrons which in turn convey a signal to a position computer, thereby relaying information to the output device.[34]

The collimator acts as an attenuation plate which only allows correctly positioned radioactive waves to contact the NaI crystals and produce an image (similar to a polarizing lens). Four fundamental collimators exist for the gamma camera: parallel, pinhole, converging and diverging. The pinhole collimator is most commonly used for parathyroid imaging. It collects radiation from a small source and then inverts and magnifies the 'image' like a pinhole camera. It can be positioned to collect oblique and antero-posterior views, which improve the accuracy of localization.[35–37] The Norman technique (described below) achieves high localization accuracy using parallel collimation.[38]

Early imaging typically occurs 5–15 minutes following administration of the radiotracer. Late imaging occurs 2–3 hours after injection, allowing adequate time for thyroid wash-out to occur. This dual-phase technique has also proven useful with Tc-99m-tetrofosmin tracer.[32] Several studies suggest that early imaging is more accurate than late imaging as the latter is subject to unpredictable wash-out from the parathyroid glands.[19,32,36] The Norman technique corroborates this finding.[36] The technique reliably localizes parathyroid adenoma in patients undergoing radio-guided minimally invasive surgery, which is useful when previous attempts at localization are unsuccessful. Several factors make the technique successful: (1) the patient is placed in the standard parathyroid operative position (neck extended with a shoulder roll); (2) the gamma camera is placed as close as possible to the patient; (3) parallel collimation is used; (4) left and right oblique anterior views are captured by moving the camera 31° from the midline (not by turning the patient's head); (5) 20 mCi intravenous sestamibi is administered; and (6) early images are captured at 5–10 minutes. Late images are acquired after 2.5 hours, although they are seldom used.

SPECT increases sestamibi sensitivity (Plate 14.1). In contrast to traditional planar imaging which uses a fixed position gamma camera, SPECT uses a mobile camera to collect images at multiple angles around the patient. The multiple images are then compiled by a computer and displayed as a 3D image (similar to positron emission tomography (PET) scan images). Sfakianakis *et al.*[39] reported high sensitivity with SPECT, although comparison with planar imaging was not mentioned. Moka *et al.*[40] reported 87–95% sensitivity with subtraction sestamibi/SPECT and 3D image rendering. Increasing size of the adenoma positively correlated with successful localization. Slater and Gleeson[41] found an increase in sensitivity from 62 to 73% using SPECT compared with low-dose (16 mCi) planar sestamibi. SPECT is also reported to improve sensitivity for ectopic lesions.[42,43] Gayed *et al.*[44] found that SPECT/CT added no clinical benefit to using SPECT alone. Some authorities feel that SPECT represents an unnecessary cost which does not justify the small sensitivity gain particularly when planar films are performed correctly.[5,33,38,45] In view of the variability of technique reported with planar sestamibi imaging, SPECT may prove a useful adjunct for parathyroid localization across institutions. Continued incremental improvement in imaging accuracy will invariably lead to improved minimally invasive parathyroid techniques.

Ultrasound

High-resolution ultrasound (US) allows anatomical evaluation of parathyroid glands (Plate 14.2). Normal parathyroid glands are not detected by any imaging modality due to their small size. However, when there is biochemical evidence of hyperparathyroidism, high-frequency US can often localize the abnormal parathyroid gland.

Ultrasound technique

The patient is positioned with the neck hyperextended using a bolster between the shoulders. A high-frequency probe (8–12 MHz) is used to search the likely parathyroid locations carefully within the thyroid bed and paratracheal tissues. The superior gland is usually found posterior to the middle third of the thyroid gland. The inferior gland usually lies near the inferior tip of the thyroid. True supernumerary glands occur in 5% of cases.[46] One to 3% of glands are found in ectopic locations such as within the thyroid parenchyma (<1%), the carotid sheath and the mediastinum. Maximum neck rotation away from the side being examined and asking the patient to swallow sometimes facilitates visualization of an enlarged gland.[47] Intrathyroidal adenomas are usually hypoechoic. They are reliably differentiated from thyroid nodules by fine needle aspiration (FNA) and the aspirate may also require PTH measurement. For high resolution, a 10 MHz (or higher) transducer probe is recommended.[48] Obese patients are more challenging to image. Although a 5 MHz transducer provides reasonable penetration in these patients, higher transducer frequency improves image resolution and sensitivity of the examination.[49,50]

A typical parathyroid adenoma appears as an oval mass with homogenous texture and low echogenicity. Hypoechogenicity is due to the uniform hypercellularity which is a feature of most adenomas due to their solid nature (although some may be cystic).[46] A more elongated and tubular appearance is also occasionally seen.[51] Colour flow Doppler may reveal a peripheral vascular arc around a portion of the gland. Patients with primary parathyroid hyperplasia may not have enlarged glands or one gland may be larger, leading to this being mistaken for an adenoma. The sensitivity of US in hyperplasia is <50%.[52] In patients with four-gland hyperplasia secondary to renal failure all four glands may be enlarged and similar in size.[52] False-positive US findings are caused by thyroid nodules, lymph nodes, oesophagus, longus coli muscle and perithyroidal veins.[46] Distinguishing between a posterior thyroid nodule and parathyroid gland can be challenging. Meilstrup[51] advocates the identification of a separating tissue plane to assist with the process. According to Hopkins and Reading,[49] false-negative findings are related to three factors: (1) small adenoma size; (2) thyroid pathology which obscures adequate visualization; and (3) ectopic location (adequate view obscured by the depth of the chest wall). Sonographer skill and diligence play an important role in successful localization.[53] In most instances, adjusting the transducer position provides additional clues to the identity of anatomical structures. When localization remains in doubt, US-guided FNA may be useful.[51,54] Parathyroid aspirates tested for PTH provide additional diagnostic confirmation.[7,54,55] In our experience, this does not compromise subsequent exploration.

Ultrasound utility

Low cost, high availability, frontline provider reimbursement (in the USA) and ease of examination have driven the utility of pre-operative US localization. It is the least expensive parathyroid localizing study.[50,56] Unfortunately, the inherent variability of US leads to a very wide range of sensitivity (27–95%).[5,32,50,53,57–59] Differences in sonographer skill and static versus dynamic image interpretation are chiefly responsible. Retro-oesophageal, retro-tracheal and mediastinal adenomas can all produce false-negative results.[52,57] Nuclear medicine studies used in addition to US increase the likelihood of successful localization.[53,59,60]

US augmented by FNA and PTH assay results in a specificity approaching 100%.[61,62] US offers the additional benefit of permitting surveillance for synchronous thyroid disease including thyroid cancer, which may occur in 6% of patients presenting with PHPT.[63]

US-guided parathyroid ablation is a treatment option for patients who refuse surgery or who are poor surgical candidates due to extensive co-morbidity. The technique, described by Lewis,[55] involves US-guided fine needle injection of pure ethanol into the adenoma. The needle is re-sited and the injection repeated until the entire adenoma is hypoechoic and there is a drop in serum PTH and calcium levels. Recurrence of hypercalcaemia is common and necessitates further treatment. The major risk of the procedure is recurrent laryngeal nerve dysfunction (temporary or permanent) due to alcohol diffusion. There is a 15% rate of temporary dysphonia and a 1% rate of permanent dysphonia.[64] This compares with 8–10% temporary dysphonia and 0–4% permanent dysphonia rates associated with traditional neck exploration.[65,66] The dysphonia rate following minimally invasive and unilateral surgery is considerably less: 0.04–1%.[67,68] US-guided laser ablation has been proposed as an alternative to ethanol injection.[69]

Other imaging techniques

Various other modalities have been used to localize parathyroid adenoma and hyperplasia. However, their consistently lower sensitivity and specificity compared with sestamibi and US and their higher cost relegate such techniques to second-line investigations. They are reserved for failed localization attempts with sestamibi, US and surgery. Each of the following techniques as well as those previously discussed may be used sequentially to provide complementary information when evaluating ectopic adenoma or in revision surgery.[70]

Computed tomography

Computed tomography (CT) may isolate large adenomas or larger hyperplastic glands[8,71] (Fig. 14.2). However, CT exposes the patient to ionizing radiation and is limited by patient swallowing and shoulder artefact.[71] Sensitivity ranges from 46 to 87% for parathyroid adenoma and it is particularly useful for ectopic gland localization.[71] CT has an increased sensitivity when combined with SPECT[44,72–74] or PET.[75]

Magnetic resonance imaging

Magnetic resonance imaging (MRI) can also be useful for parathyroid imaging. Its sensitivity for localizing parathyroid adenoma ranges from 65 to 92% for primary

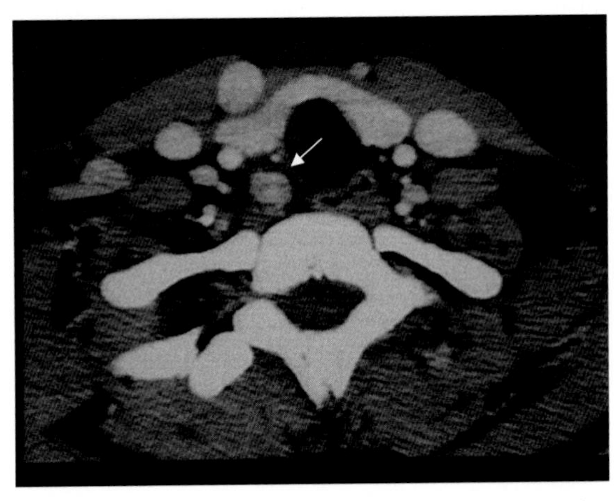

Fig. 14.2 CT. An abnormal right parathyroid gland localized by CT with contrast. http://www.med.univ-rennes1.fr/cerf/iconocerf/R/Dossier_MEDI-003685-R_0025.html

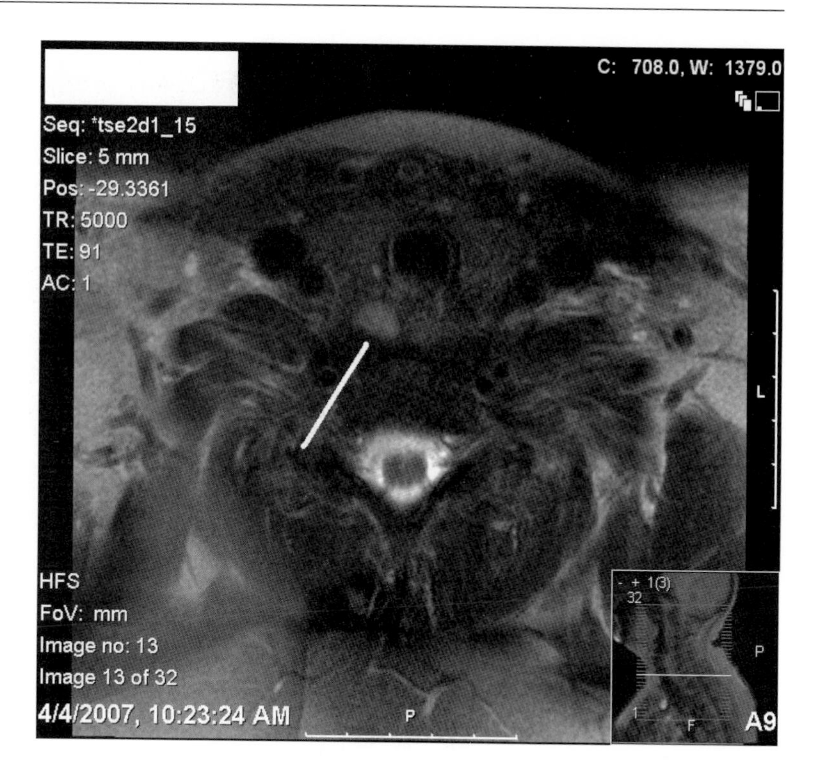

Fig.14.3 MRI. T2 axial, fat-suppressed MRI scan demonstrating a posterior, right-sided parathyroid adenoma between the right carotid sheath and the oesophagus.

cases.[71,76] This figure is lower in patients requiring re-operation due to failed parathyroid surgery, recurrent hyperparathyroidism or hyperparathyroidism after previous unrelated neck surgery.[77] Hyperfunctioning parathyroids appear iso-intense on low signal intensity T1-weighted images and demonstrate high signal intensity on T2-weighted images (Fig. 14.3). They demonstrate intense enhancement following intravenous gadolinium administration. T1 signal intensity may match T2 intensity in cystic or haemorrhagic lesions. Lower signal intensity may be seen on both T1 and T2 images in fibrotic or degenerative lesions.[71] Limitations of MRI include cost, patient claustrophobia and examination duration.[71]

Positron emission tomography

PET has not been extensively used for parathyroid localization to date (Fig. 14.4). Both fluorodeoxyglucose (FDG) and [^{11}C]methionine PET have demonstrated fairly high sensitivity and specificity for parathyroid localization.[78–81] [^{11}C]Methionine PET appears to be more sensitive than standard sestamibi or US for detecting hyperplastic disease.[82] As costs decrease and the availability of nucleotides and scanners improve, the use of PET (alone or in combination with CT) is likely to increase. This modality promises to improve preoperative parathyroid localization, and FDG uptake may be exploited to assist intra-operative detection of parathyroid adenoma.

Interventional radiology techniques

Historically, venous sampling was often utilized as a localizing modality.[83] Venous sampling requires femoral venipuncture and canalization of peri-thyroidal veins under fluoroscopic guidance. Sampled blood is analysed for PTH levels which are then compared with other sampled sites to determine which side of the neck the adenoma is located (Fig. 14.5). It is time intensive, costly and invasive, and its sensitivity for localization falls into the range of other localizing modalities (39–93%). It is useful in patients who have previously had multiple neck explorations although results are sometimes ambiguous.[84–86] A successful result is highly dependent on the experience of the radiologist performing the technique. It should therefore only be carried out in a centre with extensive experience.

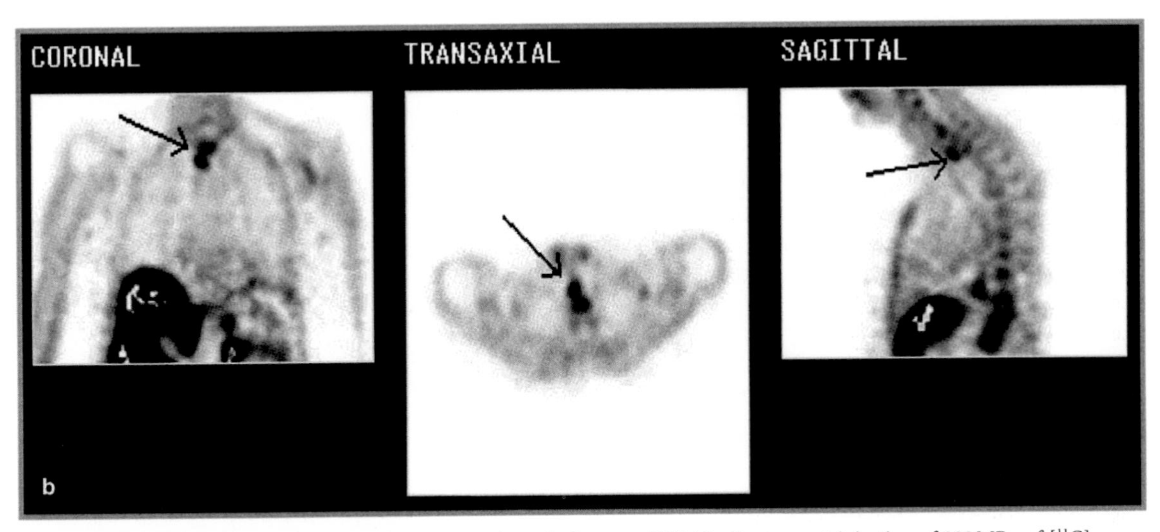

Fig. 14.4 PET. Recurrent primary HPT with retro-oesophageal adenoma. PET 10 minutes post-injection of 900 MBq of [^{11}C] methionine revealed focal tracer accumulation (arrows) suggestive of adenomatous parathyroid tissue.

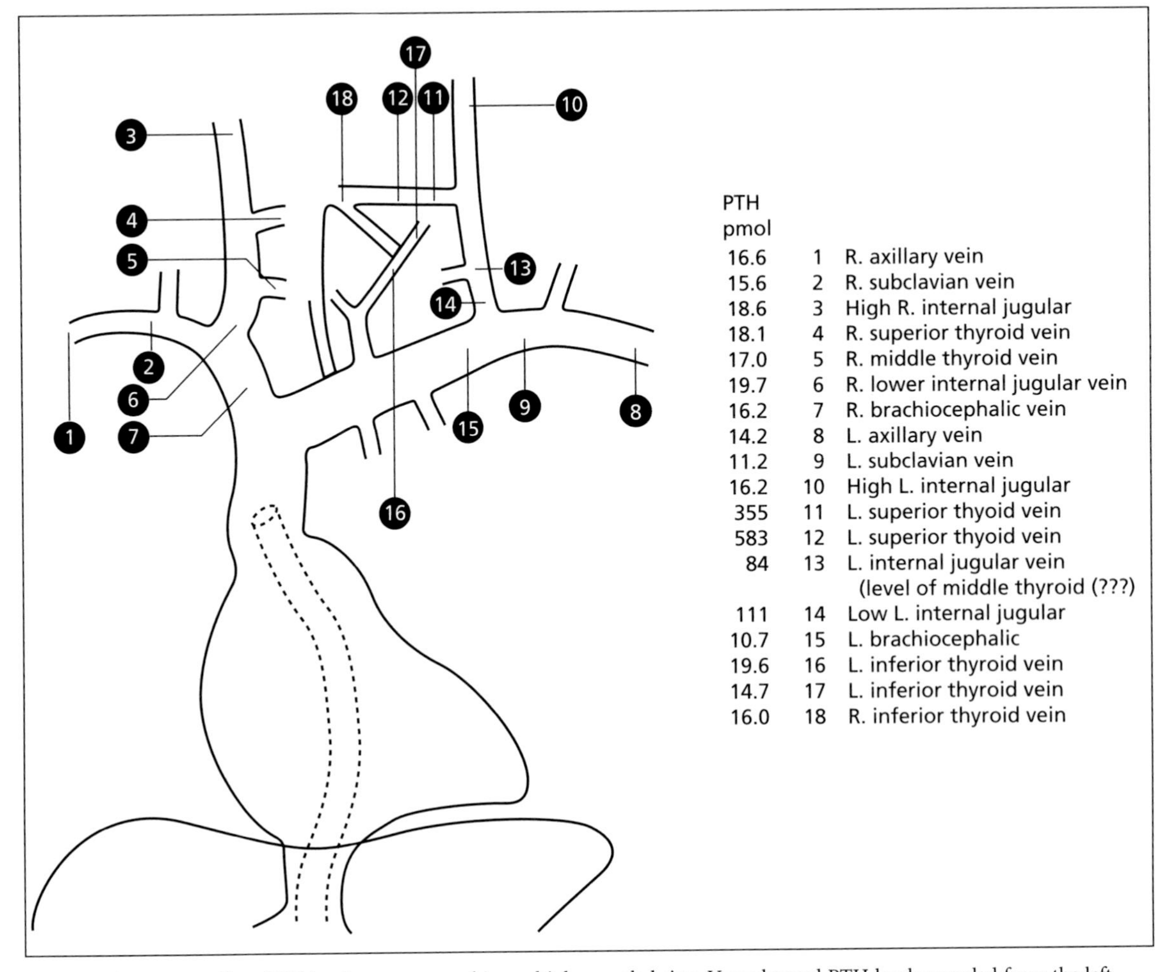

Fig. 14.5 Venous sampling. PTH levels are compared in multiple sampled sites. Very elevated PTH levels sampled from the left superior thyroid vein suggest the location of abnormal hyperfunctioning parathyroid tissue prior to re-exploration.

EVIDENCE APPRAISAL

This review chapter, by definition, should be considered Level V evidence because it is a reflection of author opinion. There are 86 referenced works in this chapter; 76/86 citations (85%) represent a low level of evidence (Oxford Centre Evidence Based Medicine Levels IV and V). We wish to highlight the following citations because they represent a higher level of evidence:

Level I: two citations[4,5] (3%)

Level II: three citations[18,31,85] (3%)

Level III: seven citations[16,21,24,29,33,41,44] (9%)

Articles such as these should be sought, whenever possible, when conducting a critical assessment of the literature. There is an obvious need for production of higher levels of evidence-based medicine articles for the diagnosis and management of hyperparathyroidism.

REFERENCES

1. Delbridge LW, Younes NA, Guinea AL, *et al.* Surgery for primary hyperparathyroidism 1962–1996: indications and outcomes. Med J Aust 1998;168:153–6.
2. Moore FD Jr, Manting F, Tanasijevic M. Intrinsic limitations to unilateral parathyroid exploration. Ann Surg 1999;230:382–8.
3. Summers GW. Parathyroid update: a review of 220 cases. Ear Nose Throat J 1996;75:434–9.
4. Denham DW, Norman J. Cost-effectiveness of preoperative sestamibi scan for primary hyperparathyroidism is dependent solely upon the surgeon's choice of operative procedure. J Am Coll Surg 1998;186:293–305.
5. Ruda JM, Hollenbeak CS, Stack BC Jr. A systematic review of the diagnosis and treatment of primary hyperparathyroidism from 1995 to 2003. Otolaryngol Head Neck Surg 2005;132:359–72.
6. Parikshak M, Castillo ED, Conrad MF, *et al.* Impact of hypercalcemia and parathyroid hormone level on the sensitivity of preoperative sestamibi scanning for primary hyperparathyroidism. Am Surg 2003;69:393–8.
7. Hortin GL, Carter AB; College of American Pathologists Point-of-Care Testing Resource Committee. Intraoperative parathyroid hormone testing: survey of testing program characterisitics. Arch Pathol Lab Med 2002;126:1045–9.
8. Gross ND, Weissman JL, Choen JI. The diagnostic utility of computed tomography for preoperative localization in surgery for hyperparathyroidism. Laryngoscope 2004;2: 227–31.
9. Hackett DA, Kauffman GL. Historical percpective of parathyroid disease. Otolaryngol Clin North Am 2004;37: 689–700.
10. Potchen EJ. Parathyroid imaging—current status and future prospects. J Nucl Med 1992;33:1807–9.
11. Price D, Okerlund MD. Parathyroid gland. In: Early PJ, Sodee DB, eds. Principles and practice of nuclear medicine, 2nd edn. St Louis: Mosby, 1995:641–51.
12. Ferlin G, Conte N, Borsato N, *et al.* Parathyroid scintigraphy with 131Cs and 201Tl. J Nucl Med Allied Sci 1981;25: 119–23.
13. Geatti O, Shapiro B, Orsolon PG, *et al.* Localization of parathyroid enlargement: experience with technetium-99m methoxyisobutylisonitrile and thallium-201 scintigraphy, ultrasonography and computed tomography. Eur J Nucl Med 1994;21:17–22.
14. Coakley AJ, Kettle AG, Wells CP, *et al.* 99Tcm sestamibi—a new agent for parathyroid imaging. Nucl Med Commun 1989;10:791–4.
15. O'Doherty MJ, Kettle AG, Wells P, *et al.* Parathyroid imaging with technetium-99m-sestamibi: preoperative localization and tissue uptake studies. J Nucl Med 1992;33: 313–8.
16. Chiu ML, Kronauge JF, Piwnica-Worms D. Effect of mitochondrial and plasma membrane potentials on accumulation of hexakis (2-methoxyisobutylisonitrile) technetium(I) in cultured mouse fibroblasts. J Nucl Med 1990;31:1646–53.
17. Piwnica-Worms D, Holman BL. Noncardiac applications of hexakis(alkylisonitrile) technetium-99m complexes. J Nucl Med 1990;31:1166–7.
18. Chen CC, Holder LE, Scovill WA, *et al.* Comparison of parathyroid imaging with technetium-99m-pertechnetate/ sestamibi subtraction, double-phase technetium-99m-sestamibi and technetium-99m-sestamibi SPECT. J Nucl Med 1997;38:834–9.
19. Taillefer R, Boucher Y, Potvin C, *et al.* Detection and localization of parathyroid adenomas in patients with hyperparathyroidism using a single radionuclide imaging procedure with technetium-99m-sestamibi (double-phase study). J Nucl Med 1992;33:1801–7.
20. Takami H, Satake S, Nakamura K, *et al.* Technetium 99m sestamibi scan is the useful procedure to locate parathyroid adenomas before surgery. Am J Surg 1996;172:93.
21. Westreich RW, Brandwein M, Mechanick JI, *et al.* Preoperative parathyroid localization: correlating false-negative technetium 99m sestamibi scans with parathyroid disease. Laryngoscope 2003;113:567–72.
22. Yamaguchi S, Yachiku S, Hashimoto H, *et al.* Relation between technetium 99m-methoxyisobutylisonitrile accumulation and multidrug resistance protein in the parathyroid glands. World J Surg 2002;26:29–34.
23. Kao A, Shiau Y-C, Tsai S-C, *et al.* Technetium-99m methoxyisobutylisonitrile imaging for parathyroid adenoma: relationship to P-glycoprotein or multidrug resistance-related protein expression. Eur J Nucl Med Mol Imaging 2002;29:1012.
24. Mehta NY, Ruda JM, Kapadia S, *et al.* Relationship of technetium Tc 99m sestamibi scans to histopathological features

of hyperfunctioning parathyroid tissue. Arch Otolaryngol Head Neck Surg 2005;131:493–8.
25. Pons F, Torregrosa JV, Fuster D. Biological factors influencing parathyroid localization. Nucl Med Commun 2003;24:121–4.
26. Arbab AS, Koizumi K, Hemmi A, *et al.* Tc-99m-MIBI scintigraphy for detecting parathyroid adenoma and hyperplasia. Ann Nucl Med 1997;11:45–9.
27. McBiles M, Lambert AT, Cote MG, *et al.* Sestamibi parathyroid imaging. Semin Nucl Med 1995;25:221–34.
28. Leslie WD, Dupont JO, Bybel B, *et al.* Parathyroid 99mTc-sestamibi scintigraphy: dual-tracer subtraction is superior to double-phase washout. Eur J Nucl Med Mol Imaging 2002;29:1566–70.
29. Neumann DR, Esselstyn CB Jr, Go RT, *et al.* Comparison of double-phase 99mTc-sestamibi with 123I-99mTc-sestamibi subtraction SPECT in hyperparathyroidism. Am J Roentgenol 1997;169:1671–4.
30. Gallowitsch HJ, Mikosch P, Kresnik E, *et al.* Technetium 99m tetrofosmin parathyroid imaging. Results with double-phase study and SPECT in primary and secondary hyperparathyroidism. Invest Radiol 1997;32:459–65.
31. Fjeld JG, Erichsen K, Pfeffer PF, *et al.* Technetium-99m-tetrofosmin for parathyroid scintigraphy: a comparison with sestamibi. J Nucl Med 1997;38:831–4.
32. Ishibashi M, Nishida H, Hiromatsu Y, *et al.* Comparison of technetium-99m-MIBI, technetium-99m-tetrofosmin, ultrasound and MRI for localization of abnormal parathyroid glands. J Nucl Med 1998;39:320–4.
33. Ruda J, Stack BC Jr, Hollenbeak CS. The cost-effectiveness of additional preoperative in ultrasonography or sestamibi-SPECT in the sestamibi-negative patient with primary hyperparathyroidism? Arch Otolaryngol Head Neck Surg 2006;132:46–53.
34. Thrall JH, Ziessman HA. Nuclear medicine: the requisites, 2nd edn. St Louis: Mosby, 2001:16–32, 363–87.
35. Arveschoug AK, Bertelsen H, Vammen B. Presurgical localization of abnormal parathyroid glands using a single injection of Tc-99m sestamibi: comparison of high-resolution parallel-hole and pinhole collimators, and interobserver and intraobserver variation. Clin Nucl Med 2002;27:249–54.
36. Arveschoug AK, Bertelsen H, Vammen B, *et al.* Preoperative dual-phase parathyroid imaging with tc-99m-sestamibi: accuracy and reproducibility of the pinhole collimator with and without oblique images. Clin Nucl Med 2007;32:9–12.
37. Ho Shon I, Bernard E, Roach P, *et al.* The value of oblique pinhole images in pre-operative localisation with 99mTc-MIBI for primary hyperparathyroidism. Eur J Nucl Med Mol Imaging 2001;28:736–42.
38. Norman J. The sestamibi scan—technical details. http://wwwparathyroidcom/Sestamibi-Technicalhtm 2007.
39. Sfakianakis GN, Irvin GL III, Foss J, *et al.* Efficient parathyroidectomy guided by SPECT-MIBI and hormonal measurements. J Nucl Med 1996;37:798–804.
40. Moka D, Voth E, Dietlein M, *et al.* Technetium 99m-MIBI-SPECT: a highly sensitive diagnostic tool for localization of parathyroid adenomas. Surgery 2000;128:29–35.
41. Slater A, Gleeson FV. Increased sensitivity and confidence of SPECT over planar imaging in dual-phase sestamibi for parathyroid adenoma detection. Clin Nucl Med 2005; 30:1–3.
42. Teigen EL, Kilgore EJ, Cowan RJ, *et al.* Technetium-99m-Sestamibi SPECT localization of mediastinal parathyroid adenoma. J Nucl Med 1996;37:1535–7.
43. Billotey C, Sarfati E, Aurengo A, *et al.* Advantages of SPECT in technetium-99m-sestamibi parathyroid scintigraphy. J Nucl Med 1996;37:1773–8.
44. Gayed IW, Kim EE, Broussard WF, *et al.* The value of 99mTc-sestamibi SPECT/CT over conventional SPECT in the evaluation of parathyroid adenomas or hyperplasia. J Nucl Med 2005;46:248–52.
45. Norman JG, Jaffray CE, Chheda H. The false-positive parathyroid sestamibi: a real or perceived problem and a case for radioguided parathyroidectomy. Ann Surg 2000;231: 31–7.
46. Hopkins CR, Reading CC. Thyroid, parathyroid and other glands. In: McGahan JP, Goldberg BB, eds. Diagnostic ultrasound: a logical approach. Philadelphia: Lippincott-Raven, 1998:1087–114.
47. Barraclough BM, Barraclough BH. Ultrasound of the thyroid and parathyroid glands. World J Surg 2000;24: 158–65.
48. Kamaya A, Quon A, Jeffrey RB. Sonography of the abnormal parathyroid gland. Ultrasound Q 2006;22:253–62.
49. Hopkins CR, Reading CC. Thyroid and parathyroid imaging. Semin Ultrasound CT MR 1995;16:279–95.
50. Koslin DB, Adams J, Andersen P, *et al.* Preoperative evaluation of patients with primary hyperparathyroidism: role of high-resolution ultrasound. Laryngoscope 1997;107:1249–53.
51. Meilstrup JW. Ultrasound examination of the parathyroid glands. Otolaryngol Clin North Am 2004;37:763–78, ix.
52. Gooding GA. Sonography of the thyroid and parathyroid. Radiol Clin North Am 1993;31:967–89.
53. Burkey SH, Snyder WH III, Nwariaku F, *et al.* Directed parathyroidectomy: feasibility and performance in 100 consecutive patients with primary hyperparathyroidism. Arch Surg 2003;138:604–9.
54. Sacks BA, Pallotta JA, Cole A, *et al.* Diagnosis of parathyroid adenomas: efficacy of measuring parathormone levels in needle aspirates of cervical masses. Am J Roentgenol 1994;163:1223–6.
55. Lewis BD, Charboneau JW, Reading CC. Ultrasound-guided biopsy and ablation in the neck. Ultrasound Q 2002;18:3–12.
56. Clark OH, Duh QY. Primary hyperparathyroidism. A surgical perspective. Endocrinol Metab Clin North Am 1989; 18:701–14.

57. Gooding G, Clark O, Stark D, *et al.* Parathyroid aspiration biopsy under ultrasound guidance in the postoperative hyperparathyroid patient. Radiology 1985;155:193–6.
58. Lane MJ, Desser TS, Weigel RJ, *et al.* Use of color and power Doppler sonography to identify feeding arteries associated with parathyroid adenomas. Am J Roentgenol 1998;171: 819–23.
59. Lumachi F, Ermani M, Basso S, *et al.* Localization of parathyroid tumours in the minimally invasive era: which technique should be chosen? Population-based analysis of 253 patients undergoing parathyroidectomy and factors affecting parathyroid gland detection. Endocr Relat Cancer 2001;8:63–69.
60. Purcell GP, Dirbas FM, Jeffrey RB, *et al.* Parathyroid localization with high-resolution ultrasound and technetium Tc 99m sestamibi. Arch Surg 1999;134:824–30.
61. Reidel MA, Schilling T, Graf S, *et al.* Localization of hyperfunctioning parathyroid glands by selective venous sampling in reoperation for primary or secondary hyperparathyroidism. Surgery 2006;140:907–13.
62. You CJ, Zapas JL. Diminished dose minimally invasive radioguided parathyroidectomy: a case for radioguidance. Am Surg. 2007;73:669–72; discussion 673.
63. Beus KS, Stack BC. Synchronous thyroid pathology in patients presenting with primary hyperparathyroidism. Am J Otolaryngol 2004;25:308–12.
64. Bennedbaek FN, Karstrup S, Hegedus L. Percutaneous ethanol injection therapy in the treatment of thyroid and parathyroid diseases. Eur J Endocrinol 1997;136:240–50.
65. Miller DL. Pre-operative localization and interventional treatment of parathyroid tumors: when and how? World J Surg 1991;15:706–15.
66. Moley JF, Lairmore TC, Doherty GM, *et al.* Preservation of the recurrent laryngeal nerves in thyroid and parathyroid reoperations. Surgery 1999;126:673–9.
67. Jacobson SR, van Heerden JA, Farley DR, *et al.* Focused cervical exploration for primary hyperparathyroidism without intraoperative parathyroid hormone monitoring or use of the gamma probe. World J Surg 2004;28:1127–31.
68. Norman J. Parathyroid surgery cure rates. http://www parathyroidcom/surgery_cure_rateshtm 2007.
69. Bennedbak FN, Karstrup S, Hegedus L. Ultrasound guided laser ablation of a parathyroid adenoma. Br J Radiol 2001;74:905–07.
70. Yusim A, Aspelund G, Ahrens W, *et al.* Intrathyroidal parathyroid adenoma. Thyroid 2006;16:619–20.
71. Ahuja AT, Wong KT, Ching ASC, *et al.* Imaging for primary hyperparathyroidism—what beginners should know. Clin Radiol 2004;59:967–76.
72. Krausz Y, Bettman L, Guralnik L, *et al.* Technetium-99m-MIBI SPECT/CT in primary hyperparathyroidism. World J Surg 2006;30:76–83.
73. Roach PJ, Schembri GP, Ho Shon IA, *et al.* SPECT/CT imaging using a spiral CT scanner for anatomical localization: impact on diagnostic accuracy and reporter confidence in clinical practice. Nucl Med Commun 2006;27:977–87.
74. Serra A, Bolasco P, Satta L, *et al.* Role of SPECT/CT in the preoperative assessment of hyperparathyroid patients. Radiol Med 2006;111:999–1008.
75. Beggs A, Hain SF. Use of co-registered ^{11}C-methionine PET and computed tomography for the localisation of parathyroid adenomas. Eur J Nucl Med Mol Imaging 2003;30:1602.
76. Saeed S, Yao M, Philip B, *et al.* Localizing hyperfunctioning parathyroid tissue: MRI or nuclear study or both? Clin Imaging 2006;30:257–65.
77. Udelsman R, Donovan PI. Remedial parathyroid surgery: changing trends in 130 consecutive cases. Ann Surg 2006; 244:471–9.
78. Beggs AD, Hain SF. Localization of parathyroid adenomas using 11C-methionine positron emission tomography. Nucl Med Commun 2005;26:133–6.
79. Hellman P, Ahlstrom H, Bergstrom M, *et al.* Positron emission tomography with 11C-methionine in hyperparathyroidism. Surgery 1994;116:974–81.
80. Neumann DR, Esselstyn CB, Maclntyre WJ, *et al.* Comparison of FDG-PET and sestamibi-SPECT in primary hyperparathyroidism. J Nucl Med 1996;37:1809–15.
81. Sundin A, Johansson C, Hellman P, *et al.* PET and parathyroid L-[carbon-11]methionine accumulation in hyperparathyroidism. J Nucl Med 1996;37:1766–70.
82. Otto D, Boerner AA, Hofmann M, *et al.* Pre-operative localisation of hyperfunctional parathyroid tissue with ^{11}C-methionine PET. Eur J Nucl Med Mol Imaging 2004;31:1405–12
83. Reitz RE, Pollard JJ, Wang CA, *et al.* Localization of parathyroid adenomas by selective venous catheterization and radioimmunoassay. N Engl J Med 1969;281:348–51.
84. Nilsson BE, Tisell LE, Jansson S, *et al.* Parathyroid localization by catheterization of large cervical and mediastinal veins to determine serum concentrations of intact parathyroid hormone. World J Surg 1994;18:605–10; discussion 10–11.
85. Jaskowiak N, Norton JA, Alexander HR, *et al.* A prospective trial evaluating a standard approach to reoperation for missed parathyroid adenoma. Ann Surg 1996;224:308–20; discussion 20–1.
86. Mariette C, Pellissier L, Combemale F, *et al.* Reoperation for persistent or recurrent primary hyperparathyroidism. Langenbecks Arch Surg 1998;383:174–9.

MULTIPLE CHOICE QUESTIONS

Select more than one optiom where appropriate.

1. Primary HPT is due to single gland disease in
A. 10%
B. 20%

C. 90%
D. 5%

2. Surgery for HPT is recommended
A. When localization imaging is positive
B. In all patients under 50 years of age
C. In all patients over 50 years of age
D. In patients with urinary 24 h calcium of less than 100 mg/%

3. Sestamibi scanning
A. May be negative in small adenomas
B. May be improved with the addition of SPECT
C. Can be used with both immediate and wash-out views
D. Can be falsely positive with thyroid Hurthle cell adenomas

4. In the pre-operative work-up of HPT, ultrasound
A. Provides structural information which may assist with sestamibi interpretation
B. Is variable in accuracy depending on the ultrasonographer
C. Always identifies hyperplasic glands
D. May serve to elevate PTH levels transiently

5. If the pre-operative sestamibi is negative one should
A. Avoid surgery
B. Consider ultrasound
C. Consider bilateral exploration
D. Check the patient's vitamin D levels

Answers

1. C
2. B
3. A, B, C, D
4. A, B
5. B, C

15 Pathological spectrum of parathyroid disease

John Lynn & Paul Lewis
Bupa Cromwell Hospital, London, UK

KEY POINTS

- Single gland disease (adenoma) is the most common pathology in primary hyperparathyroidism
- Parathyroid adenoma and carcinoma may be non-functioning
- Multiple gland disease is almost always due to chief cell hyperplasia
- Water-clear cell hyperplasia produces huge enlargement of the lower parathyroid glands
- Parathyroid carcinoma infiltrates locally but metastasis to lymph nodes is uncommon

THE NORMAL PARATHYROID

The normal adult human parathyroid is approximately the size of a grain of rice. It usually measures 5 mm in length, 3 mm in width and weighs up to 40 mg. In most adults, there are four parathyroid glands in upper and lower pairs. Five glands may occasionally be present. Rarely, in the state described as 'parathyromatosis', small clusters of glandular cells are present in the tissues around parathyroids. These clusters may enlarge in parathyroid hyperplasia, the outcome being the discovery of six, eight, ten or more glandular foci in excised tissue.

The location of the parathyroids is explained embryologically in Chapter 16. In the 8–10 mm human embryo, the parathyroids appear as thickenings in the epithelium of the third and fourth branchial pouches.[1] The lower parathyroids originate from the third branchial pouch epithelium of a parathyroid–thymus bud which moves into the chest with the developing heart. The upper parathyroids develop from the fourth pouch derivative which lies in the lateral aspect of the maturing thyroid gland and remains in the neck. The upper parathyroids therefore tend to be positioned high in the neck near the upper pole of the thyroid. In contrast, the lower parathyroids are variable in site, depending on the degree of descent of the parathyroid–thymic bud. They can be found as high as the carotid bifurcation or low in the mediastinum intimately related to the thymus.[2] Although the parathyroids may potentially occupy many positions in the neck or mediastinum, in most cases they are found within the neck, and a simple cervical exploration will be able to identify them.[3] If it becomes grossly enlarged, the upper parathyroid may be displaced downwards due to the effect of deglutition. It may be found behind the pharynx or may even descend beyond the lower oesophagus to lie in the posterior mediastinum.[4]

One of the most important points for the parathyroid surgeon to realize is that parathyroids are usually symmetrical and if a definite parathyroid has been found in a certain position on one side, the other is usually found in the mirror position on the opposite side of the neck.[2] The weight of the parathyroid, measured intraoperatively, is an important consideration in deciding whether a gland is enlarged and thus the cause of hyperparathyroidism. In general, glands heavier than 50 mg are regarded as pathologically enlarged. Various autopsy studies have shown total parathyroid weight of 120–140 mg in adults. In children and adolescents, weights are lower. The combined weight of the parathyroids at 6 months is less than 10 mg, at 1 year 20 mg, at 5 years 30–40 mg and at 10 years up to 60 mg.

The intra-operative appearance of the parathyroids is usually characteristic: their orange to yellow-brown colour contrasts well with the red-brown of the thyroid and grey-pink of lymph nodes. The parathyroid colour varies according to their fat content.

Normal histology

The normal parathyroid consists of parenchyma and supporting connective tissue. The parenchyma contains the hormone-secreting cells. The connective tissue and fat component depend on the age of the patient. Mature adipose tissue appears in the stroma, increasing in amount until middle age. According to the level of obesity, it sometimes decreases in later life.

A Practical Manual of Thyroid and Parathyroid Disease, 1st Edition. Edited by Asit Arora, Neil Tolley & R. Michael Tuttle.

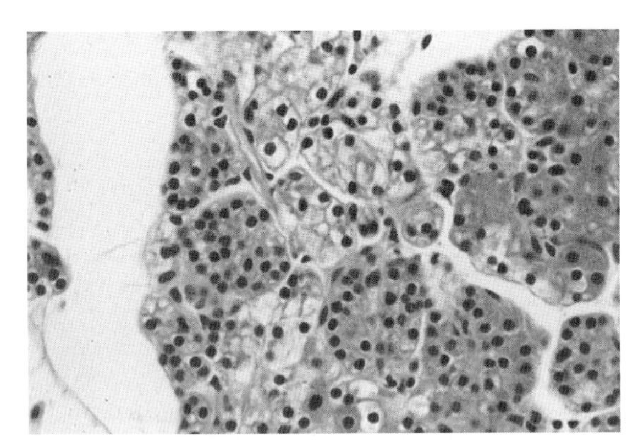

Fig. 15.1 Normal parathyroid gland consisting of chief and oxyphil cells.

In the normal adult parathyroid there are two main cell types: the chief cell and the oxyphil cell (Fig. 15.1).

A functionally more active cell type termed the 'water-clear' cell is predominant in infancy but is also found in the adult gland when there is increased parathyroid hormone (PTH) secretion. These cell types, as well as transitional forms (between chief and water-clear cells), are seen in both adenomatous and hyperplastic glands.

Chief cells are polygonal with lightly eosinophilic cytoplasm, measure about 8 μm in diameter and have a central 5 μm nucleus. It is the predominant cell type found in the adult parathyroid. Water-clear cells are larger with unstained cytoplasm rich in glycogen which is lost in tissue processing for microscopy. This is the sole cell type in the neonatal parathyroid. Oxyphil cells are larger still, with deeply staining (eosinophilic) granular cytoplasm full of mitochondria and with a small dense nucleus. They are metabolically active but non-secretory and increase in number with age, forming small nodules. This is a useful diagnostic feature found in the rim of suppressed glandular tissue at the edge of a parathyroid adenoma.

It is not uncommon for follicles to develop within a parathyroid tumour or normal parathyroid which causes difficulty when distinguishing the presumed parathyroid from a thyroid lesion. Histopathological expertise and immunostaining for thyroglobulin resolves this potential problem.

Function and size

It has already been stated that a parathyroid gland greater than 50 mg in weight is considered abnormal. However, it is debatable whether a weight of 50 mg represents the true lower limit of abnormality. There are two reasons for this. First, a parathyroid gland can be enlarged yet non-functioning. Asymptomatic, grossly enlarged parathyroids have been found weighing up to 500 mg. Secondly, experience of minimally invasive surgery (removal of a single gland localized by sestamibi scan and ultrasound) suggests an incidence of hyperplasia that does not correlate well with that found during four gland exploration. When four gland exploration entails removal of glands larger than 50 mg, it is possible that they are not actually pathological, and such cases are therefore being overtreated. The converse view is that the increasing use of minimally invasive surgery may result in the re-appearance of symptomatic hypercalcaemia due to pathologically enlarged glands being missed and subsequently becoming hyperfunctional.

PRIMARY HYPERPARATHYROIDISM

Primary hyperparathyroidism is diagnosed in patients with hypercalcaemia, inappropriate PTH levels and significant hypercalcuria. This must be in the presence of normal renal function and normal levels of vitamin D.[3]

1. Single gland disease (adenoma)
2. Double adenoma
3. Hyperplasia (multiple involvment)
4. Carcinoma
5. Microadenoma
6. Disrupted parathyroid tissue syndrome.

Parathyroid adenoma

In primary hyperparathyroidism the most frequent cause is a single adenoma.[5] This is found in women three times more often than in men. An adenoma may develop in the setting of MEN1 syndrome or MEN2 syndrome. In children, the surgeon should be aware that case management must extend beyond parathyroid pathology. Radiation to the neck has been reported to increase the incidence of parathyroid tumours.

Parathyroid adenomas vary in size from 50 mg to over 100 g. They are easily separable from the surrounding thyroid tissue, bruise very easily because of a prolific blood supply, and if not handled carefully are liable to rupture. Large calcified adenomas can be difficult to differentiate from a multinodular goitre. Indeed, when re-exploring patients who have previously failed surgery, we found that in most cases it is the larger parathyroid that has been missed, not the smaller one. Large parathyroids may have areas of haemorrhage, cystic change and calcification evident on plain X-ray. Upper parathyroid adenomas are usually situated behind the upper pole of the thyroid. As they enlarge, they may be pushed backwards behind the pharynx and oesophagus, even down into the mediastinum, while maintaining their blood supply from the neck. Enlarged lower parathyroids can be found anywhere from the carotid bifurcation, where they are usually associated with a tongue of thymic tissue, to the anterior mediastinum nestled within the thymus.[3]

Parathyroid adenomas are mainly composed of chief cells arranged in sheets or follicles, and also often contain water-clear cells or oxyphils (Plate 15.1).

Nuclear pleomorphism is commonly present and does not necessarily signify malignant potential. A rim of 'normal' (in fact suppressed) parathyroid tissue is often seen at the edge of the adenoma, but is not found in every specimen because of the vagaries of geometry and the practical limitations of histopathology.

Occasionally a pale, yellow-brown, lobulated adenoma is found to contain a large amount of fatty tissue mixed with cords and sheets of parenchymal cells. Such tumours have been described variously as lipoadenomas or parathyroid hamartomas. Lipoadenomas may or may not be functioning.

Double adenoma

Double adenomas are extremely rare.[6] In most instances a double adenoma is mistaken for asymmetric hyperplasia of all four or more glands. The diagnosis should therefore only be made if two enlarged glands are found, the remaining glands are normal or suppressed and long-term follow-up shows no recurrence of hypercalcaemia.

Microadenoma

Very rarely, parathyroid adenomas are so small that they develop in glands of normal or near normal dimension and weight, e.g. 6 mm or 50 mg. They tend to be more common in re-explorations and may account for so-called 'normal' parathyroid removal resulting in patient cure when a macroadenoma is not found.[7]

Intra-operative frozen section confirms the diagnosis, and a significant drop in intra-operative parathyroid hormone blood level measurements following removal provides confirmation of correct surgical management.

Parathyroid hyperplasia

Chief cell hyperplasia in primary hyperparathyroidism

Chief cell hyperplasia, also termed nodular hyperplasia, is accompanied by increased production of PTH which can occur in primary or secondary hyperparathyroidism. The latter arises due to renal impairment or chronic malabsorption. In primary hyperparathyroidism, chief cell hyperplasia is common in MEN syndromes 1 and 2. It should be noted that patients with MEN2B, with its typical marfanoid phenotype, have normal parathyroids and do not exhibit chief cell hyperplasia.[8]

The microscopic pattern is extremely variable and the term nodular hyperplasia is a more appropriate term than chief cell hyperplasia because of the range of cell types found (Fig. 15.2). The enlarged glands are rounded and grossly lobulated, grey or brown in colour and weigh anything from 50 mg to over 10 g. Cases of nodular hyperplasia in secondary hyperparathyroidism tend to have quite firm, hard nodules which macroscopically resemble multinodular thyroid tissue.

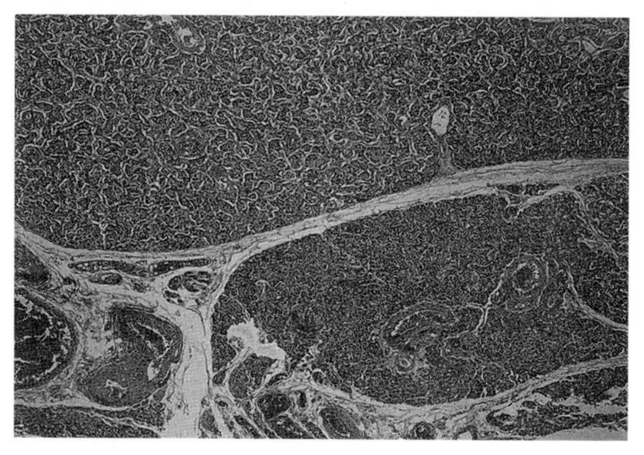

Fig. 15.2 Parathyroid chief cell hyperplasia with a multinodular pattern of growth.

Water-clear cell hyperplasia

This is an extraordinarily rare condition, and at the Hammersmith Hospital we have not seen a single case in over 500 consecutive hyperparathyroid patients surgically explored over the last 20 years. Water-clear cell hyperplasia can occur at any age, although almost half the cases arise in the sixth decade. It is a sporadic condition which is not associated with tumours of other endocrine glands. The massively enlarged glands, reportedly up to 52 g, have been described as lobulated, chocolate brown and

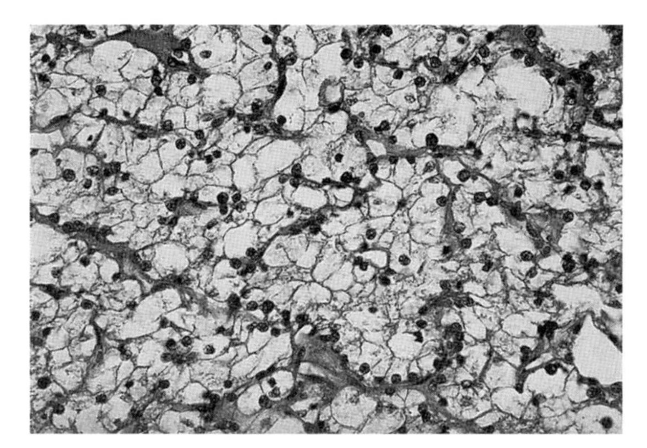

Fig. 15.3 Parathyroid water-clear cell hyperplasia. Cells are very large, optically clear and have sharply outlined cell membranes.

translucent. They can sometimes exhibit extensions into fatty tissue.[9] The upper pair are said to be 5–10 times larger than the lower pair. Large cysts and haemorrhage are reportedly common in this condition. Microscopically, uniform large (20 µm) water-clear cells with peripheral nuclei are seen (Fig. 15.3).

Parathyroid carcinoma

Parathyroid carcinoma is exceptionally rare. The National Cancer Base Incidence Cancer Review in the USA recorded only 286 cases between 1985 and 1995, which represents a mere 0.005% of all cancers during this time frame.[10] Parathyroid carcinoma presents sporadically, is associated with hyperparathyroidism jaw syndrome and also occurs in patients with end-stage renal failure.[11] It has been suggested that there is an increased incidence in patients who have had radiation to the neck, but the evidence for this is unclear. Parathyroid carcinoma occasionally develops in an adenomatous or hyperplastic gland which may be non-functioning.[12] It presents as an ill-defined neck mass which is sometimes palpable. In advanced cases, the tumour is densely adherent to adjacent soft tissues of the neck and may involve the recurrent laryngeal nerve, trachea and thyroid. The presence of voice change in a patient diagnosed with a parathyroid tumour is highly suggestive of carcinoma, particularly if there is no previous history of thyroid/parathyroid surgery. In contrast to the typical soft consistency of parathyroid adenoma, parathyroid carcinoma is lobulated, firm and stony hard. In 50% of cases there is a dense fibrous greyish capsule which makes the tumour extremely difficult to separate from contiguous structures. Growth is generally local, but metastasis to cervical lymph nodes and lungs does occur. Knowledge of the physical characteristics of parathyroid carcinoma is essential because its management is completely different from that of benign adenomas or hyperplastic benign glands. If there is evidence of direct infiltration into extraglandular structures or vascular channels, the histopathological distinction between a benign and malignant parathyroid tumour is straightforward. However, the diagnosis can sometimes be challenging. Parathyroid cancer is usually composed of chief cells arranged in solid sheets or a trabecular pattern (Plate 15.2). There is little difference between these cells and the cells in an adenoma, although sometimes the former exhibit marked nuclear pleomorphism with an increased nucleus : cytoplasm ratio. Mitotic activity is rarely prominent. Thick fibrous bands have been considered a diagnostic feature, but this also occurs in adenomas where there has been cystic degeneration. Even with specialist review, the diagnosis of parathyroid carcinoma may be in doubt, in which case the patient should be considered and treated as such.

Disrupted parathyroid tissue syndrome

Damage to a parathyroid adenoma during removal may result in implantation of glandular fragments into muscle and surrounding fat. This causes recurrence of hyperparathyroidism. The presence of multiple areas of parathyroid tissue in fat and muscle can also be mistaken for malignancy because a similar picture is seen after excision of a parathyroid carcinoma which has recurred. The entity is difficult to treat and requires wide excision of local muscle and fatty tissue. A clue to the diagnosis is the presence of talc or other birefringent material. A careful review of the previous operation notes may reveal that the adenoma or hyperplastic gland was broken at the initial surgery.

Parathyroid cysts

Parathyroid cysts result from degeneration of an adenoma or hyperplastic gland and may also have a developmental origin. They are more common in lower glands and are rarely functional. Microcysts occur in 50% of normal parathyroids. Cysts of developmental origin are thought to arise from the third branchial pouch and often contain thymus in addition to parathyroid tissue.[12]

Secondary tumours of the parathyroid

Small secondary tumours of the parathyroid are not uncommon at autopsy and have been reported in 12% of patients with malignant disease. They arise from a variety of sites including breast, skin and lungs. It is very unusual for a metastatic parathyroid lesion to present a clinical problem.

SECONDARY HYPERPARATHYROIDISM

Secondary hyperparathyroidism occurs in either chronic renal failure or intestinal malabsorption. There is an increased phosphate level and a concomitant decrease in serum calcium with a resulting stimulation of the parathyroid gland and elevated PTH.

The parathyroid pathology in secondary hyperparathyroidism is that of nodular chief cell hyperplasia. It is almost impossible to distinguish primary from secondary hyperplasia on a morphological basis alone, and a clinical history is mandatory in making this distinction. The term 'tertiary' hyperparathyroidism has been used in patients who develop autonomous parathyroid hyperfunction on a background of pre-existing secondary hyperparathyroidism. This condition has also been called non-suppressible autonomous hyperparathyroidism. Nodules develop and sometimes increase in size, suggestive of a primary parathyroid adenoma.

PARATHYROID PATHOLOGY IN THE MULTIPLE ENDOCRINE PHENOTYPE 1 AND TYPE 2

MEN1 is a rare inherited disorder with an incidence of between 0.2 and 2 per 100 000. It causes tumours in one or more endocrine glands and occurs due to a tumour suppressor gene found on the long arm of chromosome 11 (11q113). The major clinical manifestations include primary hyperparathyroidism, which occurs in 90% of patients, pancreatic endocrine tumours, which arise in 50–70% of cases, and pituitary adenomas, which occur in 30% of patients. Most patients present between the ages of 20 and 40. Unlike spontaneous hyperparathyroidism, hyperparathyroidism in the MEN1 syndrome is almost uniformly primary chief-cell hyperplasia which affects all four glands. There may be variable hyperplasia leading to asymmetrical parathyroid hyperplasia.[13]

It is not possible to distinguish whether hyperparathyroidism is spontaneous or associated with MEN1 based solely on the morphology of hyperplastic parathyroid tissue. MEN2A syndrome consists of a normal phenotype with thyroid C-cell hyperplasia and subsequent medullary carcinoma, multiple phaeochromocytomas and primary hyperparathyroidism. The pathology is usually that of a clear cell hyperplasia. The extent of hyperplasia is such that it is unusual for hyperparathyroidism to be a dominant feature in the syndrome, in contrast to MEN1. In MEN2B, patients have a marfanoid phenotype associated with medullary carcinoma of the thyroid and phaeochromocytomas. Parathyroid chief cell hyperplasia is exceedingly rare, although as the patient gets older a minimal degree of hyperplasia may develop.

HYPOPARATHYROIDISM

The most common cause of hypoparathyroidism is surgical damage to the parathyroids. This can occur in thyroid surgery, parathyroid surgery or following extensive head and neck surgery performed to excise malignant head and neck tumours. Autoimmune lymphocytic parathyroiditis rarely occurs and is another potential cause. Several congenital syndromes are also associated with hypoparathyroidism. The DiGeorge syndrome consists of hypoparathyroidism, immunodeficiency, complex heart defects and deformities of the ear nose and throat. The disorder is due to a developmental failure of the third and fourth pharyngeal pouches and results in the absence or hypoplasia of the parathyroids. The Kenney–Caffey syndrome is a bizarre syndrome of hypoparathyroidism, short stature, osteosclerosis and eye defects. Post-mortem examinations have confirmed complete absence of parathyroid tissue, suggesting that the defect is embryological. Hypoparathyroidism also occurs in the polyglandular autoimmune type 1 syndrome. This entity has a relatively high incidence in Finns and Iranian Jews.

REFERENCES

1. Gilmore JR. The embryology of the parathyroid glands, the thymus and certain associated rudiments. J Pathol 1937;45:507–22.
2. Akerstrom G, Malmaeus J, Bergstrom R. Surgical anatomy of human parathyroid glands. Surgery 1984;95:14–21.
3. Saidan Z, Lynn JA. Surgery of the parathyroids. In: Lynn JA, Bloom SR, eds. Surgical endocrinology. Oxford: Butterworth Heinemann, 1993;86–99.
4. Wang CA. The anatomic basis of parathyroid surgery. Ann Surg 1976;183:271–5.
5. Taylor GW. Surgery of hyperparathyroid disease. Br J Surg 1980;67:732–5.

6. Harkness JK, Ramsburg SR, Nishiyamarh RH, *et al.* Multiple adenomas of the parathyroids: do they exist? Arch Surg 1979;114: 468–74.
7. Liechly RD, Teter A, Suba EJ. The tiny parathyroid adenoma. Surgery 1986;100:1048.
8. Carney, JA, Roth SI, Heath H III, *et al.* The parathyroid glands in multiple endocrine neoplasia type 2B. Am J Pathol 1980;99:387–98.
9. Castleman B, Schantz A, Roth SI. Parathyroid hyperplasia in primary hyperparathyroidism—a review of 85 cases. Cancer 1976;38:1668–75.
10. Hundahl SA, Fleming ID, Fremgen AM, *et al.* Two hundred eighty six cases of parathyroid carcinoma treated in the US between 1985–1995: a National Cancer Data Base Report. The American College of Surgeons Commission on Cancer and the American Cancer Society. Cancer 1999;86:538–44.
11. Cavaco BM, Barros L, Pannett AAJ, *et al.* The hyperparathyroidism–jaw tumour syndrome in a Portuguese kindred. QJM 2001;94:213–22.
12. Carney JA. Salivary heterotopia, cysts, and parathyroid gland branchial pouch derivatives and remnants. Am J Pathol 2000;24:837–45.
13. Harach HR, Jasani B. Parathyroid hyperplasia in multiple endocrine neoplasia type I: a pathological and immunohistochemical reappraisal. Histopathology 1992;21:513–9.

MULTIPLE CHOICE QUESTIONS

Select more than one option where appropriate

1. With regard to the parathyroid glands
A. The normal gland is approximately the size of a grain of rice
B. The normal weight is 40 g
C. There may be up to 10 glands present
D. The glands develop from the second branchial arch
E. Parathyromatosis is a syndrome associated with absence of parathyroid glands

2. Histology of normal adult parathyroid glands
A. Adipose content decreases with age
B. There are two main cell types in the adult parathyroid gland
C. The water-clear cell is predominant in adulthood
D. The water-clear cell is associated with increasing levels of parathyroid hormone
E. Oxyphil cells are the sole cell type in neonatal parathyroids

3. Parathyroid adenomas
A. A solitary adenoma is the most common cause of primary hyperparathyroidism
B. Is associated with MEN2
C. May be visible on plain radiography
D. Are difficult to dissect from surrounding tissue
E. Have a poor blood supply

4. Parathyroid hyperplasia
A. Chief cell hyperplasia is associated with increased levels of PTH
B. Chief cell hyperplasia is diagnostic of secondary hyperparathyroidism
C. Never occurs in tertiary hyperparathyroidism
D. Chief cell hyperplasia is not a feature in patients with MEN2B.
E. Water-clear cell hyperplasia is associated with adrenal adenomas.

5. Parathyroid carcinoma
A. Is a common condition
B. Is easily distinguished from parathyroid adenomas
C. May result in involvement of the laryngeal nerves
D. The management is similar to that of parathyroid adenoma
E. Often have thick fibrous bands histologically

Answers

1. A, C
2. B
3. A, B, C
4. A, D
5. C, E

16 Clinical anatomy, developmental aberrations and endocrinology

Malcolm H. Wheeler

Department of Endocrine Surgery, University Hospital of Wales, Heath Park, Cardiff, UK

KEY POINTS

- Superior parathyroid glands develop from the fourth branchial pouch. Inferior parathyroid glands develop from the third branchial pouch in association with the thymus and have an increased propensity for wide distribution and ectopia
- The majority of patients have four parathyroid glands and in 60% there is complete symmetry of gland position. True supernumerary glands occur in approximately 5% of individuals
- Extracellular fluid calcium concentration is regulated within a narrow physiological range by parathyroid hormone (PTH) and 1,25-dihydroxyvitamin D_3 acting directly or indirectly on the intestine, bone and kidney
- PTH is an 84 amino acid polypeptide hormone. Its release from the parathyroid glands is tightly regulated by extracellular and intracellular calcium concentrations
- Calcium controls PTH secretion through calcium-activated channels and calcium-sensing receptors which exist on the parathyroid cell surface

INTRODUCTION

Detailed understanding and knowledge of the embryological development and anatomy of the parathyroid glands are essential prerequisites for a successful surgical strategy in patients with hyperparathyroidism. The considerable variability in size, shape, number, location and colour of these glands creates unique surgical challenges.

HISTORICAL NOTE

Sir Richard Owen, Conservator and Professor of Comparative Anatomy at the Hunterian Museum of the Royal College of Surgeons of England, first identified the parathyroid glands in 1850 whilst performing a post-mortem examination on a 15-year-old Indian rhinoceros. In 1862 he reported his findings in the *Transactions of the Zoological Society of London*, describing the gland as 'a small yellow body attached to the thyroid at the point where the veins emerge'.[1]

In 1880 the Swedish anatomist Ivar Sandstrom, born 2 years after Owen's original discovery, provided an anatomical and histological description of the human parathyroids which he named 'glandulae parathyroidae'.[2] He commented on their position, colour, size and form. With remarkable foresight he even speculated that the glands might be subject to pathological change such as tumour development.

EMBRYOLOGY

The developmental embryology and surgical anatomy of the parathyroid glands and the thyroid are intimately linked. This observation has enormous practical significance for the surgeon.[3–5]

The superior parathyroids arise from the dorsal aspect of the fourth branchial pouch endoderm and migrate inferiorly with the developing lateral thyroid lobes (ultimobranchial bodies). This relatively limited descent results in a fairly constant position adjacent to the posterior aspect of the middle third of the thyroid lobe.

The inferior parathyroids derive from the dorsal aspect of the third branchial pouch endoderm. Since the thymus arises from the ventral aspect of the same branchial pouch, it is not surprising that the inferior parathyroids and thymus develop together (parathymus complex). They share a longer caudal descent compared with the superior parathyroid glands. This unique embryological process results in a crossing of passage between the superior and inferior parathyroids (Fig. 16.1).

In the 20 mm embryo, the inferior parathyroids separate from the caudally moving thymus. This separation results in their eventual location in close relation to the inferior thyroid pole or within the thyrothymic ligament (a fibrous tract left as a vestigial structure between the tip

A Practical Manual of Thyroid and Parathyroid Disease, 1st Edition. Edited by Asit Arora, Neil Tolley & R. Michael Tuttle.

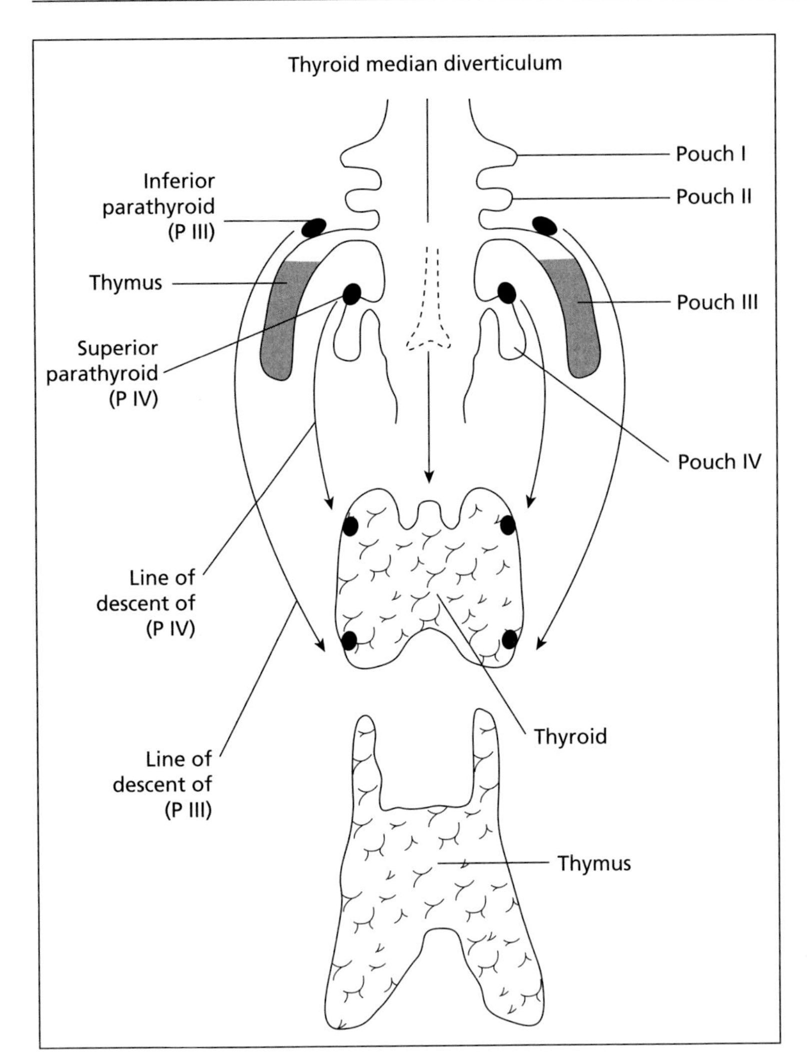

Fig. 16.1 Branchial pouch development showing the inferior parathyroid glands and thymus arising from the third branchial pouch before caudal descent. The fourth pouch gives rise to the superior parathyroids, ultimobranchial body and possibly a small thymic component. Fusion of the fourth and fifth branchial pouches constitutes the caudal pharyngeal complex.

of the thymic horn and the lower thyroid pole). Their relatively long embryological descent compared with the superior glands accounts for why they have a much greater propensity for aberrant location along the descent line. This occurs anywhere from high in the neck above the thyroid to low in the anterior mediastinum.

ANATOMY

Normal parathyroid glands are soft, pliable, discrete and compact. The majority are spherical or bean shaped, although they can also be elongated, bi-lobed or even flattened and multilobed. Their colour ranges from reddish brown in the cellular, well-vascularized gland to pale yellow in a gland with high fat content.[6] The average gland weighs 40 mg and is approximately 5 × 3 × 1 mm in dimension.[7,8]

An experienced parathyroid surgeon is able to distinguish these small glands from adjacent structures on the basis of gross appearance. The parathyroids are frequently found in fat, from which they are easily separated. In contrast, thyroid is much firmer, is often nodular and has a darker, less uniform red colour. Lymph nodes are usually multiple, firm, whitish grey and less easily separated from fat. Thymic tissue is discrete and pale yellow.

The vascular supply of the parathyroid glands has been carefully investigated. The main arterial input is an end

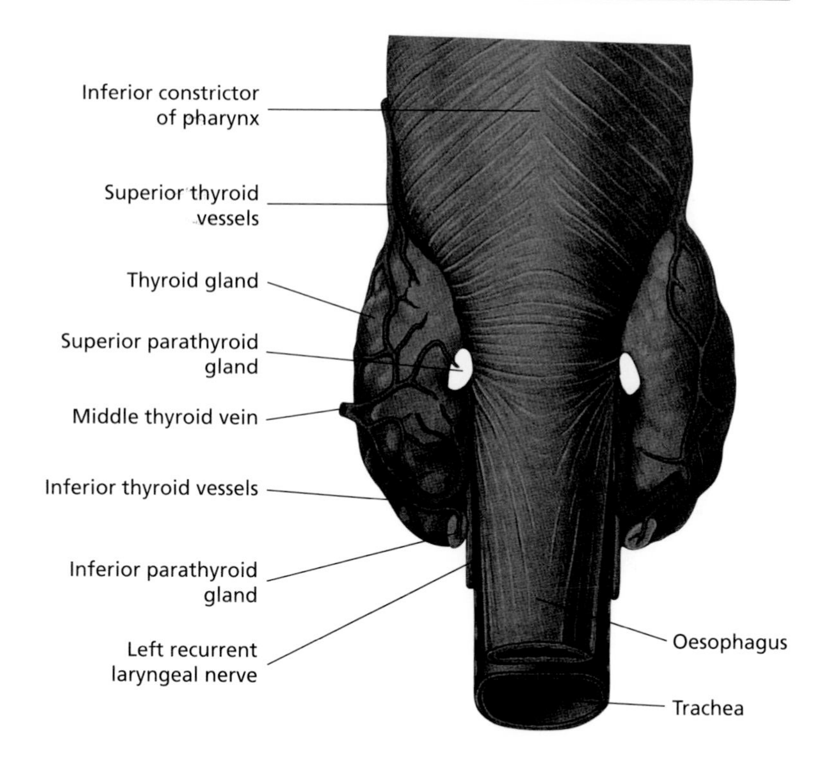

Fig. 16.2 The blood supply of the parathyroid glands.

artery type, and approximately one-third of glands are supplied by two or more arterial branches.[20] The principal parathyroid blood supply is derived from the inferior thyroid artery. A significant proportion of superior glands receive their main blood supply from either the posterior branch of the superior thyroid artery or an anastomotic loop which this vessel makes with the inferior thyroid artery. A small component of parathyroid blood supply is probably derived from the thyroid capsular vessels. Intrathoracic and intrathymic parathyroid glands receive an arterial supply from thymic vessels and sometimes receive a branch from the internal mammary artery. The venous drainage accompanies the capsular vessels and larger main thyroid veins which drain the thyroid gland (Fig. 16.2).

Autopsy studies and surgical observation confirm that almost all individuals have at least four parathyroid glands.[6,9] Fewer than four glands are reported in approximately 3% of cases, although this figure probably represents an overestimate due to the failure to identify 'missing' glands successfully. The remarkable symmetry of the parathyroids is a feature of tremendous value to the surgeon because it facilitates gland identification. Superior gland symmetry occurs in 80% of cases, whilst the inferior glands have a symmetrical location in 70%. All four glands demonstrate a symmetrical position in 60% of cases.[6] When asymmetry does occur, both parathyroids on a single side may be located either above or below the intersection of the inferior thyroid artery and the recurrent laryngeal nerve. A common asymmetry of the inferior glands is when one gland is ectopically located within the thymus.

Superior parathyroid glands

The superior parathyroids are fairly constant in position because of their limited embryological descent. More than 80% are located in an area 2 cm in diameter centred 1 cm above the intersection of the inferior thyroid artery and the recurrent laryngeal nerve[6,10] (Fig. 16.3). The superior gland often has a surrounding halo of fat and is freely mobile on the thyroid capsule. The surrounding fat probably represents atrophic thymic tissue originating from the fourth branchial pouch.[7] When the superior gland is situated more anteriorly it may be bound by the thyroid capsule and is therefore less mobile.

Superior gland ectopia is less common compared with the inferior glands. The former are located in a somewhat

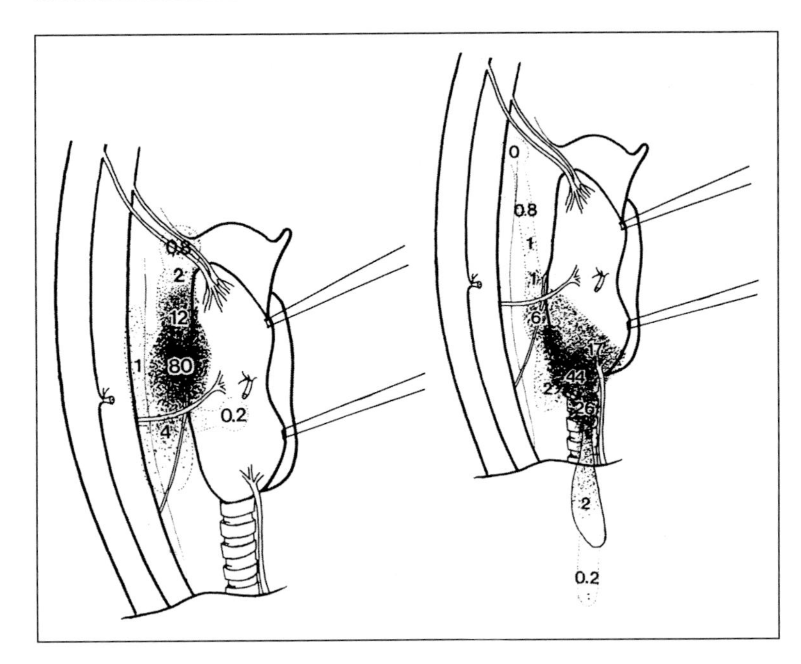

Fig. 16.3 Locations of the superior (left) and inferior (right) parathyroid glands. The more common locations are indicated by the darker shading. The numbers represent the percentages of glands found at the different locations. Observations are based on findings in 503 unselected autopsy cases. Reprinted from Surgery, 95, Åkerström G, Malmaeus J, Bergström R, Surgical anatomy of human parathyroid glands, 14–21, Copyright (1984), with permission from Elsevier.

posterior position. In descent, the superior glands tend to move posteriorly and the further caudal their migration, the more posterior their ultimate location will be. Superior parathyroid glands located in a caudal position may be partially obscured by the recurrent laryngeal nerve, inferior thyroid artery or tubercle of Zuckerkandl. Retropharyngeal or retro-oesophageal locations have also been described. A superior gland located in the posterior mediastinum alongside the oesophagus usually reflects migration of an enlarged adenomatous gland which has occurred due to oesophageal peristalsis and deglutition.[11,12]

Occasionally, superior glands are found on the posterior aspect of the thyroid upper pole or in relation to the superior vascular pedicle. Rarer still, they are located superior to the upper pole of the thyroid. The vast majority of superior glands considered to be 'intrathyroidal' are not truly so. They are better described as hidden in a cleft of nodular thyroid tissue.

Inferior parathyroid glands

The inferior parathyroids are much more likely to be widely distributed and ectopic due to their relatively long embryological migration.[6,8,9] During descent they tend to move anteriorly. The vast majority of glands are located in relation to the posterior or infero-ventral aspect of the lower thyroid pole (Fig. 16.3). Sometimes they are found at a slightly higher level close to the intersection of the inferior thyroid artery and the recurrent laryngeal nerve. A small minority migrate toward the posterior mediastinum. Approximately 25% are located within the thyrothymic ligament or posterior cervical thymic horns.[6] Approximately 4–5% occur in the anterior mediastinum located within retrosternal thymus or related to the innominate vein and ascending aorta. Only a few are located outside the thymus adjacent to the aortic arch and origin of the great vessels. An even lower position results in the inferior parathyroid being in contact with pleura or pericardium.

When the parathymus complex fails to descend fully, the inferior parathyroid may become stranded high in the neck. It is usually found with a segment of thymic tissue above the thyroid gland and superior to the superior parathyroid.[13,14] Less commonly, the gland is situated within the carotid sheath, medial to it or at the level of the mandible. The inferior parathyroid gland is truly intrathyroidal within the lower pole of thyroid in 1–3% of individuals.[15]

Supernumerary parathyroid glands

Supernumerary glands are reported in 13% of individuals. It is important to differentiate between the small rudimentary rests of parathyroid tissue derived from embryological parathyroid debris and true supernumerary glands. The former weigh less than 5 mg compared with true supernumerary glands which, on average, weigh 24 mg.

True supernumerary glands only occur in 5% of cases and occupy a location completely separate from the four normally situated glands. Two-thirds are located within the thymus or thyrothymic ligament below the thyroid gland and one-third are found close to the thyroid between two normally situated parathyroids.[6] In some individuals a fifth gland occurs due to splitting of a normal or bi-lobed gland during development. The two components lie close together and are often in direct contact with each other.

Occasionally, multiple supernumerary glands are present. They arise in pathological states with an underlying genetic disorder such as MEN1 (multiple endocrine neoplasia type 1). They also occur in renal failure-associated hyperparathyroidism in which there is an ongoing stimulatory influence. Surgically challenging ectopias are often due to the unusual location of supernumerary glands. Parathyroid glands have been found lateral to the jugular carotid complex,[16] within the piriform fossa,[17] in the vagus nerve,[18] in the aortopulmonary window[19] and deep in the thorax within the middle mediastinum. In one case, a pathological parathyroid gland was identified between the right main bronchus and right pulmonary artery. This gland, considered superior parathyroid in origin, was actually both ectopic and supernumerary.[19]

PARATHYROID ENDOCRINOLOGY

Normal human physiological cell function is dependent upon the precise regulation of the extracellular fluid calcium concentration. An extremely elegant mechanism has evolved in which the parathyroid glands play a crucial role. This involves the production and release of parathyroid hormone (PTH) which is an 84 amino acid polypeptide hormone. The circulating concentration of PTH can be precisely measured by two-site radioimmunoassay or immunochemiluminescent assay.[21]

Biological activity rests primarily with the N-terminal third of the PTH molecule (residues 1–34). The mid and C-terminal portions are devoid of PTH-like activity. The intact hormone is cleaved in the circulation between residues 28 and 48 which results in marked heterogeneity consisting of intact hormone and a range of fragments. Mid/C-terminal fragments are metabolized and cleared by the kidneys and liver. Due to intracellular degradation, the parathyroid cell secretes inactive C-terminal fragments when the extracellular calcium concentration is elevated.

PTH is secreted in response to a fall in calcium concentration. It initiates an increase and correction of calcium levels by stimulating renal reabsorption of calcium via a cyclic AMP-dependent mechanism. This effect is accompanied by decreased renal reabsorption of phosphate. It also stimulates osteoclastic activity and increases intestinal absorption of calcium. The latter occurs due to a direct stimulatory effect and indirectly via PTH stimulation of 1α-hydroxylase activity in the kidney. This in turn produces increased renal synthesis of active 1,25-dihydroxy vitamin D_3. The renal enzymatic activity is also influenced by serum phosphate and calcium levels. PTH is thought to exert its effect on peripheral target tissues via a specific receptor. Its action on the skeleton is enhanced by vitamin D_3.

The close correlation of the actions of PTH and 1,25-dihydroxy vitamin D_3 facilitate the precise regulation of extracellular calcium levels within a narrow physiological range.

The synthesis and release of PTH from the parathyroid cell is controlled by a complex and sophisticated mechanism. Calcium is the principal regulator, with an increase in extracellular Ca^{2+} inhibiting PTH release. This is in marked contrast to the stimulatory effect of calcium displayed in most other endocrine cells and systems. The control of PTH released from the parathyroids is mediated via cell surface membrane calcium receptors and other calcium-activated channels.[22,23]

The relationship between the extracellular ionized calcium concentration and PTH release is inversely sigmoidal. Physiological calcium levels are related to the steepest part of the curve, thus permitting PTH to exert powerful control over even small calcium changes[23] (Fig. 16.4). In the hypercalcaemic state of hyperparathyroidism there is a shift to the right and a decreased slope of the sigmoidal calcium/PTH response curve. Thus the set-point, defined as the calcium level at which PTH secretion is inhibited by 50%, is raised.

Changes in extracellular Ca^{2+} concentration influence the intracellular cytoplasmic calcium concentration which is the essential intracellular factor controlling PTH release.

An early rapid release of intracellular calcium from the endoplasmic reticulum may be an important component which accounts for the rise in intracellular calcium levels. The relationship between extracellular and intracellular calcium concentration is positively sigmoidal with

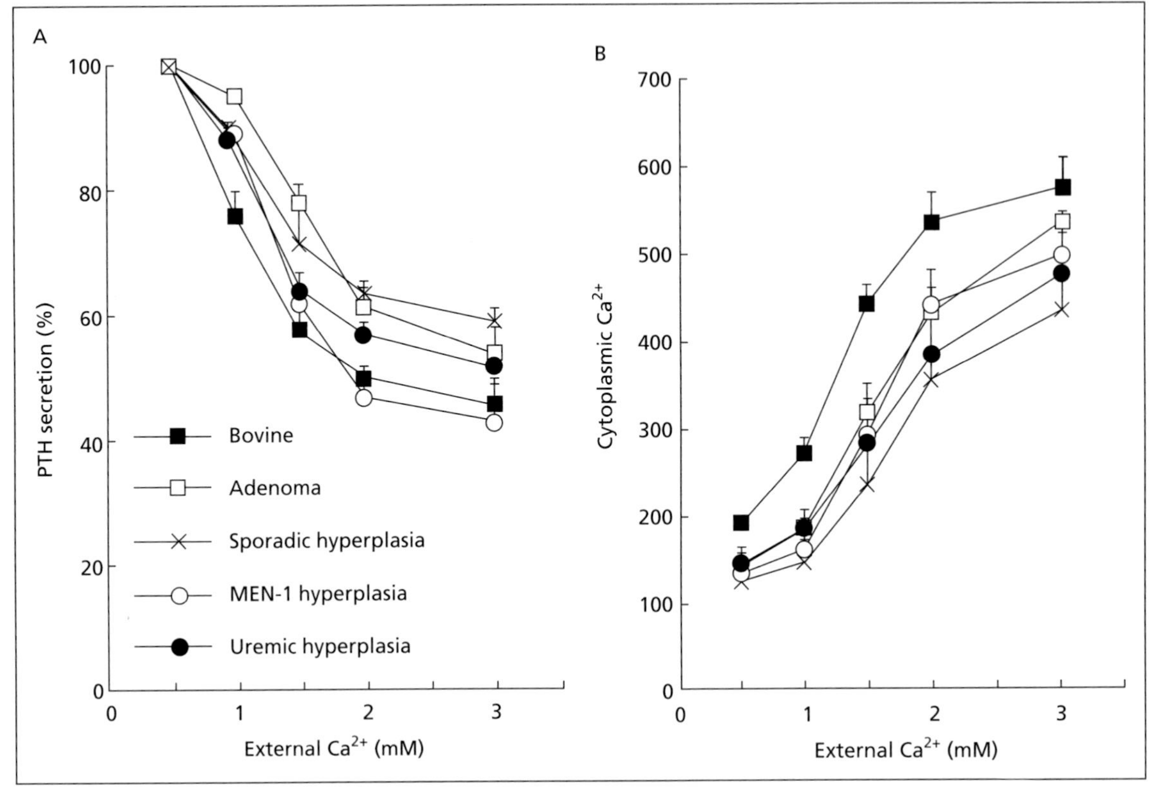

Fig. 16.4 Effects of extracellular ionized calcium on PTH release (A) and the steady-state cytoplasmic calcium concentration (B) of dispersed parathyroid cells from normal bovine glands, parathyroid adenomas ($n = 19$), hyperplastic glands of sporadic primary hyperparathyroidism (HPT) ($n = 6$), familial HPT of MEN1 ($n = 8$) and hyperplastic glands of secondary HPT ($n = 20$). PTH is expressed as a percentage of the release at 0.5 mM Ca^{2+}. Reproduced with permission from: Hellman P, Åkerström G, Juhlin C *et al.* Pathophysiology of hyperparathyroidism. In: Åkerström G, ed. *Current Controversy in Parathyroid Operation and Reoperation.* Austin: RG Landes Co (LandesBioscience.com), 1994:10.

biphasic characteristics, which suggests a receptor-mediated mechanism.[23] A 500 kDa glycoprotein has been identified as one such calcium-sensing receptor. Its expression is reduced in hyperparathyroidism, thus shedding some light on the pathophysiological derangement which occurs in this condition.[24]

Vitamin D exerts a suppressive effect on PTH mRNA transcription[25] which demonstrates yet another important aspect of the complex inter-relationship between PTH and vitamin D. A reduced expression of vitamin D receptors has been identified in parathyroid adenomas.

SUMMARY

Understanding the relatively complex embryology of the parathyroid glands enables the parathyroid surgeon to appreciate the nuances of both normal and abnormal parathyroid anatomy. This is essential for a sound basis in parathyroid surgery. In recent years, there have been significant advances in our understanding of parathyroid physiology and the derangement which occurs in hyperparathyroidism. There have also been considerable advances in knowledge of the complex inter-relationship between calcium, PTH and vitamin D_3, their regulation and the activity of calcium receptors on the parathyroid cell surface. These advances ultimately influence the role of the parathyroid surgeon and continue to pave the way for the development of new treatment strategies.

EVIDENCE APPRAISAL

The first two sections of this chapter address parathyroid embryology and anatomy.

The majority of papers cited are based on sound historical facts and extremely carefully conducted anatomical and autopsy studies. Therefore, inevitably, these papers have a high evidence base, the findings being beyond reasonable doubt. References 16, 17, 18 and 19 are to some extent based on anecdotal evidence and therefore have a lower grading.

In the Endocrinology section, several of the papers cited contain more speculative evidence, e.g. references 22 and 24. Additional data will be required before the evidence level can be moved beyond 'on the balance of probabilities'.

REFERENCES

1. Owen R. On the anatomy of the Indian rhinoceros (*Rh unicornis*, L). Trans Zool Soc Lond 1862;iv:31–58.
2. Sandström I. On a new gland in man and several mammals —glandulae parathyroideae. Uppsala Läk Förenings Förh 1879–80;15:441–71.
3. Boyd JD. Development of thyroid and parathyroid glands and the thymus. Ann R Coll Surg Engl 1950;7:455–71.
4. Embryology. In: Johnston TB, Davies DV, Davies F, eds. Gray's anatomy, 32nd edn. London: Longmans, Green and Co., 1958:183–5.
5. Sanders LE, Cady B. Embryology and developmental abnormalities. In: Cady B, Rossi RL, eds. Surgery of the thyroid and parathyroid glands, 3rd edn. Philadelphia: WB Saunders Company, 1991:5–12.
6. Åkerström G, Malmaeus J, Bergström R. Surgical anatomy of human parathyroid glands. Surgery 1984;95:14–21.
7. Gilmour JR, Martin WJ. The weight of the parathyroid glands. J Pathol 1937;44:431–62.
8. Wang CA. The anatomic basis of parathyroid surgery. Ann Surg 1976;183:271–5.
9. Gilmour JR. The gross anatomy of the parathyroid glands. J Pathol 1938;46:133–49.
10. Thompson NW. The techniques of initial parathyroid exploration and reoperative parathyroidectomy. In: Thompson NW, Vinik AI, eds. Endocrine surgery update. New York: Grune and Stratton, 1983:365–83.
11. Wheeler MH. Primary hyperparathyroidism: a surgical perspective. Ann R Coll Surg Engl 1998;80:305–12.
12. Thompson NW. Surgical anatomy of hyperparathyroidism. In: Rothmund M, Wells SA, eds. Parathyroid surgery. Basel: Karger, 1986:59.
13. Edis AJ, Purnell DC, van Heerden JA. The undescended 'parathymus': an occasional cause of failed neck exploration for hyperparathyroidism. Ann Surg 1979;190:64–8.
14. Fraker DL, Doppman JL, Shawker TH, *et al.* Undescended parathyroid adenoma: an important etiology for failed operations for primary hyperparathyroidism. World J Surg 1990;14:342–8.
15. Wheeler MH, Williams ED, Wade JSH. The hyperfunctioning intrathyroidal parathyroid gland: a potential pitfall in parathyroid surgery. World J Surg 1987;11:110–4.
16. Udekwu AO, Kaplan EL, Wu T-C, *et al.* Ectopic parathyroid adenoma of the lateral triangle of the neck: report of two cases. Surgery 1987;101:114–8.
17. Joseph MP, Nadol JB, Goodman ML. Ectopic parathyroid tissue in the hypopharyngeal mucosa (pyriform sinus). Head Neck Surg 1982;5:70–4.
18. Raffaelli M, Defechereux T, Lubrano D, *et al.* Intravagal ectopic parathyroid gland. Ann Chir 2000;125:961–4.
19. Curley IR, Wheeler MH, Thompson NW, *et al.* The challenge of the middle mediastinal parathyroid. World J Surg 1988;12:818–24.
20. Nobori MN, Saiki S, Tanaka N, *et al.* Blood supply of the parathyroid gland from the superior thyroid artery. Surgery 1994;115:417–23.
21. Curley IR, Wheeler MH, Aston JP, *et al.* Studies in patients with hyperparathyroidism using a new two-site immunochemiluminometric assay for circulating intact (1–84) parathyroid hormone. Surgery 1987;102:926–31.
22. Juhlin C, Holmdahl R, Johansson H, *et al.* Monoclonal antibodies with exclusive reactivity against parathyroid cells and tubule cells of the kidney. Proc Natl Acad Sci USA 1987; 84:2990–4.
23. Hellman P, Åkerström G, Juhlin C, *et al.* Pathophysiology of hyperparathyroidism. In: Åkerström G, ed. Current controversy in parathyroid operation and reoperation. Austin, TX: RG Landes Company, 1994:9–22.
24. Juhlin C, Klareskog L, Nygren P, *et al.* Hyperparathyroidism is associated with reduced expression of a parathyroid calcium receptor mechanism defined by monoclonal antiparathyroid antibodies. Endocrinology 1988;122:2999–3001.
25. Farrow SM, Hawa NS, Karmali R, *et al.* Binding of the receptor for 1,25-dihydroxyvitamin D3 to the 5'-flanking region of the bovine parathyroid hormone gene. J Endocrinol 1990;126:355–9.

MULTIPLE CHOICE QUESTIONS

Select more than one option where appropriate.

1. The superior parathyroid glands

A. Arise from the ventral aspect of the fourth branchial pouch

B Develop in association with the lateral thyroid lobes (ultimobranchial body)

C. Migrate inferiorly with the thymus

D. Have a relatively short caudal descent

2. The superior parathyroid glands

A. Are frequently ectopic

B. Are never located superior to the upper thyroid pole

C. Are rarely intrathyroidal
D. Can be located at a level caudal to the inferior parathyroids

3. The inferior parathyroid glands
A. Have a low propensity for ectopia
B. Are usually located in relation to the lower thyroid pole
C. Are found in the thymus in 50% of individuals
D. May be located within the carotid sheath

4. Parathyroid glands
A. Are mostly flat or bilobed
B Are firmer in consistency than the thyroid
C. Are easily dissected from surrounding fat
D. Have a mean normal weight of 80 mg
E Have a close anatomical relationship to the trachea

5. Parathyroid hormone (PTH)
A. Is secreted in response to a raised extracellular calcium level
B. Is a polypeptide containing 84 amino acids
C. Has biological activity at the C-terminal end of the molecule
D. Is cleaved at residue 60
E. Inhibits renal reabsorption of phosphate

Answers

1. B, D
2. C, D
3. B, D
4. C
5. B, E

17 Management of parathyroid disease

Paolo Miccoli, Gabriele Materazzi & Piero Berti
Department of Surgery, University of Pisa, Italy

KEY POINTS

- Treatment of primary hyperparathyroidism is predominantly surgical. Minimally invasive surgical techniques have become popular in recent years
- Minimally invasive parathyroidectomy utilizes a smaller skin incision compared with the conventional 'open' approach. Maintaining adequate access and operative field of vision is a prerequisite, and endoscopes are usually, but not always, used to facilitate this
- It is not known if the long-term results of the minimally invasive approach are comparable with the traditional open approach for bilateral parathyroid exploration
- The intra-operative 'quick' parathyroid hormone assay (qPTHa) has been widely adopted because it reduces operative time and facilitates positive localization in both the minimally invasive endoscopic and open bilateral exploration approach
- Calcimimetics effectively reduce PTH secretion in all forms of hyperparathyroidism. This group of drugs is likely to become an established therapy for secondary hyperparathyroidism associated with renal failure and for selected patients with primary hyperparathyroidism

INTRODUCTION

Primary hyperparathyroidism (PHPT) is generally considered to be rare, although recent evidence suggests that it is actually quite a common disease entity.[1] Current international guidelines suggest that medical management plays a minor role even in the asymptomatic patient. Surgical management remains the mainstay of treatment at present.[2,3] A recent prospective randomized controlled study of patients with PHPT conducted in our unit demonstrated significantly better long-term outcome in patients treated with parathyroidectomy compared with medical management or surveillance.[4] The role of surgical treatment has expanded to encompass the recent trend of minimally invasive parathyroid surgery. Perceived advantages of this technique include shorter operative time, less post-operative pain and improved cosmesis.

A Practical Manual of Thyroid and Parathyroid Disease, 1st Edition. Edited by Asit Arora, Neil Tolley & R. Michael Tuttle.

MEDICAL TREATMENT

At the time of writing, there are no approved medical treatments available for PHPT. There certainly is a role for non-surgical therapy which can successfully suppress parathyroid hormone (PTH) and normalize elevated serum calcium levels. This would be particularly useful in patients in whom surgical therapy has failed or whose co-morbidity represents an unacceptable surgical risk. Patients with metastatic parathyroid carcinoma would also benefit from such therapy. A non-surgical alternative for asymptomatic PHPT is also desirable because patients are at risk of developing progressive bone disease and renal complications.[5] Oestrogen therapy has been used with limited success to decrease serum calcium levels and increase bone mass in patients with PHPT.[6] Alendronate has also been used to increase bone mass, although neither treatment suppresses PTH.[7]

It is well established that PTH secretion by chief cells in the parathyroid gland is regulated by extracellular ionized calcium. The molecular mechanism by which this is achieved was deduced by Brown and Hebert in 1993 when they successfully cloned the extracellular calcium-sensing receptor (CaSR).[8] Genetic studies have demonstrated that the activity of this receptor determines the steady-state plasma calcium concentration in humans by regulating key elements in the calcium homeostatic system. CaSR agonists (calcimimetics) and antagonists (calcilytics) were subsequently developed in an attempt to provide potential treatment for a variety of calcium-related disorders.

Calcimimetics can effectively reduce PTH secretion in all forms of hyperparathyroidism. They are likely to become a major therapy in secondary hyperparathyroidism associated with renal failure and for treatment of certain patients with PHPT. A large variety of inorganic and organic cations have been discovered which interact with the calcium-sensitive N-terminal domain of CaSR thus mimicking the effects of calcium. These are termed type I calcimimetics. Unfortunately they exhibit substantial limitations for use in clinical practice. A second class of compounds, termed type II calcimimetics, has been developed (NPS R-467, S-467, R-568, S-568 and AMG 073).[9] These compounds, following interaction with the membrane-spanning domains of the CaSR, induce conformational changes in the N-terminal domain which increases affinity for calcium.

Pre-clinical trials of calcimimetics in animal models have demonstrated that they are effective in reducing circulating PTH, preventing progression of hyperparathyroidism, suppressing parathyroid cell proliferation and reversing osteitis fibrosa. Further clinical studies were performed using AMG 073 which has a greater bioavailability and more consistent pharmacokinetic profile than other type II calcimimetics. AMG 073 appears to be effective in reducing both PTH and calcium serum levels, with a good safety profile.[10] Studies focusing on the efficacy of AMG 073 in uraemic patients with secondary hyperparathyroidism showed a 30% reduction in PTH levels in nearly half the patient cohort. This was matched by a 5–7% reduction in both calcium and phosphate serum levels.[2,11,12]

On the therapeutic horizon are calcilytics (e.g. NPS 2143) which transiently increase PTH via inhibition of CaSR. They may therefore potentially inhibit the progression of osteoporosis (see Chapter 13).

SURGICAL TREATMENT

Indications for surgery

Parathyroidectomy is recommended for all patients with symptomatic PHPT and for asymptomatic patients who fulfil the following criteria:

- serum calcium 1 mg/dl above the normal range
- urine calcium >400 mg/24 hours
- creatinine clearance reduced by 30% compared with age-matched normal individuals
- bone mineral density T score 2.5 standard deviations below that of gender-matched controls at any site (hip, lumbar spine, forearm)
- <50 years old
- medical surveillance is not possible or desirable.[13]

Considerable controversy exists regarding the management of patients with mild, asymptomatic PHPT.

Pre-operative preparation

Most patients have moderately raised serum calcium levels and should be well hydrated pre-operatively with an overnight intravenous 0.9% saline infusion. Severe cases require specific measures to reduce calcium levels adequately. Usually this entails a forced diuresis which is achieved by intravenous infusion of 2–3 litres of 0.9% saline over 24 hours in addition to a diuretic such as furosemide. Patients with calcium levels in excess of 3.5 mmol/l require disodium pamidronate (15–30 mg in 500 ml of 0.9% saline infused over 4 hours). A dose of 60–90 mg of disodium pamidronate is justified when calcium levels exceed 4.0 mmol/l.

Intravenous phosphate has a very limited role in the management of severe hypercalcaemia due to the potential for catastrophic precipitation of calcium throughout the soft tissues and kidneys. It should therefore only be used when rapid removal of calcium from extracellular fluid is necessary, usually in the presence of severe cardiovascular complications. In this situation, 50–100 mmol phosphate may be given intravenously over 4–6 hours or as a single dose immediately before urgent surgery. Rarely, dialysis may be necessary in order to render a patient fit for surgery. There is virtually no role for mithramicin and steroids, whilst the use of calcitonin has been totally abandoned in our unit.

Pre-operative flexible nasoendoscopy by an ENT specialist is essential to record vocal cord function.

Types of operation

Wide exposure and evaluation of all four parathyroids has been the accepted surgical practice ever since 1925 when Felix Mandl performed the first successful parathyroidectomy in Vienna. The 'traditional' open approach utilizes a collar incision and involves bilateral exploration of the neck to identify all four parathyroids and remove abnormal parathyroid tissue. This approach achieves cure in 97% of cases and is associated with minimal morbidity.[14,15]

In the mid-1980s, unilateral exploration was advocated by some authorities. This approach permits removal of the single abnormal gland and visualization of a normal second ipsilateral gland. It avoids the need for contralateral exploration and its associated potential morbidity.[16,17] However, the possibility of missing a contralateral double adenoma or asymmetrical hyperplasia was an initial concern with this targeted approach. These reservations have largely been superseded due to considerable improvement in pre-operative imaging and localization studies, which have also facilitated development of the minimally invasive approach.

TRADITIONAL (OPEN) VERSUS MINIMALLY INVASIVE TECHNIQUES

Traditional parathyroidectomy

A transverse cervical incision approximately 5 cm in length is made, 2 cm above the sternal notch. Subplatysmal flaps are developed superiorly to the thyroid cartilage, laterally to the sternocleidomastoid muscles and inferiorly to the sternal notch. Exploration is directed to the side indicated by pre-operative studies. If these are negative, the right side is explored first as parathyroid adenomas most commonly arise in the right lower parathyroid gland. The strap muscles are separated along the midline and dissected laterally from the thyroid gland by blunt dissection. The middle thyroid veins are usually divided to allow anteromedial mobilization of the thyroid lobes. Meticulous haemostasis is crucial at all times, and the recurrent laryngeal nerve and inferior thyroid artery should be identified and preserved.

Minimally invasive parathyroidectomy

Minimally invasive procedures were first popularized by Michel Gagner who pioneered the endoscopic technique in 1997.[18] The term 'minimally invasive' is potentially misleading and it should not be considered a technique that only shortens the skin incision. The concept of reducing invasiveness extends to other structures whilst maintaining or indeed enhancing the operative field of vision. Endoscopes are usually used to achieve this. In addition to the endoscopic technique, other minimally invasive approaches have been described which involve small skin incisions (3–4 cm) made directly over the suspected adenoma.[24] Intra-operative nuclear mapping, first described by Norman, greatly facilitates this approach.[23] An unequivocal, positive pre-operative scintiscan localization study is mandatory. Sometimes a single, well-defined parathyroid adenoma is not identified by scintiscan. In our experience, this occurs in 10% of patients undergoing parathyroid exploration. Following pre-operative localization with ultrasound (US), they are excellent candidates for the endoscopic or video-assisted approach as radio-guided parathyroidectomy is not possible.

ENDOSCOPIC PARATHYROIDECTOMY TECHNIQUE

Several approaches have been described. The three most common techniques are:

1. endoscopic parathyroidectomy (Gagner 1996)[19]
2. video-assisted parathyroidectomy with external retraction (Miccoli 1997)[20,21]
3. videoscopic parathyroidectomy by a lateral approach (Henry 1998).[22]

Endoscopic parathyroidectomy (Fig. 17.1)

This was the first technique described for performing minimally invasive parathyroidectomy. It uses low-pressure CO_2 insufflation (8 mm Hg).[19] A 5 mm endoscope (initially 0°, switching to 30° once the subplatysmal

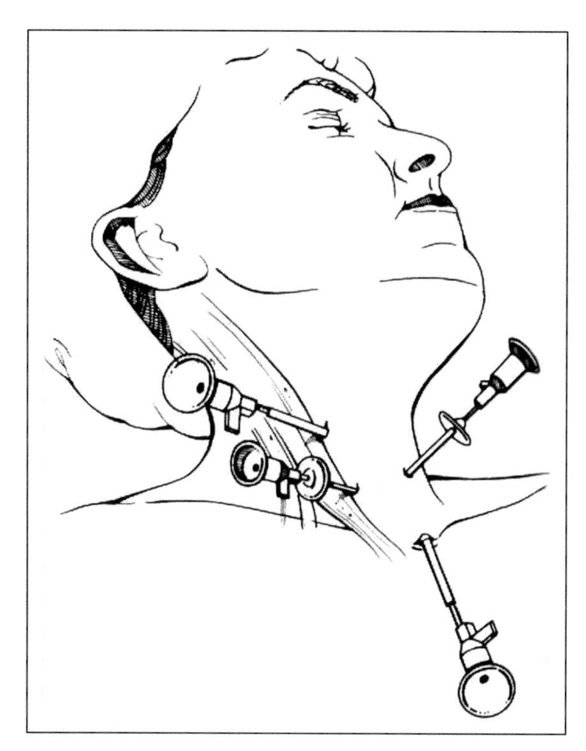

Fig. 17.1 Endoscopic parathyroidectomy. A 5 mm endoscope is inserted through a central neck trocar. Two or three additional trocars are inserted along the anterior border of the sternocleidomastoid which are required for needle-scopic instrument placement.

plane is reached) is placed through a central neck trocar with two or three additional trocars used for needlescopic instrument placement. Subplatysmal planes are dissected to obtain a good working space. The space anterior to the sternocleidomastoid is then opened and the strap muscles retracted medially to expose the thyroid gland lobes. The thyroid gland is dissected from the investing fascia and the parathyroid glands explored. Bilateral exploration is possible and, following identification and mobilization of the parathyroid adenoma, its vascular pedicle is dissected and divided between two 5 mm ligature clips. The gland is then extracted in a small sac fashioned from the fingertip of a surgical glove. Intraoperative quick parathyroid hormone assay (qPTHa) is performed 10 and 20 min after excision.

Video-assisted parathyroidectomy with external retraction

This technique does not require trocar insertion or gas insufflation. The patient's neck is not extended in the usual fashion because this position does not permit sufficient operative space deep to the strap muscles.

A transverse incision 1.5 cm long is made 2 cm above the sternal notch. Meticulous haemostasis is essential. The strap muscles are separated in the midline over a distance 3 cm longitudinally. Two retractors are used: one to lateralize the strap muscles and carotid artery on the side of the suspected adenoma whilst the other retracts the thyroid lobe medially. The thyroid lobe is mobilized from the strap muscles using small spatulas under direct vision. The middle thyroid vein is ligated and divided, exposing the thyro-tracheal groove, and a 30° 5 mm endoscope is then introduced through the incision. The rest of the procedure is performed endoscopically using small re-usable surgical instruments (spatulas, forceps, scissors and vascular clips). The video-assisted procedure requires three surgeons: primary surgeon, first assistant (holds the endoscope and spatula–aspirator) and second assistant (holds the retractors). Although only one side of the neck is usually explored, bilateral exploration is possible through the same incision. The adenoma is located and carefully mobilized with spatulas, taking care not to disrupt the capsule. Optical magnification affords the surgeon excellent visualization of the pedicle which is clipped (Plate 17.1). The excised adenoma is retrieved through the skin incision which is subsequently closed with a skin sealant whilst awaiting the qPTHa result (Fig. 17.2).

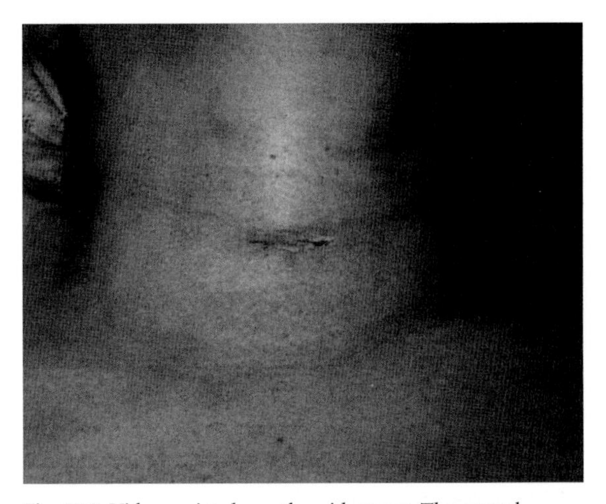

Fig. 17.2 Video-assisted parathyroidectomy. The central 1.5 cm incision is closed with a skin sealant. The cosmetic result is usually excellent.

Videoscopic parathyroidectomy by a lateral approach

In the lateral approach (originally described by Henry) a 12 mm skin crease incision is made over the medial border of the sternocleidomastoid on the side of the suspected adenoma.[12] A 10 mm trocar is inserted and, following low-pressure CO_2 insufflation, a 0° 10 mm endoscope is placed through this. Two 3 mm trocars are inserted along the medial margin of the sternocleidomastoid below and above the first trocar. Modified instruments are introduced through the smaller trocars and the adenoma is gently dissected by the primary surgeon whilst an assistant holds the endoscope. Once the gland has been completely isolated it is partly extracted and the pedicle is externally ligated using conventional forceps. Intra-operative qPTHa is essential because bilateral exploration is not possible with this technique.

INDICATIONS FOR MIVAP (MINIMALLY INVASIVE VIDEO-ASSISTED PARATHYROIDECTOMY)

The ideal candidate for MIVAP is a patient with sporadic PHPT and a single, well-localized adenoma who has not previously undergone neck exploration. Contraindications to MIVAP are classified as absolute or relative (Table 17.1).

Careful patient selection is vital to ensure a low conversion rate and achieve good patient outcome. Patient

Table 17.1 Absolute and relative contraindications to MIVAP

Relative contraindications	Absolute contraindications
Adenomas larger than 3 cm*	Large goitres
Lack of pre-operative localization†	Recurrent disease
Neck surgery on the opposite side of the suspected adenoma‡	Extensive previous neck surgery
Previous neck irradiation or small thyroid nodules§	MEN and familial PHPT
	Parathyroid carcinoma

* Depending upon their shape, even larger adenomas can be removed.
† Bilateral exploration can be performed through a central incision.
‡ A lateral access can be used.
§ Concurrent thyroidectomy is possible.

eligibility for minimally invasive parathyroidectomy depends on the selection criteria applied. The use of this approach ranges from 25% to as much as 66% in reported case series.[21,25] In our unit, the selection criteria continue to evolve and be modified as our experience develops. This probably reflects the enhancement of our technique and continued improvement in surgical instrumentation.

INTRA-OPERATIVE PTH ASSAY

This was first introduced in 1990 and represents an alternative to four-gland visualization as it confirms adequate removal of hypersecreting parathyroid tissue. Rapid intra-operative PTH assay is possible due to George Irvin's ground breaking work on the qPTHa which produces results within 12 minutes. Blood samples are obtained from a peripheral intravenous cannula prior to parathyroid exploration (basal value), during manipulation of the adenoma, and 5 and 10 minutes after removal of hyperfunctioning parathyroid tissue. Intact PTH has a half life of 2–4 minutes. Successful removal of diseased parathyroid tissue is confirmed by >50% reduction in basal PTH levels, which correctly predicts cure in 96% of cases.[26]

Role of frozen sections

The role of the pathologist in parathyroid surgery is to identify excised tissue correctly and distinguish normal from abnormal parathyroid tissue. The distinction between hyperplasia and adenoma is based on operative findings rather than pathological criteria. Definitive treatment of PHPT involves removing all hyperfunctioning parathyroid tissue. When a qPTHa is not available, all four parathyroids should be identified. Biopsy of each parathyroid is not necessary and may lead to post-operative hypoparathyroidism[27–29] Intra-operative qPTHa represents a valid alternative to frozen section during parathyroid exploration because qPTHa reliably predicts when hyperfunctioning parathyroid tissue has been removed.

COMPLICATIONS OF SURGERY

Traditional open parathyroidectomy has a 95% success rate and negligible complication rate. Potential complications include hypoparathyroidism, recurrent laryngeal nerve palsy and post-operative bleeding.

Hypoparathyroidism

The incidence of post-operative hypoparathyroidism depends on the type of the operation performed, the number of parathyroids excised and size of adenoma removed. Other factors include:

- atrophy of residual glands which occurs when there has been a long-standing single hyperfunctioning adenoma and prolonged hypercalcaemia
- hungry bone syndrome
- previous parathyroid or thyroid surgery.

A transient hypocalcaemia is more likely to occur following parathyroidectomy for hyperplasia than following excision of a solitary, small adenoma in which contralateral exploration is not performed.

Patients exhibiting clinical signs of hypocalcaemia such as peri-oral or acral paraesthesia, muscle cramps or numbness of the hands and feet are treated with oral calcium carbonate or calcium lactate. This is prescribed in divided doses up to a maximum dose of 8 g per day. Calciferol or dihydrotachysterol may also be necessary to enhance calcium absorption. Management of hypocalcaemia on the first post-operative day is summarized in Table 17.2. Oral calcium supplementation is continued following normalization of serum calcium levels until stable calcium homeostasis is achieved. Sometimes long-term supplementation is necessary, particularly following re-operative parathyroid surgery or resection of multiple gland disease.

Severe symptoms require immediate intravenous therapy with 10 ml of 10% calcium gluconate given over

Table 17.2 Management of hypocalcaemia following parathyroidectomy on the first post-operative day

Acute symptomatic	Calcium gluconate (1 g/8 hours intravenously)
Asymptomatic calcium <7.5 mg/dl*	Calcium (3 g) + vitamin D (0.5 µg) orally daily
Asymptomatic calcium 7.5–7.9 mg/dl	Calcium (1.5 g) orally daily

* Normal range: 8–10 mg/dl.

3–5 minutes. A subsequent 24 hour continuous infusion of 0.9% saline containing 30–40 ml of 10% calcium gluconate is prescribed. Intravenous calcium should only ever be administered via a central line due to the risk of small vessel thrombophlebitis.

The introduction of minimally invasive surgery with unilateral exploration and intra-operative qPTHa has resulted in a dramatic reduction of this complication.[30] Even with the traditional open approach, unilateral exploration and intra-operative qPTHa avoid the unnecessary removal of enlarged glands with normal function, thereby minimizing the risk of post-operative hypocalcaemia.[31] When hypocalcaemia does occur, it is treated with vitamin D and/or calcium supplementation.

Recurrent laryngeal nerve palsy

This is a rare complication. Most series report a rate of 1% or less in both the traditional open and minimal access approach.[32,33] The nerve is particularly vulnerable when dissection and removal of the adenoma occurs in close proximity to branches of the inferior thyroid artery. This is a particular risk during removal of a superior adenoma which has grown inferiorly and is located in the upper posterior mediastinum behind the inferior thyroid artery. The endoscopic magnification afforded by MIVAP greatly facilitates identification and dissection of the nerve when it lies in close proximity to the adenoma.

Post-operative haematoma

Haemostasis should be meticulous and drains are not required in patients undergoing first or second explorations. The incidence of haematomas requiring intervention is less than 0.5%. They are readily treated by incision and drainage or by US-guided needle aspiration.

OVERVIEW OF SURGICAL MANAGEMENT: SINGLE ADENOMA, HYPERPLASIA AND CARCINOMA

When exploring patients for PHPT there are five possible scenarios:

1. Single gland disease
2. Hyperplasia of four or more glands
3. Double adenoma
4. Carcinoma
5. No abnormal pathology found.

Single gland disease

When there is one enlarged parathyroid tumour and three normal parathyroids the abnormal parathyroid is removed. The remaining glands are identified and their location recorded. Some authorities recommend a biopsy of each normal gland with frozen section identification. The authors do not perform this because of the associated incidence of post-operative hypoparathyroidism. We prefer intraoperative qPTHa which is readily available in our unit.

Parathyroid hyperplasia

Multigland hyperplasia occurs in 10–30% of patients with PHPT. There are two types: clear-cell hyperplasia, which was described by Churchill in the 1930s, and chief cell hyperplasia, which was described by Cope in 1958. In the former, the parathyroid glands appear dark and are often irregular in shape and asymmetrical in size. Chief cell hyperplasia is the more common variant. It involves all four glands and is also associated with supernumerary glands. A parathyroid with chief cell hyperplasia is virtually indistinguishable from an adenoma because both consist predominantly of chief cells.

Three possible approaches are described for the management of parathyroid hyperplasia.

Total parathyroidectomy

The advantage of this approach is that the disease is likely to be cured. However, it does not fulfil the basic endocrine surgical concept of rendering the patient normocalcaemic.

Subtotal parathyroidectomy

This involves removal of three and a half glands. Some authorities consider this to be the best option. However, not all patients are rendered normocalcaemic and there is significant incidence of recurrence.

Total parathyroidectomy and parathyroid re-implantation

Total parathyroidectomy followed by transplantation of parathyroid tissue into the arm or sternocleidomastoid muscle is our favoured approach. It is essential that all the parathyroids are identified and removed together with the thymus. We then select the smallest gland for re-implantation. Parathyroid tissue is cooled in saline at 4°C for approximately 15 minutes which makes the tissue firm and easy to slice into 1 mm cubes. Approximately 50 mg of parathyroid tissue is transplanted into the brachialis muscle of the non-dominant arm. Alternatively, sternocleidomastoid muscle can be used. Fragments of parathyroid tissue are inserted into muscle, a small titanium clip is applied to the specific area of implantation and the incision is closed. Unused fragments of parathyroid tissue can be cryopreserved by freezing the tissue in a mixture of liquid nitrogen and dimethylsulphoxide. If further transplantation becomes necessary in the future, the frozen tissue can be rapidly thawed and is meticulously washed in tissue culture medium to remove the dimethylsulphoxide prior to re-implantation.

Parathyroid grafts become active after 1 week but may take as long as 6 months to do so. Until this happens, vitamin D and calcium supplementation is necessary. Graft survival occurs in 75–100% of parathyroid transplants.[34] Patients should have their serum calcium levels routinely monitored at 6 month intervals in view of the possibility of developing late hyperparathyroidism. Graft overgrowth and so-called 'graft-dependent' hypercalcaemia have been described in up to 15% of patients.[34] If this occurs, the graft can be excised under local anaesthetic, although parathyroid tissue often proliferates and has even been reported in enlarged axillary lymphatics.[34]

Double adenoma

Multiple adenomas occur in 5–15% of patients and double adenomas are found in at least 2% of patients with PHPT. It is unclear whether double adenomas represent a distinct pathological entity or are simply another manifestation of asymmetrical diffuse hyperplasia. The surgical management of this condition is controversial. Advocates of the 'hyperplasia theory' support subtotal parathyroidectomy or total parathyroidectomy with autotransplantation. Those who consider the double adenoma a separate disease entity advocate removal of only the clinically enlarged glands. Intra-operative qPTHa is useful in this scenario to determine the extent of parathyroidectomy.

Carcinoma

This is exceptionally rare. Patients usually have significantly elevated calcium and PTH levels. Surgical exploration reveals a solid parathyroid mass and the ipsilateral thyroid lobe may also be involved (Plate 17.2). Radical enbloc removal of the ipsilateral thyroid lobe together with the abnormal parathyroid is essential. Neck dissection for regional lymph nodes is warranted if the cervical lymph nodes appear abnormal.

Failed exploration

When four normal parathyroid glands are identified during exploration, any prominent lymph nodes in the surrounding area should be removed and sent for histology to exclude sarcoidosis. The thymus should also be excised for histological analysis to exclude a supernumerary parathyroid gland.

When a parathyroid gland cannot be found, the following steps should be taken:

- Open the thyroid capsule to inspect and palpate the thyroid gland
- Dissect the superior thymic/paratracheal tissue and perform a cervical thymectomy
- Mobilize the pharynx and oesophagus to visualise the para-/retropharyngo-oesophageal space
- Open the carotid sheath to expose the entire length of the common carotid artery in the neck
- Ligate the ipsilateral inferior thyroid artery and perform thyroid lobectomy, recording the location of any parathyroid glands successfully identified
- Abandon further exploration, check the serum calcium level for evidence of persistent hypercalcaemia and plan further localization investigations to assess the head, neck, mediastinum and thorax.

EVIDENCE APPRAISAL

The most recent guidelines emerging from different institutions regarding the optimal management of PHPT represent Level IV evidence.[2]

The data showing that alendronate increases bone mass in patients with PHPT represent Level II evidence.[7]

The recent work on CaSR agonists (calcimimetics) which show that they can effectively reduce PTH secretion in all forms of hyperparathyroidism represents Level II evidence.[10,11]

The data which suggest that there are advantages of the minimally invasive surgical approach such as reduced operative time, less painful operative course and cosmetic advantages represent Level IV evidence.[33]

REFERENCES

1. Colin R. Unilateral neck exploration for primary hyperparathyroidism. Surg Clin North Am 2004;84:705–16.
2. Bilezikian JP, Potts JT Jr, Fuleihan GE, *et al.* Summary statement from a workshop on asymptomatic primary hyperparathyroidism: a perspective for the 21st century. J Clin Endocrinol Metab 2002;87:5353–61.
3. Mack LA, Pasieka JL. Asymptomatic primary hyperparathyroidism: a surgical perspective. Surg Clin North Am 2004; 84:803–16.
4. Ambrogini E, Cetani F, Cianferotti L, *et al.* Surgery or surveillance for mild asymptomatic primary hyperparathyroidism: a prospective randomized clinical trial. J Clin Endocrinol Metab 2007;92:3114–21.
5. Silverberg SJ, Bilezikian JP. The diagnosis and management of asymptomatic primary hyperparathyroidism. Nat Clin Pract Endocrinol Metab 2006;2:494–503.
6. Farford B, Presutti RJ, Moraghan TJ. Nonsurgical management of primary hyperparathyroidism. Mayo Clin Proc 2007;82:351–5.
7. Khan AA, Bilezikian JP, Kung AW, *et al.* Alendronate in primary hyperparathyroidism: a double-blind, randomized, placebo-controlled trial. J Clin Endocrinol Metab 2004;89: 3319–25.
8. Brown EM, Gamba G, Riccardi D, *et al.* Cloning and characterization of an extracellular Ca^{2+}-sensing receptor from bovine parathyroid. Nature 1993;366:575–80.
9. Fox J, Lowe SH, Petty BA, *et al.* NPS R-568 : a type II calcimimetic compound that acts on parathyroid cell calcium receptor of rats to reduce plasma levels of parathyroid hormone and calcium. J Pharmacol Exp Ther 1999;290: 473–9.
10. Shoback DM, Bilezikian JP, Turner SA, *et al.* The calcimimetic cinacalcet normalizes serum calcium in subjects with primary hyperparathyroidism. J Clin Endocrinol Metab 2003;88:5644–9.
11. Lindberg J, Moe S, Goodman W, *et al.* The calcimimetic AMG-073 reduces parathyroid hormone (PTH), phosphorus and calcium×phosphorus product in secondary hyperparathyroidism. J Am Soc Nephrol 2003;63:248–54.
12. Drueke T, Cunningham J, Goodman W, *et al.* Short-term treatment of secondary hyperparathyroidism (SHTP) with the calcimimetic agent AMG 073. J Am Soc Nephrol 2001; 12:764.
13. Quarles L, Spiegel D, Curzi M, *et al.* The effects of one-year treatment with the calcimimetic AMG-073 on bone health in ESRD patients with secondary hyperparathyroidism (SHPT). J Am Soc Nephrol 2002;13:572A.
14. Schell SR, Dudley NE. Clinical outcomes and fiscal consequences of bilateral neck exploration for primary idiopathic hyperparathyroidism without preoperative radionuclide imaging or minimally invasive techniques. Surgery 2003; 133:32–9.
15. Clark O. What's new in endocrine surgery. J Am Coll Surg 1997;184:126–36.
16. Tibblin S, Bondeson AG, Ljungberg O. Unilateral parathyroidectomy in hyperparathyroidism due to parathyroid adenoma. Ann Surg 1982;195:245–52.
17. Wang CA. Surgical management of primary hyperparathyroidism. Curr Probl Surg 1985;22:1–50.
18. Gagner M. Endoscopic parathyroidectomy. Br J Surg 1996; 83:87.
19. Naitoh T, Gagner M, Garcia-Ruiz A, *et al.* Endoscopic endocrine surgery in the neck. An initial report of endoscopic subtotal parathyroidectomy. Surg Endosc 1998;12:202–5; discussion 206.
20. Miccoli P, Cecchini G, Conte M, *et al.* Minimally invasive, video-assisted parathyroid surgery for primary hyperparathyroidism. J Endocrinol Invest 1997;20:429–30.
21. Berti P, Materazzi G, Picone A, *et al.* Limits and drawbacks of video-assisted parathyroidectomy. Br J Surg 2003;90: 743–7.
22. Henry JF, Defechereux T, Gramatica L, *et al.* Minimally invasive videoscopic parathyroidectomy by lateral approach. Langenbecks Arch Surg 1999;384:298–301.
23. Norman J, Chheda H. Minimally invasive parathyroidectomy facilitated by intraoperative nuclear mapping. Surgery 1997;122:998–1003.
24. Goldstein RE, Blevins L, Delbeke D, *et al.* Effect of minimally invasive radio-guided parathyroidectomy on efficacy, length of stay, and costs in the management of primary hyperparathyroidism. Ann Surg 2000;231:732–42.
25. Gauger PG, Reeve TS, Delbridge LW. Endoscopically assisted, minimally invasive parathyroidectomy. Br J Surg. 1999; 86: 1563–6.
26. Irvin GL. Presidential address: chasin' hormones. Surgery 1999;126:993–7.
27. Perrier ND, Ituarte P, Kikuchi S, *et al.* Intraoperative parathyroid aspiration and parathyroid hormone assay as an alternative to frozen section for tissue identification. World J Surg 2000;24:1319–22.
28. Iacobone M, Scarpa M, Lumachi F, *et al.* Are frozen sections useful and cost-effective in the era of intraoperative qPTH assays? Surgery 2005;138:1159–64; discussion 1164–5.
29. Dewan AK, Kapadia SB, Hollenbeak CS, *et al.* Is routine frozen section necessary for parathyroid surgery? Otolaryngol Head Neck Surg 2005;133:857–62.
30. Lorenz K, Nguyen-Thanh P, Dralle H. Unilateral open and minimally invasive procedures for primary hyperparathyroidism: a review of selective approaches. Langenbecks Arch Surg 2000;385:106–17.

31. Vignali E, Picone A, Materazzi G, *et al.* A quick intraoperative parathyroid hormone assay in the surgical management of patients with primary hyperparathyroidism: a study of 206 consecutive cases. Eur J Endocrinol 2002;146:783–8.
32. Udelsman R. Six hundred fifty-six consecutive explorations for primary hyperparathyroidism. Ann Surg 2002;235:665–72.
33. Miccoli P, Berti P, Conte M, *et al.* Minimally invasive video assisted parathyroidectomy: lesson learned from 137 cases. J Am Coll Surg 2000;191:613–8.
34. Senapati A, Young AE. Parathyroid transplantation. Br J Surg 1990; 77:1171–4.

MULTIPLE CHOICE QUESTIONS

Select the single most appropriate option.

1. Surgery is indicated in patients with asymptomatic primary hyperparathyroidism when
A The serum calcium level is 1 mg/dl above the reported normal range
B. The serum calcium level is 2 mg/dl above the reported normal range
C. Creatinine clearance is reduced by 15% compared with age-matched normal individuals
D. Bone mineral density T score is 1.5 standard deviations below a sex-matched control

2. Primary hyperparathyroidism is caused by:
A. A single benign parathyroid tumour (parathyroid adenoma)
B. Two or more enlarged glands (parathyroid hyperplasia)
C. Parathyroid cancer
D. All of the above conditions

3. Parathyroid hyperplasia can be treated by:
A. Total parathyroidectomy
B. Subtotal parathyroidectomy
C. Total parathyroidectomy and reimplantation of parathyroid tissue
D. All of the above

4. Recurrent nerve palsy after parathyroidectomy is rare in all the series (both traditional operations and endoscopic approaches) with a rate of:
A. 3%
B. 0.01%
C. 0.1%
D. 1%

5. In the case of a negative parathyroid exploration:
A. Abandon further procedure, follow-up the patient for evidence of persistent hypercalcaemia and plan further localization studies
B. Proceed with sternotomy and mediastinal exploration at the time of the initial exploration
C. Perform endoscopic minimally invasive mediastinal exploration at the time of the initial exploration
D. None of the above

Answers

1. A
2. D
3. D
4. C
5. A

Index